Lecture Notes in Biomathematics

Managing Editor: S. Levin

49

Rhythms in Biology and Other Fields of Application

Proceedings, Luminy 1981

Edited by M. Cosnard, J. Demongeot and A. Le Breton

Springer-Verlag
Berlin Heidelberg New York Tokyo

Lecture Notes in Biomathematics

Managing Editor: S. Levin

49

Rhythms in Biology and Other Fields of Application:

Deterministic and Stochastic Approaches

Proceedings of the
Journées de la Société Mathématique de France,
held at Luminy, France, September 14–18, 1981

Edited by M. Cosnard, J. Demongeot and A. Le Breton

Springer-Verlag
Berlin Heidelberg New York Tokyo 1983

Editors

Alain Le Breton
Michel Cosnard
Jacques Demongeot
IMAG
Laboratoire d'Informatique et de Mathématiques Appliquées de Grenoble
BP 68, 38402 St Martin d'Hères Cédex, France

ISBN 3-540-12302-4 Springer-Verlag Berlin Heidelberg New York Tokyo
ISBN 0-387-12302-4 Springer-Verlag New York Heidelberg Berlin Tokyo

Printing and binding: Beltz Offsetdruck, Hemsbach/Bergstr.
2146/3140-543210

Preface

This volume contains most of the talks presented at the Journées de la Société Mathématique de France entitled "Rhythms in Biology and other fields of application - Deterministic and Stochastic Approaches" held in Luminy from the 14th to the 18th of September 1981.

The aim of our meeting was to bring together scientists from different disciplines to discuss a common topic and to stimulate exchanges between participants. We hope that this goal was reached.

This volume is divided into four chapters. In each one the papers are arranged in alphabetical order by first author.

Chapters one and two contain papers devoted to description or modelling of rhythmic biological phenomena. Chapters three and four deal with models for the study of rhythms involving the use of deterministic or stochastic tools capable of fruitful transfer to Biology.

We are pleased that these Proceedings appear in a series which constitutes an interface between Biologists and Mathematicians.

We are indebted to all who provided us with their help, particularly the Centre International de Rencontres Mathématiques (C.I.R.M.) at Luminy, the Société Mathématique de France (S.M.F.), the Délégation aux Relations Universitaires Internationales (D.R.U.I.) and the Laboratoire d'Informatique et de Mathématiques Appliquées de Grenoble (I.M.A.G.).

Special thanks are due to Mrs. A. Litman for her dedication and her efficiency throughout the organization of this meeting.

Grenoble, December 1982.

M. COSNARD
J. DEMONGEOT
A. LE BRETON

CHAPTER 1

EXPERIMENTS AND MODELLING IN BIOLOGY

CHAPTER 2

THEORETICAL STUDY OF BIOLOGICAL MODELS

CHAPTER 3

Deterministic modelling of rhythms

CHAPTER 4

STOCHASTIC MODELLING OF RHYTHMS

CHAPTER 1

EXPERIMENTS AND MODELLING IN BIOLOGY

SIMULATION OF THE ENTRAINMENT OF THE RESPIRATORY RHYTHM BY TWO CONCEPTUALLY DIFFERENT MODELS

P. Baconnier, G. Benchetrit, J. Demongeot and T. Pham Dinh.

Laboratoire de Physiologie (Médecine) and Laboratoire I M A G
Université Grenoble – B. P. 53X – 38041 Grenoble FRANCE.

1. INTRODUCTION

The location in the central nervous system of the respiratory rhythm is now well established. Indeed, elimination of ventilation related sensory inputs does not abolish the respiratory rhythm. Transection experiments delimit the location of the respiratory rhythm generator to the lower brainstem. The question actually under debate is : how is the respiratory rhythm generated ? (7)

During each respiratory cycle take place 1/ <u>an inspiration</u> which corresponds to a) the entrance of the air in the lungs, b) the contraction of diaphragmatic muscles c) the phase of activity on the phrenic nerves which are the main output of the respiratory centers and which innervate the diaphragmatic muscles. The duration of inspiration (T_I) may be determined by measuring either the time during which air entered the lungs or the duration of the activity on the phrenic nerves. Although these two values are not exactly identical there exists a close relationship between them. The volume of air admitted during each inspiration is the tidal volume (V_T).

2/ <u>an expiration</u> which corresponds to a) the exit of the air from lungs b) the rest of diaphragmatic muscles c) the non activity phase on the phrenic nerves. The duration of expiration (T_E) may be determined by two ways as above. It may be noticed that expiration is apparently passive. Indeed, the exit of the air from lungs is slowed, and there exists in the respiratory centers neurones which pulse during expiration although no activity is recorded on the phrenic nerves. The duration of each cycle (T_T) is defined as the sum of T_I and the following T_E .

A descriptive study of the above variables (T_I , T_E and T_T) has been performed on series of respiratory cycles recorded on the phrenic nerves of cats (2), (3). Using statistical time series analysis, it has been shown that in series of T_I s, each T_I was not independent of the preceding T_I , and an autoregressive model of order 1 yielded a good fit at first approximation. The same was with the series of T_E and T_T. In addition, there exist relations between a T_E and the preceding T_I .

Biological rhythms are known to be generated by non linear oscillators (11) . Among the properties of these oscillators is their ability to be entrained by external rhythmic inputs (13) . On anesthetized cats, we have shown that central respiratory rhythm may be entrained by a periodic stimulation (4) . Sensory inputs issued from the lung stretch receptors, sensitive to lung inflations were used to periodically stimulate the respiratory centers. Indeed, inflating lungs causes an inhibition of inspiration, or a lengthening of expiration according to the time of its occurrence in the respiratory cycle (5). The threshold of the stimulation depends also on the timing of the stimulation in the cycle (6). In our experiments, respiratory centers were deefferented from the lungs (phrenic nerves were sectionned) and the animals were ventilated by a pump with adjustable parameters (inflation and deflation times – I and E –, and inflating flow Q). The central respiratory rhythm was measured by re - cording the activity of the central end of the phrenic nerves; the pump provided the periodic stimulation. By changing the period T of the pump it was possible to entrain the central respiratory rhythm in a fairly large range of frequencies. The patterns of entrainments (phase difference) were different, depending on the period of entrainment.

Two models have been elaborated in order to simulate entrainment of the respiratory rhythm. The first one, is based upon the idea that respiration is made of series of events, each comprising an inspiration and an expiration. This model simulates the action of the pump by using quantitative data on the effect of inflation on inspiratory and expiratory durations (6), (9) . The second model is based upon a continuous conception of respiration : inspirations and expirations being different phases of the same phenomenon. The periodic stimulation is represented here by a forcing function mimicking the action of the pump.

2. DISCRETE MODEL

2. 1. Building of a boolean dynamical system with non constant delays

To describe the model, we shall use two right-continuous boolean valued functions $R(t)$ and $P(t)$, which will represent respectively the respiratory state of the cat and the state of the pump at the time t :

$$R(t) = \begin{cases} 0, \text{ during expiration} \\ 1, \text{ during inspiration} \end{cases} \qquad P(t) = \begin{cases} 0, \text{ during deflation} \\ 1, \text{ during inflation} \end{cases}$$

The temporal relations between $R(t)$ and $P(t)$ are given, as for the classical boolean dynamical systems (12), by the delays between the ends of inspirations and expirations and respectively the ends of inflations and deflations.

We suppose that $P(t)$ is periodic with period T and that the inflation time is constant, equal to I and that : $P(0) = P(I) = 1$, $R(0) = 0$.

Let $t_0 = \inf (t>0; R(t) = 1)$ then the delays are given by :

$$S_1 = \inf (t>t_o ; R(t) = 0) - I$$

$$t_1 = \inf (t>S_1 + I ; R(t) =1) - T$$

$$\vdots$$

$$S_i = \inf (t>t_{i-1} + (i-1) T ; R(t) = 0) - (i-1) T - I$$

$$t_i = \inf (t>S_i + (i-1) T + I ; R(t) = 1) - iT$$

The figure below shows the first 3 cycles and the corresponding delays :

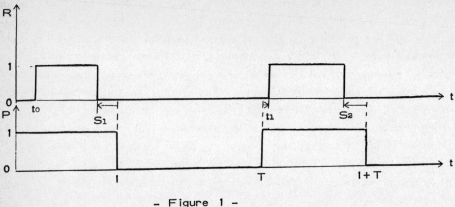

- Figure 1 -

Unlike the classical boolean dynamical systems, delays are non constant; (S_i, t_i) depends on (S_{i-1}, t_{i-1}) through an iteration operator H :

$$\begin{bmatrix} S_i \\ t_i \end{bmatrix} = H \begin{bmatrix} S_{i-1} \\ t_{i-1} \end{bmatrix}$$

The building of H is based on a previous model described in (6) and using physiological data. Briefly, the first equation is obtained by writing :

$$(1) \qquad S_i = t_{i-1} + T_{I\,i} - I$$

where $T_{I\,i}$, the ith inspiratory duration, is limited by two extreme values m and M, and is given by an inspiratory cut-off function f. Let $t_{i-1}^T \in]\,I - T,\ I\,]$, $t_{i-1}^T \equiv t_{i-1}$ (mod T) and $f(t_{i-1}^T)$ is the abscissa of the point of intersection of (i) the linear function $t \mapsto (t+t_{i-1}^T)Q$ representing the increasing respiratory volume during inflation and (ii) the hyperbolic function $t \mapsto k/t - h$ representing the cut-off (fig. 2). Then,

$$(2) \qquad T_{I\,i} = \max(m, f(t_{i-1}^T)) \quad \text{if} \quad -t_{i-1}^T < f(t_{i-1}^T) \leq \min(I-t_{i-1}^T, M)$$
$$= M \qquad\qquad\qquad \text{otherwise}$$

Observe that if the abscissa $f(t_{i-1}^T)$ is such that $t_{i-1}^T + f(t_{i-1}^T) \notin [0, I]$ then $T_{I\,i} = M$

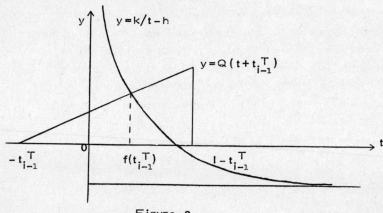

- Figure 2 -

By substitution, using (1) and (2), one can express S_i as a function of t_{i-1}.
The second equation is obtained from :

(3) $\quad t_i = S_i + T_{E_i} - (T - I)$

where T_{E_i}, the ith expiratory duration is related to T_{I_i} (6) with a possible lengthening (9) depending on $\quad \varphi(t_{i-1}^T) = \max(0, D(t_{i-1}^T))\quad$ where D is the maximal deviation between the expected and the actual respiratory curve. The expected curve is
supposed to be polynomial of degree 4 :

$t \mapsto \quad (k/T_{I_i} - h)(y-1)^2(Ay^2+2y+1)\qquad$ if $\quad 0 < y = \dfrac{t - T_{I_i}}{aT_{I_i} + b} < 1$

$t \mapsto \quad 0 \qquad$ otherwise

and the actual curve, when it corresponds to passive expiration, is a decreasing exponential :

$t \mapsto \quad I\,Q\,e^{-c(t-I+t_{i-1}^T)}\qquad$ when $\quad I-t_{i-1}^T < t < T-t_{i-1}^T$

$t \mapsto \quad (t+t_{i-1}^T)\,Q\qquad$ when $\quad T_{I_i} < t < I-t_{i-1}^T$

$t \mapsto \quad (t+t_{i-1}^T - T)\,Q\qquad$ when $\quad T-t_{i-1}^T < t < T+I-t_{i-1}^T$

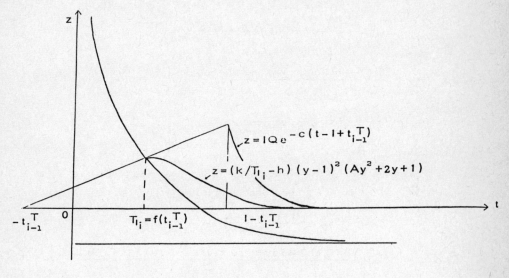

$$z = IQ\,e^{-c(t-I+t_{i-1}^T)}$$

$$z = (k/T_{I_i} - h)(y-1)^2(Ay^2+2y+1)$$

- Figure 3 -

Let $(T_{I_i} + \psi(t_{i-1}^T))$ be the time in the interval $[T_{I_i}, (1+0.7a)T_{I_i}+0.7b]$ for which the
deviation between the two curves is maximum; we have :

(4) $\qquad T_{E_i} = aT_{I_i} + b + \dfrac{\varphi(t_{i-1}^T)}{k/T_{I_i} - h}\left(\alpha\,\dfrac{\psi(t_{i-1}^T)}{aT_{I_i} + b} + \beta\right)$

By substitution, using (1) and (4), one can express t_i as a function of t_{i-1}.

2. 2. Study of the fixed point of H

We note that the iterative system H can be reduced to an unidimensional iterative

system as in (8) $\qquad t_i = t_{i-1} - T + F(t_{i-1}^T)$,

where $F(t_{i-1}^T) = T_{I_i} + T_{E_i}$, T_{I_i} and T_{E_i} being given by the relations (2) and (4).

We get one-to-one entrainment for the system if and only if t_i converges to t_* as i

goes to infinity. This implies that t_* is a fixed point of the above unidimensional

iterative system. Equivalently t_*^T is the solution of $T = F(t_*^T)$. We consider first

the case the threshold is not reached for equation (2). Then we have, denoting t_*^T

by x :
$$T = (1+a) f(x) + b + \frac{\varphi(x)}{(f(x) + x) Q} (\alpha \frac{\psi(x)}{af(x)+b} + \beta)$$

In practice, the polynomial expiratory curve was such that either $\psi(x) = 1 - f(x) - x$

or $\psi(x) = 0.7 (a f(x) + b)$. For the usual values of parameters, $0.7[ak/(QI+h)+b]<T-1$

and it can be shown that the latter possibility is excluded. Hence,

$$(5) \qquad T = (1+a) f(x) + b + [\frac{1}{f(x)+x} - (\frac{1-f(x)-x}{a f(x)+b} - 1)^2 (A (\frac{1-f(x)-x}{a f(x)+b})^2 +$$

$$2 (\frac{1-f(x)-x}{a f(x)+b}) + 1)](\alpha \frac{1-f(x)-x}{a f(x)+b} + \beta)$$

We remark that :

a) $f(x) = \dfrac{-(Qx+h) + \sqrt{(Qx+h)^2 + 4kQ}}{2 Q}$ is a decreasing function of x,

because $f'(x) = \dfrac{1}{2} (-1 + \dfrac{Qx + h}{\sqrt{(Qx+h)^2 + 4kQ}})$

b) $f(x) + x = (k/ f(x) - h) / Q$ is an increasing function of x.

Hence the right hand side of the equation (5) is a decreasing function of x, if

$u(x) = [1 - f(x) - x] / [a f(x) + b]$ is a decreasing function of x . Let us denote $f(x)$

by y, we have :
$$u(x) = v(y) = \frac{(IQ+h) y - k}{Q y (ay+b)}$$

and $\qquad v'(y) = \dfrac{(IQ+h) y (ay+b) - ((IQ+h) y - k) (2ay+b)}{Q y^2 (ay+b)^2}$

Since $y < M$, if the condition $IQ < \dfrac{2k}{M} - h$ holds, then $v' > 0$; hence v is increa-

sing in y and u is decreasing in x . In practice, the above condition is fulfilled.

Consider now the case where the threshold value is reached in equation (2) : $T_{I_i} = M$.

As above, either $\psi(x) = 1-M-x$, or $\psi(x) = 0.7 (aM+b)$. The first case leads

to an equation similar to (5) with M in place of $f(x)$. The second case leads to the

following equation :

$$T = (1+a) M+b+ [Q \frac{w}{k/M-h} - (0.7-1)^2 (A (0.7)^2 +2 (0.7)+1)](0.7 \alpha + \beta),$$

where $w = (x + (0.7a+1)M+0.7b) (mod T)$, if the last is in $[0,1]$, $w=0$ otherwis

The above right hand side is an increasing linear function of x . To conclude,

F(x) has the following form :

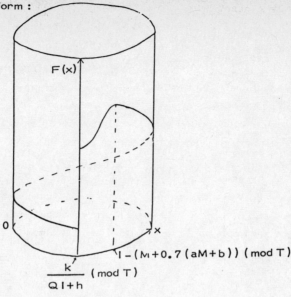

- Figure 4 -

In these conditions, there is an unique locally attractive fixed point x_0 for the iterations : $t_i^T = t_{i-1}^T - T + F(t_{i-1}^T)$, if and only if $0 > F'(x) > -2$

This last inequality gives the conditions on parameters which we have to satisfy to obtain the local convergence of the iterations.

2. 3. Numerical properties of the boolean model

Simulations have been carried out corresponding to various experimental conditions. On figure 5 are represented results of an experiment and the corresponding simulation for 3 different successive entrainments at periods 3.67 , 3.17 and 2.67 sec. It can be seen that a) entrainment occurs for the same values of T and, at T =2.17, entrainment is no longer observed in the experiment as in the simulation, b) the shift of the inspiration toward inflation while T decreases, which is observed in the experiment, is well simulated by the model.

Comparing the (T_i, T) plots obtained from experiments and simulations (Fig. 6) one can observe a discrepancy : simulated T_i is saturated at a given T level while experimental T_i always increases with T. The saturation of T_i in simulation results is intrinsic to the model : it comes from the upper bound M imposed on T_i .

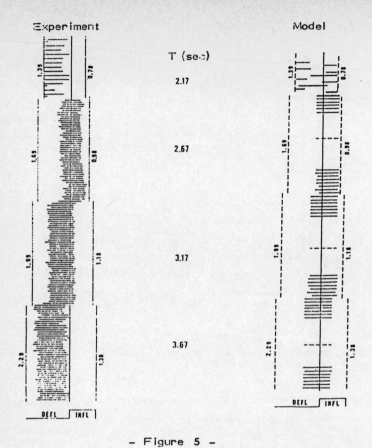

- Figure 5 -

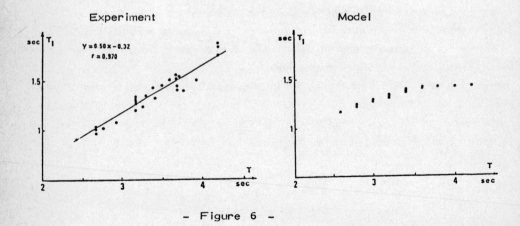

- Figure 6 -

3. CONTINUOUS MODEL

The second model is based on the theory of differential dynamical systems. It is well known that some non linear differential systems could exhibit sustained oscillations and hence can be used as models of biological oscillators.

Let us begin with a brief recall on some fundamental notions on differential systems. We will consider only the simple case of a system of two variables defined by the equations :

$$(1) \qquad \frac{dx}{dt} = f(x, y) \qquad\qquad \frac{dy}{dt} = g(x, y)$$

the solution of this system provides two functions of time $x(t)$, $y(t)$. If we plot the points of coordinates x, y on a plane, called the phase plane, then we obtain a trajectory, describing the evolution of the system. For certain systems there exists a limit cycle, that is a closed trajectory, corresponding to a periodic solution such that any other trajectory tends to approach it as the time goes to infinity. It is this type of differential systems which interests us since it corresponds to an oscillator.

3. 1. Connection between model and experiments

We will assume that the variables x, y of our theoretical oscillator are hidden unobservable variables and may not have any physiological meaning. One reason is that only the beginnings of the inspiration and the expiration are observed and they may not be the relevant variables. Another reason is that a model with explicit physiological variables would have to be built on some assumptions on the rhythm generating mechanism, which is largely unknown.

To interpret the inspiratory and expiratory durations, we divide the phase plane into two regions, the inspiratory and the expiratory regions. If the representative point of the differential system is in the inspiratory region, we say that the oscillator is in the inspiratory phase and the same is with the expiratory region. Thus the beginnings of the inspirations and of the expirations are the passage times on the separatrix of the two regions. For simplicity, we will take as separatrix a straight line passing through the unstable stationary point of the system. This point is taken as the origin of the axes and the separatrix, the x's axis.

We need to define the stimulation, that is the action of the pump. A simple way to introduce the stimulation is to add a forcing term on the right hand sides of (1) . For simplicity, it is not unrealistic to assume that the stimulations in our experimental situations are of impulsional type, that is their effect is concentrated in a short lapse of time. The forcing function is thus a sequence of pulses, each pulse produces a displacement of the representative point of the system along a certain vector. The direction of this vector should be parallel to the separatrix since if it is not the case, then it may happen that a stimulation occurring just after the beginning of an expiration could bring the representative point of the system into the inspiratory region, and hence starts a new inspiration. This situation, however, has never been experimentally observed.

3. 2. Entrainment of an oscillator defined by a differential system

The differential model of oscillator can successfully explain the entrainment phenomenon (1), (11), (13), with the help of the notions of isochron and the phase response curve.

Consider a radius starting from the origin and intersecting the limit cycle at an unique point M_0. Let t_1, t_2, ... denote the passage times at this radius, of a trajectory starting at M. Then the phase of M relative to M_0 is defined as $T_T - \lim t_n \pmod{T_T}$ T_T being the description time of the limit cycle. An isochron is then defined as the set of all points having same phase. An example of oscillator with its system of isochrons of phases increasing by step of $T_T/10$ is shown in figure 7. Such a system is quite useful to visualize the temporal behavior of the oscillator : the time to travel along a trajectory from an isochron to the next is $T_T/10$.

expiratory region

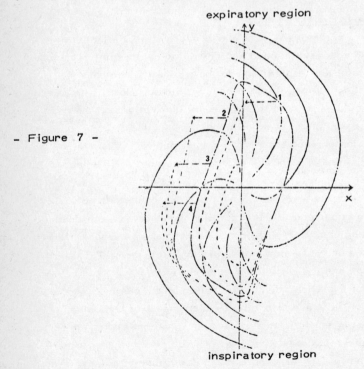

- Figure 7 -

inspiratory region

Suppose that the oscillator is stimulated periodically with period T. Let 1, 2, ... denote the successive positions of the representative point of the system when the stimulus occurs (Fig. 7). As a first approximation, we shall consider that the points 1, 2, ... are on the limit cycle and hence can be specified by their phases $\varphi_1, \varphi_2, ...$

11

The relation between φ_{n+1} and φ_n can be seen to be :

(2) $\varphi_{n+1} = \varphi_n + S(\varphi_n) + T - T_T \pmod{T_T}$

Here $S(\varphi)$ is the phase shift caused by the stimulus :

$$S(\varphi) = \text{phase of } M' - \varphi$$

where M' is the position of the representative point after the stimulus have been applied when the system was at M of phase φ.

The graph of $-S(\varphi)$ against φ, called the phase response curve, is quite useful to construct the sequence $\{\varphi_n\}$. One-to-one entrainment occurs if $\varphi_n \longrightarrow \varphi^*$, a fixed point of the iterations (2) or equivalently, a solution of :

(3) $-S(\varphi^*) = T - T_T \pmod{T_T}$

However, in order that φ_n converge to φ^*, the starting φ_1 should be sufficiently close to φ^* and the slope of the phase response curve should be between zero and two (fixed point theorem). Typically, the phase response curve has an increasing and a decreasing part, and hence (3) admits at most a solution φ^* at which the slope of the phase response curve is positive. This means that when the system is entrained, the stimulus occurs at phases in the interval of increase of $-S(\varphi)$. If we assume that experimentally the pump acts mostly at the start of the deflation, then the stimulus always occurs in the expiratory phase. Thus the increasing part of the phase response curve has to coincide more or less with the expiratory phase.

The maximum entrainment range is contained between the maximum and minimum phase shifts. Experimentally, this range is quite large implying that the slope of the increasing part of the phase response curve is rather close to two, its maximum value.

3. 3. Model description and simulation results

Based on the above considerations we reach the conclusion that an adequate model of oscillator should have its isochrons turning around the origin (see Fig. 2). This insures that : (i) the phase shift range is large, (ii) the maximum phase delay is obtained toward the end of the expiration and the maximum phase advance is obtained toward the beginning of the expiration, and (iii) the time needed to travel through the inspiratory region increases with the "mean distance" from the trajectory to the origin. Note that properties (i) –(iii) agree with experimental results.

To build a model of oscillator having the above characteristics we start from the Van der Pol equations which has been already used in modelling of the respiratory system (10). We modified the Van der Pol equations to :

$$\frac{dx}{dt} = y , \qquad \frac{dy}{dt} = - h(y)x - g(y)$$

The function h should be positive for small $|y|$ and negative otherwise, and $y g(y) > 0$ in order that the system admit sustained oscillations. From heuristic considerations, we decided that $|h(y)|$ and $|g(y)|$ should not increase too fast with $|y|$, and therefore we consider the functions :

$$h(y) = a \frac{1-y^2}{1+by^2}$$

$$g(y) = \begin{cases} y \dfrac{1+cy}{1+dy} & y > 0 \\[2mm] y \dfrac{1-c'y}{1+d'y^2} & y < 0 \end{cases}$$

the forcing term being $P(t) = Q I e^{-5t/3}$, $0 < t < T$, $P(t) = P(t+T)$, to mimick the deflation of the pump. Here $Q I$ is proportional to the pulmonary volume at the start of the deflation. Note that the time is measured in relative units for which the period of the oscillator is about 15. The parameters a, b, c, d, c', d', and Q are adjusted by trial and comparison between simulated and experimental entrainment characteristics. The obtained values are $a = .5$, $b = .3$, $c = .1$, $d = 2.5$, $c' = .3$, $d' = .48$, $Q = .5$ giving the following results :

T	I	DI	T_i	ED
11	4.3	4.81	4.34	1.85
12	4.6	4.32	4.82	2.86
13	4.9	3.84	5.36	3.80
14	5.2	3.34	5.91	4.75
15	5.5	2.88	6.48	5.64
16	5.8	2.40	7.06	6.54
17	6.1	1.96	7.66	7.38
18	6.4	1.48	8.23	8.29
19	6.7	0.98	8.79	9.23
19.5	6.85	0.61	9.03	9.86

Simulation results in arbitrary units

T: pump period; I : inflation time; DI : time difference between the beginnings of deflation and inspiration; T_i : inspiratory duration; ED : time difference between the beginnings of expiration and deflation.

Figure 8 shows the limit cycle and the system of isochrons of the retained model. Figure 9 shows the trajectories of the system when entrained (T = 11, 14, 17, 19.5 with T = 11 corresponding to the innermost trajectory). Figure 10 illustrates the convergence to entrainment. Figure 11 and 12 compare the experiment (a) and simulation (b) results. In figure 11 (b), the graphs of $-P(t)$ are shown below the bars representing the inspirations.

- Figure 8 -

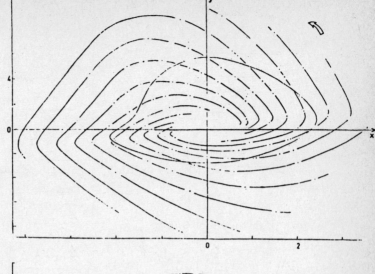

- Figure 9 -

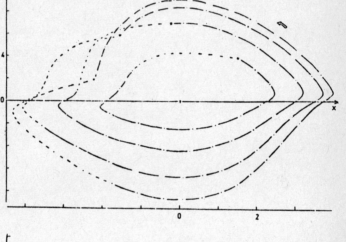

- Figure 10 -

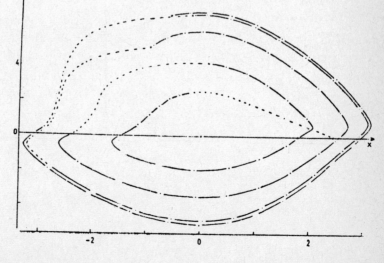

14

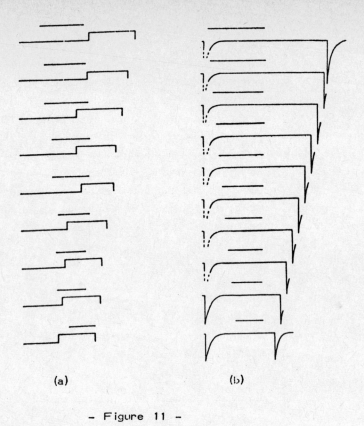

(a)   (b)

- Figure 11 -

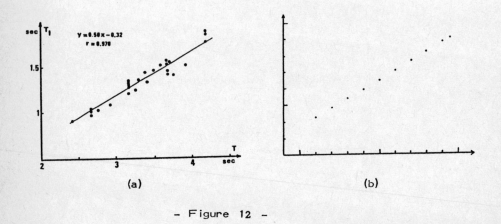

(a)   (b)

- Figure 12 -

4. CONCLUSION

The two model approaches have been complementary. The boolean model predicted possibilities of entrainment provided the values of T and of the parameters satisfy certain conditions. Numerical values of these parameters taken from physiological data satisfied the conditions required by the model for entrainment. However, there exist discrepancies between the model and experiments, especially on the pattern of entrainment. The differential dynamical system gave a better fit with the experiments and showed the usefulness of attributing to the respiratory rhythm generator a continuous oscillatory behavior in order to explain its entrainment characteristics. Both models may be useful to study the entrainment of respiratory rhythm generator either functionning in different physiological conditions or with different stimulations.

REFERENCES

1. BACONNIER, P., G. BENCHETRIT, J. DEMONGEOT and T. PHAM DINH, Etude des phénomènes d'entrainement : application au système respiratoire. in Sém. Ec. Biol. Théor. Ed. by H. Le Guyader and T. Moulin, ENSTA, Paris pp. 483-503, (1981).

2. BENCHETRIT, G. La périodicité respiratoire – Essai d'interprétation par une méthode statistique. Thèse de Sciences, Grenoble (1974).

3. BENCHETRIT, G. and F. BERTRAND. A short-term memory in the respiratory centers : statistical analysis. Respir. Physiol. 23 : 147-158, (1975).

4. BENCHETRIT, G. Some oscillator properties of the respiratory centers : entrainment by periodic lung inflations. (in preparation).

5. BREUER, J. Die Selbststeuerung der Atmung durch den Nervus vagus. Sitzber. K. K. Akad. Wiss. Wien 58 : 909-937, (1868).

6. CLARK, F. J. and C. Von EULER. On the regulation of depth and rate of breathing. J. Physiol. (London) 222 : 267-295, (1972).

7. COHEN, M. I. Neurogenesis of respiratory rhythm in the mammal. Physiol. Rev. 59 : 1105-1173, (1979).

8. GLASS, L., C. GRAVES, G. A. PETRILLO and M. C. MACKEY. Unstable dynamics of a periodically driven oscillator in the presence of noise. J. Theor. Biol. 86 : 455-475, (1980)

9. KNOX, C. K. Characteristics of inflation and deflation reflexes during expiration in the cat. J. Neurophysiol. $\underline{36}$: 284-295, (1973).

10. LINKENS, D.A. Modulation analysis of forced nonlinear oscillations for biological modelling. J. Theor. Biol. $\underline{77}$: 235-251, (1973).

11. PAVLIDIS, T. Biological oscillators : their mathematical analysis. Academic Press New York (1973).

12. THOMAS, R. Application of boolean analysis to identification of stationary states for continuous systems. (in this book)

13. WINFREE, A. T. The geometry of biological time. Biomathematics $\underline{8}$. Springer Verlag New York (1980)

GLYCOLYTIC OSCILLATIONS : AN ATTEMPT TO AN "IN VITRO" RECONSTITUTION

OF THE HIGHER PART OF GLYCOLYSIS

MODELLING AND EXPERIMENTAL APPROACH

J. Demongeot

IMAG BP 53 X

38 041 Grenoble Cédex France

N. Kellershohn

EPCM - GR 13 CNRS

91 405 Orsay   France

1. Introduction : historical background

The oscillatory properties of the glycolysis have been discovered about twenty years ago in intact yeast cells by L.N.M. Duysens and J. Amesz in a "princeps" paper (Biochim. Biophys. Acta 24, 19 (1957) ; cf. also (4)) and after in cytoplasmic extracts of yeast, containing all glycolytic metabolites and enzymes in quasi in vivo conditions (5). More recently, several attempts were made in order to reconstitute in vitro simple systems built from glycolytic reactions, with the aim to observe non trivial dynamical behaviours (oscillations,multisteady states)(11,12,20). The essential feature of dynamical properties of these studied biochemical systems is, like in the well-known oscillatory chemical ones, the presence of non-linear self-regulated kinetics (10) in an open system far from equilibrium.

Because the complexity in the coupling and rate laws of enzymatic reactions in biochemical systems, the necessity appeard of a theoretical approach based on a simplifying modelling in order to find the main features of the regulatory mechanism. The basic ideas for building these models were :
1) to take into account the role of effectors (inhibitors or activators), which counteract the usual activation by substrates in a metabolic pathway
2) to find a subsystem of the glycolysis which is minimal in the following sense : a subsystem of an oscillatory system of reactions is minimal, if it does not keep this oscillatory character by suppressing any of its reaction steps.

The first models by E.E. Sel'kov (21) and A. Goldbeter & R. Lefever (9) involved a minimal subsystem centered on the non-linear and regulated phosphofructokinase (PFK) reaction with a retroactivation by one of its products (adenosine diphosphate, denoted by ADP), coupled with a sink of this product. This simple mechanism was sufficient to generate oscillations ; a more realistic view was given in

(6) by taking into account the allosteric properties of the PFK. However, recent molecular studies concerning the structural and functional properties of the yeast PFK (15-17, 22-24) have leaded to more sophisticated models (6-8), which are better related to the real system. Moreover, another very powerful PFK activator (fructose-2,6-biphosphate, denoted by $F2,6P_2$) has been discovered two years ago, suggesting the existence of a second PFK specie (PFK2) (25) ; in this paper, we are trying to show what brings the introduction of this new activator in previous models, concerning their oscillatory properties.

2. Interaction between modelling and experiments

Progress in the understanding of the molecular mechanism which generates oscillatory behaviour in glycolysis needs collation of theoretical and experimental informations according to the following logical frame :
- the existence of oscillations in yeast extracts, modulated by an input rate of glucose substrate and addition of other metabolites of the glycolytic pathway (adenylates, hexophosphates) leads to the hypothesis of an oscillations generating mechanism at the molecular level. Moreover, the disappearence of oscillations by supplying yeast extracts with substrates below the PFK reaction in the glycolysis and phase shift considerations between successive metabolites (13) pointed out the key role of the PFK.
- the possibility to obtain oscillations with a simple model centered on the PFK reaction (9, 21) showed that we could try to reconstitute an in vitro oscillatory subsystem around PFK and that it was necessary to get more precise experimental data on structural, kinetic and regulatory aspects of this enzyme studied in vitro.
- these recently obtained molecular data have been introduced in extended models retaining oscillatory properties, in a good qualitative agreement with the observed oscillations in yeast extracts. The use of stability diagrams of these models allowed us to make qualitative predictions concerning possible oscillations of the reconstituted system.
- the corresponding experiments have shown recently a certain agreement with these predictions, but also certain discrepancies suggesting later improvements in the modelling.

This to and fro motion between modelling and experiments will continue until all important regulatory factors will be taken into account.

3. An attempt of an experimental reconstitution of the high part of glycolysis

The reconstituted system involves reactions catalysed by hexokinase (HK), PFK, aldolase (ALD), triosephosphate isomerase (TIM), glyceraldehyde-3-phosphate dehydrogenase (GPDH) and 3-phosphoglycerate kinase (PGK). Besides these enzymes, initial reaction mixture contains adenosine triphosphate (ATP), the dinucleotide NAD^+ and inorganic phosphate in a pH 6.8 PIPES Standard buffer (1,4 piperazine diethane sulfonic acid /K_2HPO_4/NH_4Cl/dithiothreitol). Recycling of NAD^+ which is reduced in the GPDH reaction is performed by lactate dehydrogenase (LDH) in presence of pyruvate in excess. Moreover, appreciable amounts of adenylate kinase (ADK) allow to generate adenosinemonophosphate (AMP), in a quasi-equilibrium, which is the most powerful activator of PFK after the $F2,6P_2$. ATP and ADP consumption stoichiometries show that this reconstituted system is autonomous towards adenylates.

The enzymatic coupled system is placed under constant stirring and suplied with fructose-6-phosphate (F6P) or fructose (FRU) (or even glucose (GLU), with previous addition of phosphoglucoisomerase (PGI)) at a constant input rate by means of a calibrated perfusion pump. Fluorescence of NADH involved in the coupled GPDH-LDH reactions is recorded by a data acquisition system coupled to a Wang 2200 desk calculator, as a signal detector for flux variations through the enzymatic system. The behaviour of the coupled enzymatic system below PFK reaction was tested, in presence of NAD^+, P_i and pyruvate, by injecting pulses of a fructose-1,6-biphosphate ($F1,6P_2$)/ADP mixture (1:2 ratio) ; after reaching a maximum, NADH fluorescence decreases and returns to its initial level. When there is no rate limiting step in the sequence of reactions catalysed by ALD/TIM/GPDH/PGK, fluorescence decreasing is only controlled by LDH activity. Provided that PFK activity remains rate limiting, the whole reconstituted system allows $F1,6P_2$ elimination as it is produced and the PFK catalysed reaction may be considered as an open sub-system. When pulses of $F1,6P_2$ are injected in the reconstituted system, area mesured under the fluorescence variation curves are proportional to total F6P concentrations. With a constant supply of F6P, which is increased sequentially from low values of input rate, the system reaches (after a transient period) steady states in NADH concentrations which are proportional to the input rate. F6P and ATP titration at steady states obtained for different and increasing values of fructose input rate ("input characteristic") shows that unstable steady state may be obtained in this reconstituted system for moderate values of fructose flux (.1 to .2 mM/mn). Under such conditions, this in vitro reconstituted enzymatic system presents a temporal behaviour which is characteristic of a self-regulated system. However, steady state seems to be always of the stable focus type or, if unstable, surrounded by a very small limit cycle, and attempts to obtain oscillations of large amplitudes, as in yeast cell extracts, led to failure (1,2,18,19). Some credible reasons may be advanced to account for this behaviour discrepancy, in connection to model studies and experimental data obtained upon functional properties of yeast PFK. We will study this point in the following sections.

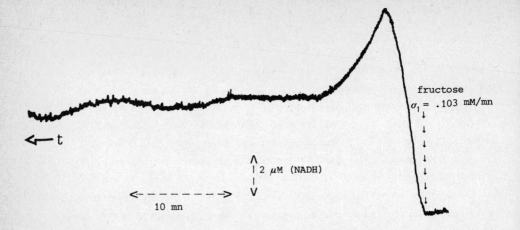

fructose
$\sigma_1 = .103$ mM/mn

$\wedge$
| 2 μM (NADH)
|
V

$\leftarrow$ - - - - - - - $\rightarrow$
10 mn

$\leftarrow$ t

Figure 1 (after (1))

Response of the coupled enzymatic system to a constant input rate of fructose (concentration of fructose : 1M) ; the curve gives the variations of NADH fluorescence

4. Modelling of the high part of glycolysis

4.1. The first models

The models by E.E. Sel'kov (21) and A. Goldbeter & R. Lefever (9) were based on a retroactivation of the PFK reaction by one of its products, for example by ADP (see (6) for a retroactivation by AMP) ; the input rate σ_1 for F6P was suppo- sed to be constant and the sink of ADP was denoted by σ_2 :

$$\xrightarrow{\;\sigma_1\;} \underset{a}{F6P + ATP} \xrightarrow[v(a,a_2)]{PFK^{\oplus}} \underset{a_2}{F1,6P_2 + ADP} \xrightarrow{\;\sigma_2(a_2)\;}$$

The differential system S_1 governing the kinetics of this minimal sub- system of the glycolysis was given by :

$$\begin{cases} \dfrac{da}{d\theta} = \sigma_1 - v(a,a_2) \\[3mm] \dfrac{da_2}{d\theta} = \rho(v(a,a_2) - \sigma_2(a_2)), \end{cases}$$

where a and a_2 correspond respectively to the normalized concentrations of F6P and ADP :

$$a = [F6P] / K_{R,F6P} \qquad a_2 = [ADP] / K_{R,ADP}$$

($K_{R,F6P}$ and $K_{R,ADP}$ denoting the dissociation constants for ATP and ADP respectively, with respect to the active form R of the allosteric enzyme PFK)

- θ is a normalized time : $\theta = t \, V_m/K_{R,F6P}$, where V_m is the maximal rate of the PFK reaction
- ρ is a proportionality constant : $\rho = K_{R,F6P}/K_{R,ADP}$
- σ_1 is the normalized input rate of F6P :
$$\sigma_1 = V_o/V_m, \text{ where } V_o \text{ is the input rate of F6P (mM/mn)}$$
- $v(a,a_2) = \dfrac{a(Lc(1+ca)^{n-1} + (1+a)^{n-1})}{L(1+ca)^n + (1+a)^n}$, if we consider the allosteric kinetics as

a K-system, where c is the non-exclusion coefficient of F6P ($c<1$) and where :
$$L = L_o(\frac{1+da_2}{1+a_2})^n, \; L_o \text{ being the allosteric equilibrium constant}$$
in absence of activator and d being the non-exclusion coefficient of ADP ($d<1$)
- $\sigma_2(a_2)$ is the decay function of ADP.

The system S_1 has a unique stationary state and the normal mode analysis shows that a necessary and sufficient condition of instability for this state is given by the following inequality :
$$(1) \quad -\frac{\partial v}{\partial a} + (\frac{\partial v}{\partial a_2} - \frac{\partial \sigma_2}{\partial a_2}) \geqslant 0$$
We can see in (1), that the oscillatory behavior is only caused by the positivity of $\frac{\partial v}{\partial a_2}$, which corresponds to the activation by ADP.

4.2. Previous generalizations

In previous papers (1,2,3,6,7,8), we have studied certain generalizations of the classical model above :

4.2.1. Activation by AMP

Because AMP is a more powerful activator of the PFK than ADP and because the existence of AMP is ensured by the ADK reaction, we have introduced the ADK equilibrium in the subsystem : the new system has two steady states, a state with high energy charge, which is stable or surrounded by a limit cycle, and a state with low energy charge, which is always unstable (if we denote by a_1 and a_3 respectively the concentrations of AMP and ATP, the energy charge is defined by :
$$\zeta = \frac{a_3 + a_2/2}{a_1+a_2+a_3} \quad \text{and } \zeta > 1/2 \text{ in the case of high energy}$$
ge and $\zeta < 1/2$ in the case of low energy charge). If we multiply the rate term v by $a_3/(K_m+a_3)$, where K_m is the Michaëlis constant of ATP for the both forms R and T of the PFK, we have a system nearer than the real system ; the stability of the high energy state has been studied in stability diagrams such as that given Figure 2.
We have also shown that :
- a part of the limit cycle could be in the low energy region of the state space (in these conditions, the concentration a_2 has two maxima in a period).

- there was a region in the parameter space, in which the high energy state was un-unstable and the limit cycle did not exist (in this case, the concentration a goes to infinity and the concentration a_3 goes to zero).

- if we considered the ADK reaction as a reversible reaction, but not at equilibrium, this had a stabilizing effect on the high energy state.

In the last generalization, the reaction scheme was the following :

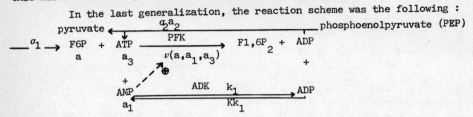

The sink of ADP was supposed to be realized here by the PEP reaction (we assumed that it was of the first order for a_2).

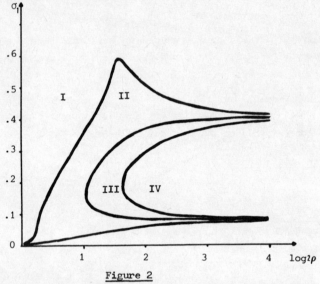

<u>Figure 2</u>

stability diagram in the case where AMP is activator and the ADK reaction is suppo-sed to be at equilibrium (I : stable node ; II : stable focus ; III : unstable focus ; IV : unstable node ; the concerned state is the high energy charge steady state. The parameters have the following values : $n=4$, $L_o=3\ 10^3$, $K=.5$, $c=.02$, $a_1+a_2+a_3=190$, $K_m=2$, $K_{R,AMP}=.01mM$, $d=0$, $\sigma_2=.01$, allosteric kinetics being supposed to be a K-V system, with constant .1 ; $K_{R,F6P}$ is variable).

The differential system S_2 corresponding to the reaction scheme above is given by the two following equations, when the ADK reaction is assumed to be at equi-librium :

$$\begin{cases} \dfrac{da}{d\theta} = \sigma_1 - v(a,a_1,a_3) \\ \dfrac{d\gamma}{d\theta} = \rho(\sigma_2 a_2 - v(a,a_1,a_3))/2, \end{cases}$$

where $\rho = K_{R,F6P}/K_{R,AMP}$, $v(a,a_1,a_3) = \dfrac{a_3}{K_m + a_3} \dfrac{a(Lc(1+ca)^{n-1} + 0.1\ (1+a)^{n-1})}{L(1+ca)^n + (1+a)^n}$

and $L=L_o(\frac{1+da}{1+a_1}1)^n$. We have also : $\sigma_2=v\,K_{R,AMP}/V_m$, where v is the rate constant of the sink of ADP ; $a_1=[AMP]/K_{R,AMP}$, $a_2=[ADP]/K_{R,AMP}$, $a_3=[ATP]/K_{R,AMP}$

$$- a_1+a_2+a_3=A,\text{ where A is a constant ; } X=A\zeta$$
$$- a_1a_3 = Ka_2^2$$

4.2.2. Slow transition between the two allosteric conformations R and T

We have shown that the introduction of a slow transition between the two forms R and T (active and inactive respectively) of the allosteric enzyme PFK had a stabilizing effect on the high energy steady state (6).

4.2.3. Addition of the hexokinase reaction

By adding the hexokinase reaction before the PFK reaction, we have also a stabilization of the high energy steady state :

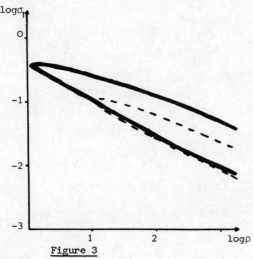

Figure 3

stability region of the high energy steady state in the same case as 4.2.1.(——) and after adding the hexokinase reaction (- - -)(the parameters have the following values : σ_1 denotes the maximum rate of the hexokinase reaction supposed to be michaëlian ; the Michaëlis constant of ATP in the hexokinase reaction was chosen equal to .15 mM ; fructose was supposed in excess ; $K_{R,F6P}$=.2mM, all other parameters having the same values as in 4.2.1., except for $K_{R,AMP}$ which was here variable and for σ_2 supposed equal to $K_{R,AMP}$).

4.3. A new generalization

If we introduce the second kind of PFK producing the $F2,6P_2$, which is the most powerful activator of the first kind of PFK, we obtain the reaction scheme described in the Figure 4 :

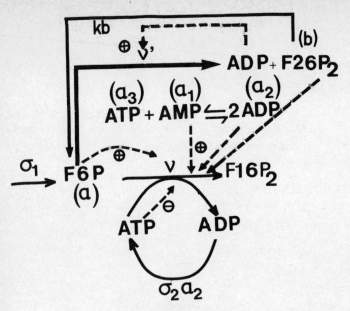

Figure 4

reaction scheme in the case of the coexistence of two kinds of PFK (ν' denotes the kinetic term corresponding to the second PFK, b denotes the normalized concentration of $F2,6P_2$ and the symbols $\oplus$ and $\ominus$ signify respectively an activation and an inhibition). We have added a possible hydrolysis of the $F2,6P_2$.

The differential system S_3 governing the kinetics is given by :

$$\frac{da}{d\theta} = \sigma_1 - v(a,a_1,a_2,a_3,b) - v'(a,a_3) + kb$$

$$\frac{db}{d\theta} = \rho'(v'(a,a_3) - kb)$$

$$\frac{d\chi}{d\theta} = \rho(\sigma_2 a_2 - v(a,a_1,a_2,a_3,b) - v'(a,a_3))/2,$$

where ρ' is a proportionality constant : $\rho' = K_{R,F6P}/K_{R,F2,6P_2}$

- b is the normalized concentration of $F2,6P_2$: $b = [F2,6P_2]/K_{R,F2,6P_2}$,

$K_{R,F2,6P_2}$ being the dissociation constant of $F2,6P_2$ considered as an activator of the first PFK.

- $k = v' K_{R,F2,6P_2}/V_m$, where v' is the rate constant of the hydrolysis of the the $F2,6P_2$ supposed to be of the first order.

- the equilibrium constant L is here given by :

$$L = L_0 \left(\frac{1+da_1}{1+a_1}\right)^n \left(\frac{1+d'a_2}{1+e'a_2}\right)^n \left(\frac{1+d''a_3}{1+e''a_3}\right)^n \left(\frac{1+fb}{1+b}\right)^n$$

where $d'=K_{R,AMP}/K_{T,ADP}$, $e'=K_{R,AMP}/K_{R,ADP}$, $d''=K_{R,AMP}/K_{T,ATP}$, $e''=K_{R,AMP}/K_{R,ATP}$, $f=K_{R,F2,6P_2}/K_{T,F2,6P_2}$; we have : $d'/e' < 1$, $d''/e'' > 1$ and $f < 1$, because ADP and F2,6P$_2$ are activator and ATP is inhibitor.

- v has the same expression as in 4.2.1., after replacing L by its new expression

- v' is defined by :

$$v'(a,a_3) = \frac{V'_m}{V_m} \frac{a_3}{K_m+a_3} \frac{a(L_0 c(1+ca)^{n-1} + 0.1 (1+a)^{n-1})}{L_0(1+ca)^n + (1+a)^n} ,$$

where V'_m denotes the maximum rate of the second PFK reaction (the other kinetic parameters being supposed to be the same as for the first PFK).

S_3 has two steady states : the low energy state is always unstable and the high energy state is stable or unstable ; in this state, the following relations are avalaible :

$$\begin{cases} a_2 = (-A+\sqrt{A^2+4(4K-1)\,\chi\,(A-\chi)})/(4K-1) \\ a_1 = (A-a_2-\sqrt{(A-a_2)^2-4Ka_2^2})/2 \\ a_3 = (A-a_2+\sqrt{(A-a_2)^2-4Ka_2^2})/2 \end{cases}$$

These relations allow us to calculate the terms $J(i,j)$ of the jacobian matrix of S_3 ; its characteristic equation can be written as :

(2) $(s-J(1,1))(s-J(2,2))(s-J(3,3)) = detJ - J(1,1)J(2,2)J(3,3)$
$$+ s(J(1,2)J(2,1)+J(1,3)J(3,1)$$
$$+J(2,3)J(3,2))$$

We have :
$$-2detJ=k\rho\rho'(\frac{\partial v}{\partial a}\frac{\partial v'}{\partial \chi} - \frac{\partial v}{\partial \chi}\frac{\partial v'}{\partial a}) -\rho\rho' \sigma\frac{da}{2d\chi}2(\frac{\partial v}{\partial b}\frac{\partial v'}{\partial a} + \frac{\partial v}{\partial a})$$

We have also : $\frac{da}{d\chi}2 < 0$, $\frac{da}{da_2}1 > 0$ and $\frac{da}{da_2}3 < 0$; hence, if $\frac{\partial v}{\partial \chi}$ is negative, $detJ < 0$.

Then, by considering the two curves whose equations are given by the left hand side of (2) (a cubic C) and by the right hand side (a straight line D), a necessary condition of instability (which is also sufficient if $\sigma\frac{da}{2d\chi}2 - \frac{\partial v}{\partial \chi} - \frac{\partial v'}{\partial \chi} < 0$) is given by:

(3) $\omega_C < \omega_D$, where ω_C and ω_D are the slope at the origin respectively for C and D. The Figure 5 shows the respective positions of C and D, when C has three negative roots. The inequality (3) can be written as :

(4) $\frac{\partial v+v'}{\partial a} \sigma_2 \frac{da}{d\chi}2 - \rho'k(\rho(\frac{\partial v+v'}{\partial \chi} - \sigma\frac{da}{2d\chi}2) + \frac{\partial v}{\partial a}) - \rho'\frac{\partial v}{\partial b}(\rho\frac{\partial v'}{\partial \chi} + \frac{\partial v'}{\partial a}) > 0$

The comparison between inequalities (1) and (4) is interessant : in (1), we must have a large activation by a_2 ; here also we must have a large activation by b, but only if the term $\rho\frac{\partial v'}{\partial \chi} + \frac{\partial v'}{\partial a}$ is negative : hence we need a sufficiently large activation by ADP, AMP and a sufficiently large inhibition by ATP to have this negativity ; there is a curious effect of balance for the F2,6P$_2$:

- if the other effectors of the first PFK are not sufficiently powerful, the role of F2,6P$_2$ is stabilizing

- if the other effectors are sufficiently powerful, F2,6P$_2$ reinforces largely

their action. We have then a multiplicative effect of the effectors leading
to a destabilization of the high energy steady state ; but in order to obtain
this multiplicative effect, we need a sufficient action by the other adenylates effectors (inhibition for ATP substrate and activation for ADP and AMP
products).

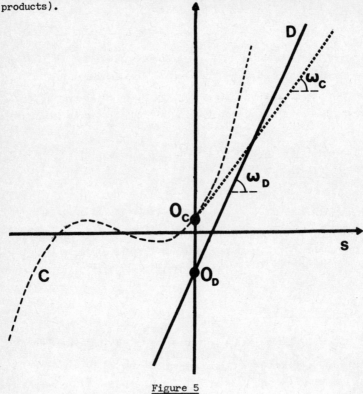

Figure 5

relative positions of the cubic C and the straight line D, in the case where
all roots of C are negative.

If the third root of C is positive, we must replace in the inequality (4)
the right hand side by an appropriate number λ, which is strictly positive.
Remark : the condition above $\frac{\partial \tau}{\partial X} < 0$ is realized, if the action by effectors is larger
than the activation by ATP substrate, which is in general the case.

5. Conclusion

5.1. Relations between models and experiments

There is a good qualitative agreement between the evolution of the values
of the oscillations periods in the model S_2 and in the experiments made in cellular
extracts (19) ; we are also finding in certain conditions two maxima in a period of
the oscillatory concentration of ADP as in certain experiments (see Hess B. & Boiteux
A. in Biological and biochemical oscillators, Chance B. et al. eds, 229, Acad. Press,

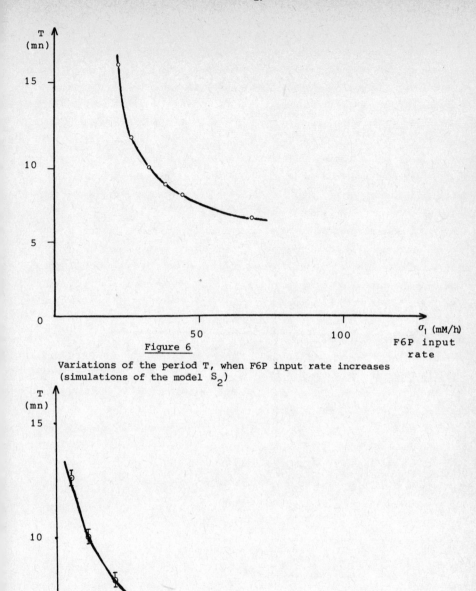

Figure 6

Variations of the period T, when F6P input rate increases
(simulations of the model S_2)

Figure 7

Variations of the period T, when the glucose input rate increases
(experimental data obtained in cellular extracts (19))

New York (1975)). We have also a good prediction by the model S_2 of the behavior observed in the reconstituted system : in Figure 1, we have damped oscillations for the value σ_1 = .103 mM ; in this case, the stability diagram of the figure 2 shows a stable focus, because the real value of $\log\rho$ is equal to 0.5.

The main discrepancy is due to the fact that we can observe oscillations in cellular extracts, when the input rate σ_1 is equal to .1 mM. Two explanations are possible :

1) there is in cellular extracts the two kinds of PFK described above ; then the multiplicative activation effect due to the $F2,6P_2$ causes an enlargement of the unstability region ; this effect could explain the difference of behaviour between the cellular extracts and the reconstituted system.

2) the conditions of application of the classical allosteric kinetics are the following : the concentrations of the substrates and effectors must be very larger than the concentration of enzyme ; in fact, these conditions are not realized in vivo, because the concentrations for example of PFK and F6P are approximatively the same : 0.24 mM (see Sols A. & Marco R. in Current topics in cellular regulation $\underline{2}$, 227-275 (1970)) ; in order to take into account this observation, we must replace, in the kinetic term v the concentrations a, a_1, ... by the concentrations $\underline{a}$, $\underline{a}_1$, ... of the free fractions of the substrate and of the effectors.

5.2. A possible improvement of the models

Let us give some indications about the determination of the free fractions of the substrate and of the effectors ; if we use the Dalziel's equations (see Dalziel K. FEBS Letters $\underline{1}$, 346-348 (1968)), we have in the case of only one substrate s and one activator a, if we denote by Rs_ia_j the more general complex :

$$\underline{s} = s - (Rs + Rsa + \ldots + Rsa_j + \ldots + Rsa_n)$$
$$- 2(Rs_2 + Rs_2a + \ldots + Rs_2a_j + \ldots + Rs_2a_n)$$
$$\ldots\ldots\ldots\ldots\ldots\ldots\ldots\ldots\ldots\ldots\ldots\ldots\ldots\ldots\ldots\ldots$$
$$- i(Rs_i + Rs_ia + \ldots + Rs_ia_j + \ldots + Rs_ia_n)$$
$$\ldots\ldots\ldots\ldots\ldots\ldots\ldots\ldots\ldots\ldots\ldots\ldots\ldots\ldots\ldots\ldots$$
$$- n(Rs_n + Rs_na + \ldots + Rs_na_j + \ldots + Rs_na_n)$$
$$- (Ts + Tsa + \ldots + Tsa_j + \ldots . Tsa_n)$$
$$\ldots\ldots\ldots\ldots\ldots\ldots\ldots\ldots\ldots\ldots\ldots\ldots\ldots\ldots\ldots\ldots$$
$$- n(Ts_n + \ldots + Ts_na_j + \ldots + Ts_na_n)$$

Hence the free fraction $\underline{s}$ of the substrate can be written as :

$$\underline{s} = s - nR(\underline{s}/K_R(1+\underline{s}/K_R)^{n-1}/((1+\underline{s}/K_R)^n + L_o/(1+\underline{a}/K_{R,a})^n))$$
$$- nT(\underline{s}/K_T(1+\underline{s}/K_T)^{n-1}/((1+\underline{s}/K_T)^n + L_o/(1+\underline{a}/K_{T,a})^n)),$$

where R (resp. T) is the total concentration of the form R (resp. T), K_R and K_T (resp. $K_{R,a}$ and $K_{T,a}$) are the dissociation constants of the substrate (resp. the activator) for the forms R and T ; this results from the expression of the concentration for the complex Rs_i :

$$Rs_i = \binom{n}{i}(\frac{s}{K_R})^i R$$

We have also the same expression for Ra_j and Rs_ia_j :

$$Rs_ia_j = \binom{n}{i}(\frac{s}{K_R})^i Ra_j = \binom{n}{i}\binom{n}{j}(\frac{s}{K_R})^i(\frac{a}{K_{R,a}})^j R$$

Because we have a dual expression for $\underline{a}$ as function of $R,T,\underline{s},a$ and $\underline{a}$, the two implicit equations allow us to calculate $\underline{s}$ and $\underline{a}$ by a method of successive approximations. If we put these values $\underline{s}$ and $\underline{a}$ in the kinetic term ν, we obtain a system S_2' which is different of S_2 ; for example, in the case where the allosteric kinetics is simple (c=0, d=0 and the form T being completely inactive), we have for ν the following expression :

$$\nu(\underline{s},\underline{a}) = \frac{Ds(1+s)^{n-1}}{(1+s)^n + \frac{L_o}{(1+a)^n}} \quad ,$$

where D denotes the concentration of enzyme. If ADP is chosen as activator, a differential system analogous to the system S_1 is given by :

$$\begin{cases} \frac{d\underline{s}}{d\theta} = \sigma_1 - \nu(s,a) \\ \\ \frac{d\underline{a}}{d\theta} = \rho(\nu(s,a) - \sigma_2 a), \end{cases}$$

where D equal to 1, if θ is a normalized time. For this new system S_1', a necessary and sufficient condition of instability is given by :

$$(5) \quad -\frac{\partial \nu}{\partial \underline{s}} + \rho(\frac{\partial \nu}{\partial \underline{a}} - \sigma_2\frac{\partial a}{\partial \underline{a}}) \geqslant 0$$

We can show easily that (5) leads to the inequality :

$$(6) \quad -\frac{\partial \nu}{\partial \underline{s}} + \rho(\frac{\partial \nu}{\partial \underline{a}} - \sigma_2(1+n\frac{\partial \nu}{\partial \underline{s}}) - \frac{n\sigma_1}{s(1+a)}\frac{\partial \nu}{\partial a} - \frac{n\sigma_1 a}{(s(1+a))^2}(\frac{1}{a}+\frac{nL_o}{(1+s)^n(1+a)^n})) \geqslant 0$$

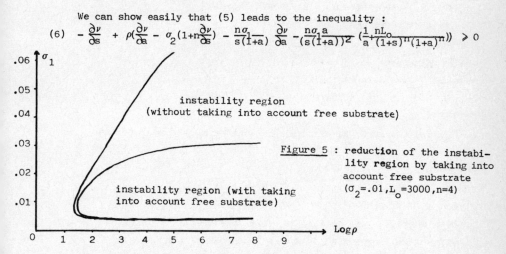

Figure 5 : reduction of the instability region by taking into account free substrate (σ_2=.01, L_o=3000, n=4)

We are now in a new step of the modelling : after a first approach, the discrepancies between models and experiments have suggested certain improvements ; this return to the modelling will perhaps allow us to make better predictions, essentially in the case of cellular extracts.

References :

(1) ANEB M.

Thesis Orsay (1980)

(2) ANEB M. & KELLERSHOHN N.

in Ben Hamida F. & al. eds ; Ecole franco-africaine de biologie moléculaire

vol. II, 187 (1980)

(3) ANEB M. & KELLERSHOHN N. (to appear)

(4) CHANCE B., ESTABROOK R.W. & GHOSH A.

Proc. Natl. Acad. Sci. U.S.A. 51, 1244 (1964)

(5) CHANCE B., HESS B. & BETZ A.

Biochem. Biophys. Res. Commun. 16, 182 (1964)

(6) DEMONGEOT J. & SEYDOUX F.J.

in Delattre P. & Thellier M. eds ; Elaboration et justification des modèles

vol. II, 519.

Maloine Paris (1979)

(7) DEMONGEOT J.

Lect. Notes in Biomaths 41, 40 (1981)

(8) DEMONGEOT J.

in Paulré B. ed. ; System dynamics and analysis of change, 151

North Holland Amsterdam (1981)

(9) GOLDBETER A. & LEFEVER R.

Biophys. J. 12, 1302 (1972)

(10)HEINRICH R., RAPOPORT S.M. & RAPOPORT T.A.

Progress in Theor. Biol. 32, 1 (1977)

(11)HERVAGAULT J.F.

Thesis Compiègne (to appear)

(12)HERVAGAULT J.F. & THOMAS D.

Eur. J. Biochem. (to appear)

(13)HESS B. & BOITEUX A.

in Järnefelt J. ed. ; Regulatory functions in biological membranes, 148

Elsevier Amsterdam (1968)

(14)HIGGINS J.

Biochemistry 51, 989 (1964)

(15)LAURENT M. & SEYDOUX F.J.

Biochem. Biophys. Res. Commun. 78, 1289 (1977)

(16)LAURENT M., CHAFFOTTE A.F., TENU J.P., ROUCOUS C. & SEYDOUX F.J.

Biochem. Biophys. Res. Commun. 80, 646 (1978)

(17)LAURENT M., SEYDOUX F.J. & DESSEN P.

J. Biol. Chem. 254, 7515 (1979)

(18) PUISSANT H.

Thesis Angers (1979)

(19) PUISSANT H. & KELLERSHOHN N. (to appear)

(20) SCHELLENBERGER W., ESCHRICH K. & HOFMANN E.

Adv. in Enzyme Regulation 19, 257 (1981)

(21) SEL'KOV E.E.

Eur. J. Biochem. 4, 79 (1968)

(22) TIJANE M.N., SEYDOUX F.J. , HILL M., ROUCOUS C. & LAURENT M.

F.E.B.S. Letters 105, 249 (1979)

(23) TIJANE M.N., CHAFFOTTE A.F., SEYDOUX F.J., ROUCOUS C. & LAURENT M.

J. Biol. Chem. 255, 188 (1980)

(24) TIJANE N.N., CHAFFOTTE A.F., YON J.M. & LAURENT M.

F.E.B.S. Letters (to appear)

(25) VAN SCHAFTINGEN E., HUE L. & HERS H.G.

Biochem. J. 192, 897 (1980)

MEDICAL EXPLORATION

OF SOME RYTHMIC PHENOMENA :

A TOPOLOGICAL SEMEIOLOGY

Y.L. KERGOSIEN

Institut des Hautes Etudes Scientifiques

91440 Bures sur Yvette, France.

ABSTRACT : We modelize the process of medical exploration in
the setting of Elementary Catastrophe Theory and mapping
controls. Morphologic exploration leads in this way to some
topological pattern recognition devices that we then apply to
the electrocardiologic study of the periodic data of Body
Surface Potential Mapping. Dynamical systems are proposed to
be explored by coupling them with controlled families of
systems ; a priori hidden parameters of the state space are
shown to be measurable in the case of sleep training experiments.

KEY WORDS : CATASTROPHE THEORY, PATTERN RECOGNITION, SEMIOLOGY,
RADIOLOGY, BODY SURFACE POTENTIAL MAPPING, SYSTEM COUPLING.

INTRODUCTION

The territory that the physician explores is the space of available tests
or questions, just as for the experimentalist it is the space of experimental
protocoles. In order to fulfill some optimality conditions (patient state and
comfort, cost, time...) the protocole of exploration has to be hierarchically
organized (in fact as a kind of generalized catastrophe), and at each step of
the investigation gross identifications on the results have to be made in order
to relate these to a small set of further investigations, or diagnosis, or the-
rapeutic alternatives. We shall generalize these aspects of radiologic interpretation to general morphological investigations and then sketch some possible
extensions to the study of dynamical systems.

I. THE MORPHOLOGY OF MAPPING CONTROLS

FUNDAMENTAL EXAMPLE : STANDARD RADIOLOGY

Let us examine the first successive steps of the interpretation, restricted to its geometric aspects, of a standard radiograph : from a function defined on the two-dimensional film (the optical density) we want to find some characteristics of the radiographed object. The radiologic opacity of this object is a piecewise constant function defined on $\mathbb{R}^3$, we assume the discontinuities to occur on a smoothly embedded compact two-dimensional manifold that we call the contrast surface (C.S.). The X-rays are emitted from a point and impress the film according to the cumulated opacities of the volumes they crossed. On the film, the radiologist sees lines that roughly correspond to the set of target singular points of the conical projection that maps the C.S. on the film and the center of which is the X-ray source (fig.1). From this target singular set, we want to find some properties of the C.S., i.e. to put it in some class of an equivalence relation (see KERGOSIEN 1977, 1979 for details and a discussion of the hypotheses).

For a given object, the radiograph depends on operating conditions (position of the object relatively to the source and the film, deformations of the object) that constitute a topological space D. As the C.S. is not directly visible, the first step of the examination consists in taking a radiograph with a poor control on the operating conditions. It is this lack of control that facilitates the interpretation of this first picture : we can assume that any property that is generic for D is true here (a property of the elements of of a topological space is called generic in this set if it is true for the points of residual subset, i.e. a countable intersection of open dense subsets, that is an open dense set in a Baire space such as the D that we consider). In particular, the embedding of the C.S. has the following generic property (Whitney) : the projection of the C.S. on the film is topologically (C^p) stable, its target singularity is locally made of three types of curve germs (see fig.) : (1) smooth parts of curves coming from the projection of folds of the C.S., (2) normal crossings coming from the generically superimposed projections of two folds of the C.S., (3) cusps coming from the projection of a "pleat" of the C.S. The first sign (tangential incidence) has been used from the beginning of radiology. The second one is known as the silhouette sign and has recently been used in a very efficient way (see FELSON), but its justification, needing the present theory, has been a puzzle for radiologists : it is possible to construct counterexamples to the silhouette sign, that is patterns of normal

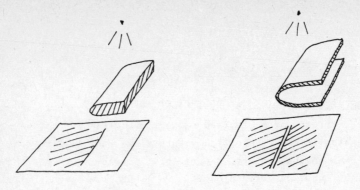

Fig. 1 : Two modes of formation of the radiologic line : a) classical, b) double contrast technique.

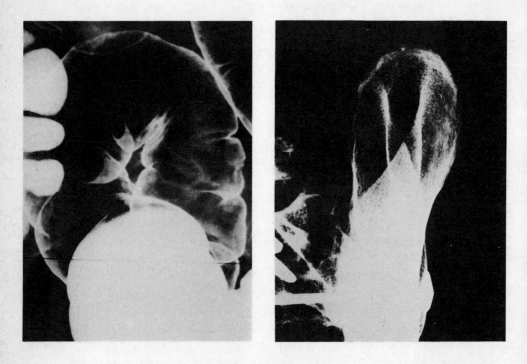

Fig. 2 : Appearance of lines, crossings, and cusps on radiographs. Left : swallow tail sections on a colon (double contrast technique). Right : cusps on an oblique incidence of ilium (see KERGOSIEN 1977 for details), radiograph here taken on a dry bone but this pattern is stably seen during intra-veinous urographies.

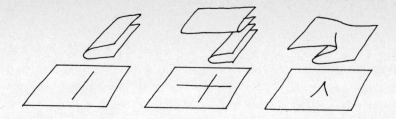

FIG.3 : The three signs of generic standard radiology : curve from a
fold, crossing from two folds, cusp from a "pleat".

crossings that do not come from the superimposition of separate folds, or separate folds intersected by the same ray that do not generate a crossing, but in
order to stabilize such situations one needs an amount of control that is not
available in practice ; they therefore have no chance to occur. The third sign
is new as a sign and we started to use it. From these local signs, the radiologist reconstructs a germ of the C.S. over the target singularity and then has
to pick the good answer among a discrete set of possible prolongations to a
global C.S., what he does with the help of his anatomic knowledge or other
radiographs.

Two methodologic features should be noticed : (1) Both the completeness
of this set of signs and the meaning of these rely on genericity assumptions
that, by restricting in a negligible way only the context of interpretation,
brings a discrete classification on morphologies. (2) From the initial data
(the opacity function defined on $\mathbb{R}^3$), data reduction extracted first a mapping
from a 2-manifold to $\mathbb{R}^3$ (image : the C.S.), then a mapping from a 1-manifold
to $\mathbb{R}^2$ (image : the curve on the film), each time considering sharp variations,
as opposed to the averaging and integration processes that are so often used
in the presentation of data. The first extraction uses a property of biological
objects, the second one is done by the eye but also uses the properties of an
artifical projection (a mere section of the C.S. would not permit such a recons-
truction). An advantage is that the interpretation can be localized and hierarchically organized as opposed to scanning techniques that need to consider the
same whole set of measurments in order to reconstruct the opacity at any point,
what is beyond the capabilities of the human brain.

With a single radiograph, the only amount of control we have is the capability of moving our eyes on the film to detect curves. But with some expense,
we can explore the object under a bigger control, i.e. restrict D to a member
of a family of subspaces the parameters of which we control. For instance, we

can control the position of a rigid object under the X-rays and observe the
qualitative changes of the radiograph. The extension of the exploration consists in structuring the new dimensions of the control. A careful choice of the
position of the object will now show new types of singularities such as the beek
to beek (see THOM) or tangent lines, but we can still assume some genericity
for the shape of the object, what limits again the number of local types. Let
us fix a point of the object and take $\mathbb{P}^2$, the 2-manifold of non oriented directions in $\mathbb{R}^3$, as the control space,(assuming the rays to be parallel). We shall
then observe some of these new patterns for positions of the object corresponding to curves in $\mathbb{P}^2$: they need only a 1-dimensional control to be observed
(and come from special points of the C.S. that lie on curves), the other ones
occur for isolated points of $\mathbb{P}^2$: they need the full 2-dimensional control to
appear (and come from isolated points of the C.S.). The set of directions for
which non stable patterns occur is called the obturation set, it is a stratified
closed subset of the control space $\mathbb{P}^2$, in correspondance with the set, called
the singular set of the control, of points of the C.S. that generate these unstable patterns. To sum up, the extension of the control permits to observe
more and more patterns, that are associated to higher codimensional strata and
thus had no chance to appear before.

THE FORMALISM OF MAPPING CONTROLS

We merely extend E.C.T. to a morphologic problematics, replacing changes
in the asymptotic states of gradient dynamical systems by changes of types (C^p
or else) of mappings. All the formalism is C^p.; let A, B, C, be manifolds ; a
mapping control from A to B is a mapping $F : A \times C \to B \dot{\times} C$ (where $B \dot{\times} C$ stands for
a certain fiber bundle with fibre B and base C) morphism of fiber bundles that
leaves C fixed. A is the source, B the target, C the control space. One can
thus define for any $c \in C$ a mapping f_c from A to B and such that $F(,c) = (f_c,c)$.
Two controls F and G are C^p equivalent if there exist diffeomorphisms h and k of
$A \times C$ and $B \dot{\times} C$ respectively, commuting with the bundle projections on C, and
such that $k \circ F = G \circ h$. A set of controls being given the topology induced by
the one of $C^p(A \times C, B \dot{\times} C)$, a control is stable in it if it has a neibourhood of
equivalent controls. We call contour diagram the subset of $B \dot{\times} C$ that is the
union of the singular values of all the f_c ; obturation set of the control the
set of points of C such that f_c is not stable (or, better in some cases : such
that any neibourhood contains a point with non equivalent f_c) ; singular set of
the control the set of points $x \in A$ such that there exist a $c \in C$ for which the
germ of f_c at $f_c^{-1}(f_c(x))$ is not structurally stable (see KERGOSIEN 1981 for
details).

In this setting, the constitution of a qualitative semiology thus follows the steps : (1) find some equivalence relation on controls such that the corresponding stability is generic in the set of controls, (2) describe the features of the stable controls : local properties of their obturation sets, singular sets and contour diagrams, (3) from the properties of a given stable control, deduce some information on the operating conditions it involved, i.e. relate classes of controls to other features of the operating conditions.

Example : Multiprojective types of plane curves. Let us consider for a curve a circle smoothly imbedded in $\mathbb{R}^2$. Given a point O in $\mathbb{R}^2$, the orthogonal projection of the curve on a line passing through O is controlled by the direction of the line. The set of such directions is the one-dimensionnal projective space, $\mathbb{P}^1$, and is equivalent to a circle. A is the curve, B the line, A×C a cylinder, B×C a Moebius strip. The control depends on the embedding and its stability is generic in the space of smooth embeddings of a circle in $\mathbb{R}^2$ (operating conditions). For such a stable control, the diagram of contours exhibits only cusps and normal crossings, no two of them occuring for the same direction. Cusps correspond to inflexions of the curve and crossings to double tangents

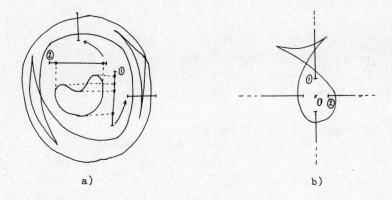

a)   b)

Fig.4 : a) A way of drawing a diagram of the contours of a curve as seen from different directions (from infinitely remote points).This diagram, drawn on a cylinder, exhibits the identification properties of the double covering of a diagram drawn on a Moebius strip. b) Getting the contours from sections of the polar transform of the curve ; O center of the inversions (a second inversion should be performed on each section, that glues the two ends of the segment by mapping infinitely remote points on O).

(fig.4). In fact, the diagram of contours is equivalent to the polar transform (transformée par polaires réciproques) of the curve (the plane becomes equivalent to a Moebius strip when it is compactified into $\mathbb{P}^2$ and a point removed). The obturation set is the set of directions of double tangents and tangents at the inflexion points, the singular set contains inflexion points of the curve and points of contact of double tangents. A class of smooth equivalence of such controls is called a multiprojective (m.p.) type of embedding. M.p. types provide a rather refined, though qualitative, classification of plane curves. In fact, the diagram of contours can be used in pattern recognition to code such shapes into series of symbols and compare them to each other, to establish a morphological distance between them (counting the minimum number of codimension one "bumps" necessary to transform one type into another), to extract features (subsequences of symbols), to write formal metaphors and study the constraints on them, etc... The mapping control tools thus transform gross classifications of the contour diagrams into finer ones for curves.

Example : Multidistance types of plane curves. For the same curve, we can control the distance function to a point of the plane by the position of this point. The control space is the plane itself, and for each value of the control, the distance is a mapping of the curve on $\mathbb{R}^+$. The smooth stability of such controls is generic in the space of smooth embeddings of the circle in the plane. The obturation set is the evolute of the curve and has generically only cusps (corresponding to the vertices of the curve) and normal crossings (doubly osculating circles). The contour diagram, in $\mathbb{R}^3$, shows stable swallow tails. Restricting the classification to smoothly equivalent types of obturation sets gives a new classification of curves, comparable to the use of the cut-locus (the symmetric axis of Harry BLOOM), but more refined. The symbolic coding formerly mentionned can also be used for the evolute.

Example : Radiology. For a simpler study, we only consider orthogonal projections of a smoothly embedded compact 2-dimensionnal submanifold of $\mathbb{R}^3$ on a
plane that passes through a fixed point O and the direction of which is controlled by the 2-dimensionnal projective space $\mathbb{P}^2$ (the conical character of the projections of real radiology, however, must be taken into account to assure that the symmetry properties of the body will not stabilize higher codimensionnal singularities on strict profile radiographs). The equivalence relation on controls has to be loosened into a quasi-smooth formalism involving blow-ups (see KERGOSIEN 1981) in order to avoid moduli, i.e. continuous variations of the smooth type, and to provide generic stability. We still get a finite number of local types of image, corresponding to diverse strata of the obturation set and the singular set, the points of the latter being characterised by

properties that are expressible in terms of classical differential geometry :
e.g. the beek to beek and lip patterns (see THOM for these terms) occur at
parabolic points of the surface, also the swallow tail patterns appear at points
of the surface where the geodesic curvature of one asymptotic line is null. The
global obturation set make understandable the changes in the radiologic image
of the same object when it is rotated (fig.). From it, one can deduce much

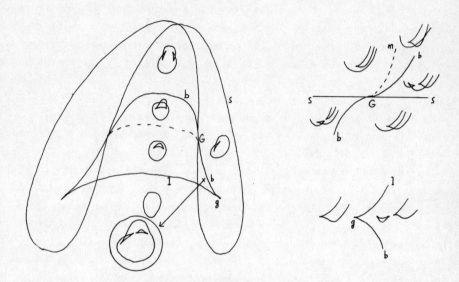

Fig.5. Left : How the obturation set can account for the changes in the radiologic image of a rotated object ; b, l, s, g, G, m, refer respectively to beek
to beek, lip, swallow tail, gouttière, godron, and multilocal strata. Right :
Details of the unfolding of the godron (top) and gouttière (bottom).

information about the differential geometry of the object. We now use this
method to create a semiology (i.e. a system of signs or an interpretation procedure) on the data of another medical investigation, basing the data reduction
on singularisation rather than on averaging or sampling.

II.

INTERPRETATION OF SOME PERIODIC DATA : BODY SURFACE POTENTIAL MAPPING.

Body surface potential mapping (B.S.P.M.) is a refinement of electrocardio-
graphy (E.C.G.). The human body can be considered as a juxtaposition of media
of different conductivities, the surrounding air being an insulator. The heart
generates electric currents that are supposed to reach equilibrium instantane-
ously but that vary with the physiologic state of the heart in a periodic way.
The electric potential (relatively to a reference zero) is measured every 2

milliseconds at more than a hundred leads scattered on the body surface ; a set of synchronous measurments is called a sample. The amount of data for a single cycle is thus huge, and things get even worse when one studies the effects of respiration, pathology, drugs, etc... Among the problems that arise on the way to the clinical use of this exam : to display a nice map of a sample requires some interpolation that takes much computing time and the artefacted leads have to be detected ; on what basis should one select fewer samples for a deeper study ? (the danger is here to skip some interesting instants) ; if the effects of the inhomogenous conductive medium are removed by solving an inverse problem (what involves a lot of computation), are the standard chest conductivity data fitted to the actual patient ? How can this exam be related to the standard E.C.G. pathology ?

The set of samples can be considered as discretizing a C^p function defined on the skin surface, i.e. a mapping $v : S^2 \to \mathbb{R}$, controlled by the time that describes a circle S^1. The mapping control is thus $V : S^2 \times S^1 \to \mathbb{R} \times S^1$. Let us assume this control to be C^p ; in order to check the genericity of the C^p stability of this control, we have to know the set of operating conditions, i.e. the set of possible generators and conducting media. Let us recall that once a generator and a medium are known, the equilibrium potential on the body surface is deduced from a second specie Fredholm equation the kernel of which is related to the medium, and the second member to both the generator and the medium ; it is therefore easier to check genericity and stability properties (what involves perturbations)relative to (or coming from) the set of generators than relatively to the set of media. Here must come some assumptions on the phenomenon : we can assume the generator to lie in a space of distributions with punctual support situated inside the chest (multipole representation of early approaches), or in the space of functions (electric potentials) defined on a sphere representing the epicardium,etc... For some of such assumptions, the C^4 stability of the control, restricted to the instants of non null gene-rator, is generic whatever the medium taken in a reasonable class, but for many settings the problem is still open ; however, the examination of real data seems to justify the hypothesis of stability of the control in the case of the recorded phenomenon by showing the features of stable controls, that we now describe. The contour diagram is a curve in $\mathbb{R} \times S^1$ (a cylinder), with only cusps and normal crossings (we study only parts during which the generator is not at rest). To draw this diagram, one plots, for each sample, the values of the peaks, wells, and saddles of the skin potential. Cusps of it correspond to saddle-node patterns on the potential maps of the related instants ; cros-sings come from the presence of two extrema that have the same values (fig.6).

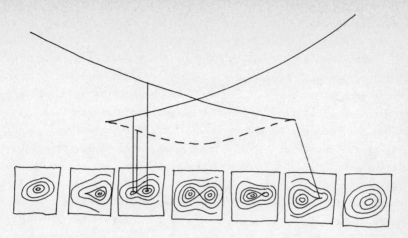

Fig.6 : Interpretation of a swallow tail section pattern of the contour diagram in terms of singularities of potential maps. Plain curves : peak values, dotted curve : saddle point values.

A nice feature of this representation is that although the locus of peaks and saddles jumps from one lead to   another, its potential value varies much more progressively and one gets very continuous curves on the contour diagram. One can thus avoid any interpolation and the processing becomes very fast.

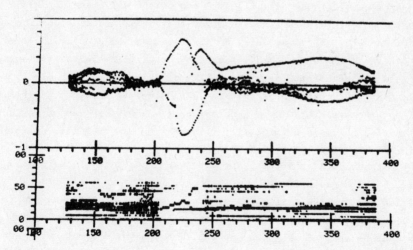

Fig.7 : Computer display of the contour diagram of the body surface potentials of a normal subject (time unit : 2 ms, logarithmic scaling of the potentials). The diagram is readable despite numerous artefacts. One recognises the P wave, QRS complex with its swallow tail (saddle point values are not plotted) in the positive wave, and the T wave. The lower part of the screen displays projections of the extrema (thick lines : maxima) on the belt, plotted against time.

Defective leads generally disrupt the continuity of the curve and are detected at first sight. What one sees is a set of waves (fig.7), the timing of which identifies them with the classic P, QRS, and T waves of the E.C.G., thus permitting the use of standard E.C.G. signs such as the QRS duration, but with a slight difference : the T wave is often seen, especially with a logarithmic scale of potential, to start as soon as before the end of the QRS (the different curves decompose, loosely speaking, what is added in the E.C.G. plotting). The continuity of the curves permits to track these even at low potential values where an instant filter would not discriminate them from noise. The quick processing of data permits to extend the control to respiration : the typical swallow tail sections on the QRS wave are then seen to increase or decrease and even disappear according to the state of the chest, what gives them an anatomic signification. Such an embedding in a larger control as a way of interpreting some features (the swallow tail sections of the contour diagram) of the restricted control, signification being conceived as the position in a control space, is what will constitute our second step about B.S.P.M.. At the end of this first step, we can deduce from the single diagram some qualitative facts about what we would get controlling (choosing) both the position of the lead and the time. We now want to extend the interpretation to a control in which some pathology can be understood.

Let us now restrict the set of generators to the different dipoles of a given module and located at a fixed point of the chest, and consider the skin potential now controlled by the oriented direction of the dipole, to get a new mapping control $V : S^2 \times S^2 \to \mathbb{R} \times S^2$. Assume a set of possible conducting media that garantees the genericity of C^p stability of this control, or else allow small multipolar perturbations of the dipole to occur (to get the genericity of stability, but the breaking of the symmetry of the generator makes the interpretation of the control more artificial). This setting is not quite realistic, but it follows an approximation widely used for E.C.G. interpretation ; it certainly does not fit the data quantitatively but enlightens some of their qualitative features. The contour diagram is now in $\mathbb{R} \times S^2$, locally as $\mathbb{R}^3$; its "worst" singularities are swallow tails. The electric activity of the heart during a cycle is modelized, the strengh of the dipole being neglected, by a mapping of S^1 in the control space S^2. In this setting, the contour diagram of an actual B.S.P.M. data is interpreted as the intersection of the 3-dimensionnal contour diagram of the new control with a cylinder the base of which is the image of S^1 in S^2 (fig.8). This accounts for the fact that the occurence of swallow tail sections on the standard contour diagram depends on the trajectory of the generator dipole. Indeed, besides the increase of QRS duration, the lack of these swallow tail patterns was a striking feature of the contour diagrams of the

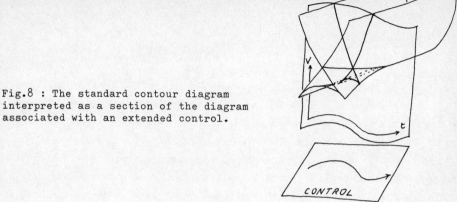

Fig.8 : The standard contour diagram
interpreted as a section of the diagram
associated with an extended control.

left bundle branch block cases that we observed. As in this case the trajectory
of the dipolar part of the cardiac generator is different, this disappearance
is consistent with the hypothesis, supported by the effect of breathing and the
repetition of the pattern with the same location (singular set) for the jumps
of wells and then peaks at different instants of the cycle, that on certain
normal patients, the swallow tails are due to the presence of the right lung
on the trajectory of the dipole rather than to the appearance of a new focus
of electric activity ; this waiting for the completion of this study and the
results of heavier explorations that will make clear the respective parts of
the medium and the generator in the appearance of multiple peaks or wells.
Even as an effect of the medium, this pattern on the contour diagram still
interests Cardiology, then becoming a topographic clue about the behaviour of
the cardiac generator. This also shows how B.S.P.M. can be conceived as a way
of exploring the chest with the aid of the heart generator, just as the method
of earth exploration. For a S^2 control, the singular set is the set of curves
on the skin where saddle-node patterns of the potential occur, with saddle-double node points on them. They are smooth and their saddle-double node strata
correspond to cusps on the obturation set.

This presentation of data is seen to contain much information, and it
seems that even if heavier means are used, such as the solution of the inverse
problem giving an epicardial potential for each sample, this tool will still
be useful to study the new results, as the study of the movements of an anima-
ted map is very difficult unless the time coordinate is spatially represented
to turn movements into shapes, what brings dimensionnal problems. On the theo-
rical side, the experimental observability of such patterns as cusps gives

clues on the justified physiological hypotheses, i.e. the spaces that can modelize the generators and media : they should make the stability of these patterns generic.

III.

DYNAMICAL SYSTEM EXPLORATION.

Let us outline what could be a similar protocole to explore dynamical systems. There will be a problem for the definition of equivalences, as in the recent past many properties of vector fields were found to be non generic ; genericity may also loose here a part of its experimental relevance by contradicting its "intuitive" probabilistic interpretation. But in a given set of vector fields there are often regions where open sets of structurally stable vector fields are separated by stratified sets : we could require the control to remain within them. As a control of a system, we choose the coupling of it with a family of systems (that we call stimulations) parametrized by the control space. This fits many experimental procedures, but also the behaviour of a system under coupling is often the only pertinent data to study higher level phenomena although the qualitative classification of systems that is established by coupling them with a given system is generally hardly related to the usual qualitative classifications of isolated systems. The space of stimulations is very large, especially because of the non autonomous ones, and we should find a hierarchical approach to it. An other new feature is here the importance of the notion of state, what calls for Catastrophe Theory in order to predict the actual occurence of sudden changes of the state under coupling, according to the history of the system, what a bifurcation diagram alone does not tell. This introduces the experimentally important problem, that we only mention, of the existence and usability,for a given system, of a preparatory coupling protocole that will bring it to a certain state whatever its past couplings.

Stable state exploration.

Let us interpret the graphic methods of ecologic system analysis as presented by Robert M.MAY : to find the equilibria of a growing system coupled to a grazing one (fixed population of grazers), one plots against the mass of vegetation the rate of growth of this vegetation and the rate of grazing of the herbivores. Equilibria occur at the intersection points of the two curves, either stable or unstable (cf. MAY). Assume that we can control continuously the shape of one curve, getting for instance a two dimensionnal family of linear characteristics : the sharp changes of state of the coupled system occur only if the linear characteristic is tangent to the other one. The catastrophe set (in the control space) is thus the polar transform of the non linear characte-

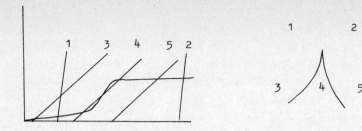

Fig. 9 : The incidence relations of the lines with the S-shaped curve (left)
summarized by the catastrophe set in the space of lines (right). The associated controlled coupling of systems exhibits hysteresis (cf. MAY).

ristic ; it is the piece of the contour diagram that we would draw from this
characteristic to study its multiprojective type. Cusps of the catastrophe set
are associated to inflexions of the characteristic (fig.9) and under our control, the state is here submitted to the hysteresis effects described in E.C.T.
The qualitative behaviour of the explored system under our particular control
is thus described by the m.p. type of its characteristic ; but, for instance,
the coupling with a three parameter family of circular characteristics (restricting the circles to what is included in a small studied region) would involve multi-distance types : the type of classification that is experimentally
established upon systems depends on the type of the couplings that are used.

In general, however, the use of a mapping control instead of a family of
curves is not so simple and only E.C.T. can be used. Let us mention another
analogon of the radiologic interpretation for a dynamical system : assume that
a heavy point slips on a given rigid smooth surface surrounding it and placed
in a black box, so that we hear only its sudden moves when we incline the box.
This action on the box is equivalent to coupling the system with another one,
e.g. a constant magnetic field acting on the point (but the exclusive action
of a 3 parameter family of central fields would involve m.d. types of surfaces).

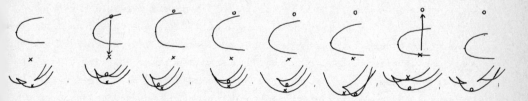

Fig.10 : Hysteresis in the equilibrium of a heavy point on a surface near a
godron. As the surface is inclined, it is simultaneously turned around a vertical axis so as to show the beek to beek pattern at jumps of the point.
Top : the movement seen from above, relatively to the parabolic line.

Then generically we can tell something about the shape of the surface from the
set of the positions at which we hear a sound : the point jumps when it reaches
a parabolic line on the surface, that we can reconstitute from the catastrophe
set in the control space (target singularity of the Gauss mapping) somewhat
as in radiologic interpretation. Moreover, hysteresis effects unfold from
"godron" points (fig 10) that correspond to cusps of the catastrophe set, besides
defined by radiologic properties ; also, the height functions have there the
same behaviour as the B.S. potential functions near (on the skin and for the
control) the saddle-double node strata.

<u>Periodic coupling.</u>

Let us consider a vector field X on a manifold M that we call the state
space. As a stimulation, we add to this vector field a non autonomous vector
field. Fortunately, natural phenomena and experimentation often involve a
simpler class of stimuli, in the form of instant (periodic or not) endomorphisms
E of the state space (cf. for instance PAVLIDIS) ; we assume these endomorphisms
to be obtained from autonomous vector fields by multiplication by a time-depen-
dent function on which a limit process is performed as in distribution theory,
and we shall restrict ourselves to periodic simple stimulations, i.e. the same
endomorphism performed periodically on M, the vector field X acting during the
intervals of length T separating two successive stimuli. In this class, the case
of a periodic projection on a submanifold, such as a periodic voltage clamp
experiment, involves for instance endomorphisms of a line segment and shows
the possibility of "chaotic" behaviour for a stimulated two dimensionnal vector
field. More generally, one studies $P = E \circ F(T)$, where F is the flow associated
to X. Under P, the state may travel rather far away relatively to the effect
of E, especially when F(T) is close to the identity, what may occur for instance
when T is close to the period of an eventual orbit of X. The behaviour of such
systems is very rich, and we shall only try to emphasize some methodological
points.

A way of simplifying things is to identify systems by looking at their
asymptotic states, for instance fixed points of P, what will bring us close to
the equilibrium considerations of the previous section. One can then vary E and
T and do some Catastrophe Theory, looking for sudden jumps of the state of the
discrete time system P when the control progressively alters E and T ; but it
is even better to deduce information on the subset of M where the jumps occur,
that we call again singular set. For instance, controlling in M the position
of a stable node of P with two parameters, M being 2-dimensionnal, cusp catastrophe situations quite similar to the godron case can be seen : the node
cannot go everywhere on the state space and jumps when reaching certain lines,

where it becomes a saddle-node ; these lines, the singular set, are comparable
to the parabolic lines of our previous sounding surface, smooth and in correspondance with the catastrophe set (to build trivially the analogy, just notice
that a high frequency small stimulation has almost the effect of adding a constant vector field to X, but other cases may involve longer trajectories under
X, possibly close to orbits of X, not to mention periodic points of P that we
excluded from this discussion). This is to insist on the need for considering
hysteresis effects, or their generalisations, in the study of locking phenomena,
lockings on the same periods possibly corresponding to very different physiologic functionnal states. The kind of study just mentionned can of course go
further with the alternation of different endomorphisms,etc... In a way, it
modelizes perception by the capability for the systems to perform rythm recognition.

These deductions on the system and the behaviour of the state under coupling, made from the catastrophe set, may however be limited in the absence of
experimental data concerning the state itself ; on the other hand, what is
known about the evolution of the system may be limited to a single parameter.
This case is not hopeless, as indirect evidence can often be found, as shown,
for instance, by the case of sleep training experiments. When time clues are
suppressed, subjects incease their nyctemeral periods, alter the phase relations
of their temperature and sleep oscillations, and show subharmonic phenomena
after about five weeks (cf. CZEISLER & al.). To fix ideas, let us quickly (and
loosely, because we do not take into account duck phenomena) modelize sleep

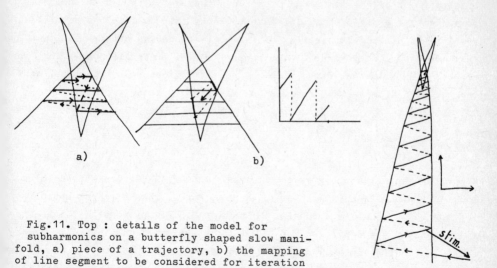

Fig.11. Top : details of the model for
subharmonics on a butterfly shaped slow manifold, a) piece of a trajectory, b) the mapping
of line segment to be considered for iteration
and its graph. Right : the state space and its
slow manifold with two coordinates, the stimulation.

and awakening, the only observables that we shall consider, by fold catastrophes, and simulate subharmonics with a butterfly shaped slow manifold (fig.11). We intend to study only the location and stabilisation of the state during the training, that we suppose to consist in the periodic occurence of an endomorphism. If, in this setting, one coordinate of the state on the slow manifold is taken to be normal to the folds, to describe the nyctemeral oscillation of the state (at the training frequency when the locking is established), another one should be related to the delay from the end of the training to the appearance of subharmonics, and physiologically expresses the slow adaptation of the system to the training. For instance, the study of the relation between this delay and the period of the training is quite accessible to experimentation and should be taken into account in any modelling option (the qualitative modelling of subharmonics needs of course to be checked by complex stimulation protocoles). The conditions of stabilisation under coupling, that depend on rather refined quantitative particularities of the vector field, should be explored through this parameter, for which, for instance, hysteresis under the control of the training frequency should be looked for. Besides experimental hints,this short example shows that a system, even if subject to chaos when isolated, with the subsequent difficulties for qualitative analysis, may take very easily (time clues are experimentally very difficult to eliminate) a behaviour for the study of which standard methods still work. It also shows that even for such an isolated system, the study can be focused on early phenomena, reached soon after the end of coupling, that may be much more relevant to normal physiology than asymptotic behaviours (the latter eventually giving more insight on the composition of the system and thus on pathology) ; this distinction is made possible by the use of a qualitative property (the chaotic character of subharmonics) to distinguish regions of the state space, as opposed to its classical use to define regions of the control space. It finally shows that for these studies, experimental data, such as indirect evidence on the state, can be collected even from rare observables by the use of proper protocoles.

ACKNOWLEDGEMENTS.

The experimental radiologic work was done during 1975-76 in the Radiology department of Pr.LEDOUX-LEBARD, hôpital Cochin, Paris, thanks to the support of its head and the help of Pr.A.BONNIN. Studies on B.S.P.M. were done in the Physiology and Biophysics department of Dalhousie University, Halifax N.S., in the group of Dr.E.D.SMITH, in 1979-80, on a grant from the Nova Scottia Heart Foundation ; we thank Pr.G.KLASSEN for arranging our invitation and Pr.R.ROSEN for welcome in the Red House. Our interest in system training was stimulated by

conversations with Pr.O.QUEIROZ on Plant Physiology and the data of Pr.E.D.
WEITZMAN were revealed and made available to us by Pr.J.BIRMAN.

REFERENCES.

CZEISLER C.A., WEITZMAN E.D., MOORE-EDE M.C., ZIMMERMAN J.C., KNAUER R.S. :
     "Human sleep : its duration and organization depend on its circadian
     phase", preprint.

FELSON B. : "Chest Roentgenology", W.B.Saunders Company (1973).

KERGOSIEN Y.L. : "Introduction de la Topologie en Médecine", thèse de Médecine,
     Paris (1977).

KERGOSIEN Y.L. : "L'utilisation de modèles topologiques en Médecine", Actes du
     colloque Elaboration et Justification des Modèles, ed.P.Delattre and
     M.Thellier, tome 2, pp. 551-564, Maloine, Paris (1979).

KERGOSIEN Y.L. : "La famille des projections orthogonales d'une surface et ses
     singularités", C.R. Acad. Sciences Paris, t.292 (1er juin 1981), Série
     I-929-932.

MAY R.M. : "Tresholds and breakpoints in ecosystems with a multiplicity of
     stable states",Nature, Vol.269, pp.471-477 (6 October 1977).

PAVLIDIS T. : "A mathematical model for the light affected system in the Droso-
     phila eclosion rythm", Bull. Math. Bioph., Vol.29 (1967), pp.291-310.

THOM R. : "Stabilité structurelle et Morphogénèse", Benjamin et Edisciences,
     Paris (1972).

SPATIO-TEMPORAL ORGANIZATION IN IMMOBILIZED ENZYME SYSTEMS

J.P. KERNEVEZ *, E. DOEDEL **, M.C. DUBAN *,
J.F. HERVAGAULT *, G. JOLY * AND D. THOMAS *

* U. T. C., BP 233, 60206, Compiègne, France

** Computer Science Department, Concordia University,
1455 de Maisonneuve Blvd. w., Montréal, Québec H3G 1M8

ABSTRACT

This paper discusses temporal ans spatial structures in immobilized
enzyme systems.

The reactions considered consume two substrates, S and A, and are
inhibited by exceeding S and activated by A. The coupling of diffusion
and enzymatic reaction is first studied in a simple model which exhibits a time-periodic behavior. A complete description of stable and
unstable steady states, together with stable and unstable orbits, is
obtained through numerical methods of continuation. Then these methods
are employed to find oscillations in a Phosphofructokinase system.

Sustained oscillations are experimentally observed for the parameter
values thus obtained.

This study of biochemical rhythmicity concludes with mathematical
considerations about families of periodic solutions, and algorithms
of continuation for calculating them.

Our analysis of spatial patterns in immobilized enzyme systems first
describes how polarity arises in a simple model.

Then, motivated by Stuart Kauffman theory of morphogenesis, we study
a diffusion-reaction model governed by two coupled P.D.E.s. Kauffman's
proposition that a uniform (reaction-diffusion) mechanism may act

throughout development to determine the locations of successive developmental commitments is justified by the sequence of patterns obtained in our model as size grows.

Using numerical methods for continuation and bifurcation of solutions,
together with the finite element method, we obtain a complete picture
of the stable and unstable steady state solutions as size varies.

I. INTRODUCTION

Enzymes are molecules which catalyze the biochemical reactions of metabolic pathways. We restrict ourselves here to reactions in which
two sustrates S and A are consumed :

$$S + A \xrightarrow{\text{Enzyme E}} Products$$

and which are inhibited by exceeding S and activated by A. Many enzyme
kinetics involving two substrates share this property.

As a first example the enzyme uricase catalyzes the consumption of
uric acid (S) and oxygen (A), with the velocity term

$$(1.1) \quad r(S,A) = V_M \frac{A}{K_A + A} \frac{S}{K_S + S(1 + S/K_{SS})}$$

where S and A are substrate concentrations, K_A, K_S and K_{SS} are parameters characteristic of the enzyme uricase and V_M is a parameter
proportional to its concentration in the reacting medium.

Since $K_A \gg A$ we take, instead of (1.1),

$$(1.2) \quad r(S,A) = V_M \frac{A}{K_A} \frac{S}{K_S + S(1 + S/K_{SS})}$$

It is this example that we have in mind when dealing with structuration in space in paragraphs 6 and 8.

As a second example, with a rate of reaction slightly more complicated
(see § 3), the enzyme Phosphofructokinase (PFK) catalyzes the consumption of ATP (S) and F6P (A). We have this example in mind while

dealing with time periodic phenomena, although in § 2 we adopt for convenience the simpler velocity term (1.2) to exemplify what we call the S-A system.

Of course in § 3 the PFK system is studied with its exact measured velocity term (3.1).

General accounts of oscillatory phenomena in biology are given in [1, 2, 3] . [4] is devoted more specifically to oscillatory enzymatic reactions.

Oscillating glycolysis represents the best known example of oscillations in a metabolic pathway. See rewiews [4, 5, 6, 7] .

It has been experimentally observed in the cytoplasm of yeast cells, in more dilute cell-free extracts of yeast, beef heart muscle and rat skeletal muscle, and in ascite tumor cells. These observations have pointed out the crucial role played by the enzyme Phosphofructokinase (PFK). Many models have been elaborated, all based upon the kinetic behavior of PFK, acting either alone or coupled with other enzymes involved in the glycolytic pathway. However, few attention has been paid to the influence of diffusion phenomena on non-linear enzyme kinetics, although there is strong experimental evidence that living cell is highly compartmentalized. In paragraphs 2 and 3 we analyze the coupling of metabolite diffusion and enzyme reaction in the case respectively of the S-A system and of Rabbit Muscle Phosphofructokinase.

The main result is the experimental observation of oscillations in a model PFK system (§ 3). From the mathematical point of view the appearance of oscillations is usually related to Hopf bifurcation [8, 9] .

§ 4 contains a mathematical analysis of the branch of periodic solutions continuing a given periodic solution as some parameter varies.

§ 5 gives the principle of numerical methods of continuation of periodic solutions and gives numerical results.

Pattern formation in chemically reacting and diffusing systems and its possible role in morphogenesis have been pointed out by Turing in 1952 [10] . Many authors have developed reaction diffusion models showing pattern formation [10, 11, 12   ]. We present in § 6 a particularly simple two-cell system in which polarity appears.

Then § 7 presents S. Kauffman model of sequential developmental commitments in embryos. In § 8 we analyze the steady states of a similar model, coupling S-A kinetics (1.2) and diffusion of the substrates.

We find that the field of concentrations shows, as size grows, sequential patterns according to Kauffman propositions.

2. OSCILLATIONS IN THE S - A SYSTEM

2.1.   0 - DIMENSIONAL MODEL

An inactive membrane (i.e. without enzyme activity) separates a reservoir containing a solution of S and A, at fixed concentrations S_0 and A_0, and a well- stirred reactor containing enzyme E. The substrates S and A diffuse through the membrane from the reservoir to the reactor, where they are consumed. The concentrations S and A in the reactor are governed by the two O.D.E.s.

$$(2.1) \begin{cases} v_R \dfrac{ds}{dt} = \dfrac{D_S \Sigma}{L} (S_0 - S) - v_R \, r\,(S,A) \\[2mm] v_R \dfrac{dA}{dt} = \dfrac{D_A \Sigma}{L} (A_0 - A) - v_R \, r\,(S,A) \end{cases}$$

where v_R = reactor volume, D_S and D_A = diffusion coefficients and L and Σ = membrane thickness and contact area.
These equations can be rewritten

$$(2.2) \begin{cases} \dfrac{ds}{dt} = s_0 - s - \rho\,R\,(s,a) \\[2mm] \dfrac{da}{dt} = \alpha\,(a_0 - a) - \rho\,R\,(s,a) \end{cases}$$

where $s = S/K_S$, $a = a/K_S$, the new unit of time is

$$(2.3) \quad \theta = \frac{v_R}{v_M}\,\frac{L^2}{D_S} \quad (v_M = L\Sigma = \text{membrane volume}),$$

$$(2.4) \quad \rho = \frac{v_M}{K_A}\,\theta,$$

$$(2.5) \quad \alpha = D_A/D_S$$

and

$$(2.6) \quad R\,(s,a) = a\,s\,/\,(1 + s + ks^2), \quad (k = K_S/K_{SS}).$$

2.2.   NUMERICAL ANALYSIS OF (2.2)

For $\rho = o$, (2.2) admits the steady-state $s = s_o$, $a = a_o$. This steady-state solution can be continued as ρ varies, thus yielding a family

(2.7) $s = s (\rho)$, $a = a (\rho)$

of solutions of the algebraic system

$$(2.8) \quad \begin{cases} s_o - s - \rho R (s,a) = o \\ \alpha (a_o - a) - \rho R (s,a) = o \end{cases}$$

parameterized by ρ. This branch of solutions is represented in figure 2.1, full (resp.dashed) lines corresponding to stable (resp.unstable) foci. The nature of the steady state is easily found by inspecting the eigenvalues of the Jacobian matrix

$$(2.9) \quad \begin{bmatrix} -1 - \rho R_s & -\rho R_a \\ -\rho R_s & -\alpha - \rho R_a \end{bmatrix}$$

where $R_s = \partial R / \partial s$ and $R_a = \partial R / \partial a$.

The points separating arcs of stable and unstable foci are Hopf bifurcation points, from which branches of periodic solutions emanate. Numerical methods of continuation enable to move along these branches, thus obtaining arcs of stable orbits (✱✱✱) and arcs of unstable orbits (✱✱✱) as described in figure 2.1. Only one point (say the one for $t = o$) represents each orbit. We see in figures 2.1, 2.2 and 2.3 the possibility of an hysteresis cycle with stable oscillations as ρ decreases and stable foci as ρ increases.

For continuation of steady states, see [13, 14] . For continuation of periodic solutions see [15] .

3. OSCILLATORY BEHAVIOR OF A PHOSPHOFRUCTOKINASE SYSTEM

3.1. DESCRIPTION OF THE ENZYME REACTION

Rabbit Muscle Phosphofructokinase (E.C.2.7.1.11) catalyzes the consumption of ATP and F6P :

$$ATP + F6P \xrightarrow{\quad PFK \quad} Products.$$

This reaction was modelled by Pettigrew and Frieden $\begin{bmatrix} 16 \end{bmatrix}$.
Their kinetic model was adopted by Hervagault in $\begin{bmatrix} 17, 18, 19 \end{bmatrix}$ with the reaction rate

$$(3.1) \quad \begin{cases} R(s,a) = \dfrac{0.76 \ u \ v^3}{v^4 + w \ x^4} \\[2ex] u = 0.1 \ s \ a \\[2ex] v = 1 + s + 0.5 \ a + u \\[2ex] w = y^4 \\[2ex] y = (504 + 95 \ s) \ / \ (504 + 1.9 \ s) \\[2ex] x = 1 + s + 0.0025 \ a + 0.0025 \ u \end{cases}$$

Here s and a denote dimensionless ATP and F6P concentrations :

$$(3.2) \quad s = \begin{bmatrix} ATP \end{bmatrix} / K, \quad a = \begin{bmatrix} F6P \end{bmatrix} / K, \quad K = K_{MgATP} = 5 \ \text{micromoles}.$$

This reaction is characterized by a very strong inhibition by excess substrate.

Figure 3.1 shows the measured reaction rate (relative to a standard assay activity) at pH = 6.9 and temperature 18° C [20] .□ , ■ , ○ and ● correspond respectively to F6P = 0.2, 0.5, 1. and 2. millimoles.

3.2. THE ZERO-DIMENSIONAL MODEL

corresponds to an open dialysis bag and is governed by equations (2.2) where R (s,a) is given by (3.1). Numerical analysis of system (2.2), (3.1) was effected by two methods.

The former was to search out parameter values s_o, a_o and ρ satisfying conditions for a steady-state of (2.2) to be an unstable focus
[17] . The latter was to continue a steady-state solution as one of
these parameters varies, until finding an arc of unstable foci. The
underlying assumption was that a branch of periodic solutions could
emanate from a Hopf bifurcation point separating arcs of stable and
unstable foci, as shown in figure 3.2.
Both methods provide the same values of the parameters, for example

$$(3.3) \quad s_o = 121., \qquad å_o = 200. \qquad \text{and} \quad \rho = 450.$$

The value of α, imposed by the diffusional properties of the (ossein
gelatin) membrane, was

$$(3.4) \quad \alpha = 0.6.$$

Solving equations (2.2), (3.1) with the parameter values (3.3) and
(3.4) gives a stable orbit, with a period on the order of 1/6.
The unit of time Θ, which is also the characteristic time for diffusion in our model, is given by (2.3). For our experimental set up the
parameter values were

$$(3.5) \quad v_R/v_M = 100, \quad L = .015 \text{ cm}, \quad D_s = 7.6 \ 10^{-4} \text{ cm}^2 \text{ h}^{-1},$$
whence
$$(3.6) \quad \Theta = 29.6 \text{ hours.}$$

Thus the actual period of oscillations was on the order of 5 hours.
Such a period may seem to be very large to experimentalists acquainted
with glycolytic oscillations. However one must be aware of the fact
that equations (2.2), (3.1) represent a model system in which the
period is about 1/6, but with a unit of time Θ which can be tuned at
will by changing the ratio v_R/v_M. Thus, all other parameters (s_o, a_o,
ρ and α) being the same, the actual period, $\Theta/6$, depending upon Θ,
may range from a few seconds to several hours or days.

3.3.   EXPERIMENTAL RESULTS : With the parameter values (3.3),
(3.4) and (3.5), our experimental set up showed oscillations as represented in figure 3.3 [20] . In figure 3.3 NADH concentration
(representing the activity of the reaction) is plotted versus time,
first for $a_o = 150$ (curve 1, no oscillation), then for $a_o = 200$

(curve 2, oscillations !). Curve 2 shows that sustained oscillations with a period of approximately 5 hours were observed during more than three cycles.

3.4.   DISCUSSION   [20]

It is interesting to observe the behavior of an enzyme having a great biochemical interest, such as PFK, when its reaction is interacting with diffusion of the metabolites. The compartmentalization inherent in our model corresponds to what is expected to exist within living cells. We have shown that oscillations can exist with simple bioche-mical conditions, by only incorporating mass transfers. Since biolo-gical systems are highly structured and compartmentalized, oscillations arising from associated transfer phenomena and enzyme reactions are likely to occur.
We have also shown that a given biochemical system can exhibit sus-tained oscillations with periods ranging from, say, a few seconds to several hours or days.

3.5.   OSCILLATORY PHOPHOFRUCTOKINASE : ONE-DIMENSIONAL MODEL

If PFK molecules are uniformly immobilized within a membrane separa-ting two compartments, the ATP and F6P concentrations are governed by the partial differential equations :

$$(3.7) \begin{cases} \dfrac{\partial s}{\partial t} - \dfrac{\partial^2 s}{\partial x^2} + \sigma R\,(s,a) = 0 \\[4mm] \dfrac{\partial a}{\partial t} - \alpha\,\dfrac{\partial^2 a}{\partial x^2} + \sigma R\,(s,a) = 0 \qquad 0 < x < 1 \\[4mm] s\,(0,t) = s(1,t) = s_0 \quad ; \quad a\,(0,t) = a\,(1,t) = a_0. \end{cases}$$

where

$$(3.8) \quad \sigma = \dfrac{V_M}{K_A}\,\Theta\,, \qquad\qquad \Theta = L^2 / D_S,$$

L being the membrane thickness.

Numerical experiments were done with the parameter values

(3.9) $\sigma = 4000.$, $\alpha = 0.2$, $s_o = 326.$, $a_o = 1570.$,

showing oscillations in this distributed system with a period of $0.6\ \theta$.
However these are purely numerical results. In fact it was observed
[21] that the kinetic properties of PFK are markedly modified by
immobilization within an artificial membrane. In particular the inhibition by excess substrate disappears.

The interest of the zero-dimensional model is to make possible the
interaction of metabolite diffusion and enzyme reaction without molecular modifications.

4.   CONTINUATION OF A PERIODIC SOLUTION

Consider the autonomous system

(4.1) $\frac{dy}{dt} + f(y,\lambda) = 0,$ $y(o) = y(T)$

where y, $f \in \mathbb{R}^n$ and λ is a real parameter.

This system can be rewritten

(4.2) $\frac{dy}{d\tau} + \rho f(y,\lambda) = 0,$ $y(o) = y(2\pi)$

where

(4.3) $\rho = T/2\pi$ and $\tau = t/\rho$.

By a solution to (4.2) we mean a pair (y,ρ) of a 2π-periodic function
y and a "period" ρ. Let (y_o, ρ_o) be such a solution for $\lambda = \lambda_o$.
Then, under suitable assumptions, this solution can be continued by
a family of periodic solutions as the parameter λ is changed.

Remark 4.1. Since (4.2) is an autonomous system, time τ, parameter
used as a referent for determining $y(\tau)$ is defined up to an arbitrary
phase shift ϕ,i.e. if $y(\tau)$ satisfies (4.2), so does $y(\tau - \phi)$ for every
ϕ.
To remove this undeterminancy remark that the distance between two
neighboring orbits corresponding to λ_o and λ respectively can be

defined as inf $J(\phi)$ where

(4.4) $J(\phi) = \int_0^{2\pi} \|\, y(\tau,\lambda) - y(\tau-\phi,\lambda_0)\|_{\mathbb{R}^N}^2 \, d\tau,$

define ϕ_0 through $J'(\phi_0) = 0$ where

(4.5) $J'(\phi) = 2\int_0^{2\pi} ((y(\tau,\lambda) - y(\tau-\phi,\lambda_0), \frac{dy}{d\tau}(\tau-\phi,\lambda_0)\,))d\tau$

and shift from τ to $\tau - \phi_0$ on the orbit corresponding to λ, thus obtaining the synchronization condition

(4.6) $\int_0^{2\pi} ((y(\tau,\lambda) - y_0(\tau), \xi_0(\tau)\,)) \, d\tau = 0$

where

(4.7) $\xi_0 = dy_0/d\tau.$

Remark 4.2. It is easy to check that

(4.8) $T_0\, \xi_0 = 0$

where

(4.9) $T_0 = d/d\tau + \rho_0\, f_y(y_0,\lambda_0)$

is a linear operator acting on 2π-periodic functions.

Assumptions 4.1

(4.10)   Kernel (T_0) = span ξ_0 and $\xi_0 \notin$ Range T_0.

Proof of existence of an arc of periodic solutions passing through (y_0,ρ_0,λ_0)

We apply the Implicit Function Theorem to the mapping

(4.11) $(y,\rho,\lambda) \longrightarrow (\frac{dy}{d\tau} + \rho f(y,\lambda), \int_0^{2\pi} ((y - y_0,\xi_0)) \, d\tau\,).$

We only have to check that the linear mapping

(4.12) $(\hat{y},\hat{\rho}) \longrightarrow (T_0\hat{y} + \hat{\rho}f(y_0,\lambda_0), \int_0^{2\pi} ((\hat{y},\xi_0)) \, d\tau)$

is an isomorphism, or, equivalently, that the relations

(4.13) $T_0\hat{y} + \hat{\rho}\, f(y_0,\lambda_0) = 0$ and $\int_0^{2\pi} ((\hat{y},\xi_0)) \, d\tau = 0$

imply that

(4.14) $\hat{y} = 0$ and $\hat{\rho} = 0.$

But $\hat{\rho}\, f(y_0,\lambda_0) = -(\hat{\rho}/\rho_0)\, \xi_0 \in$ Ker T_0 while, from the first relation in (4.12), $\hat{\rho}\, f(y_0,\lambda_0) \in R(T_0).$

Thus, applying the second assumption in (4.9), we have $\hat{\rho} = 0$. Hence, from the first equation in (4.12), we get $\hat{y} = k\xi_o$ which, brung into the second equation in (4.12), gives :

$$k \int_o^{2\pi} \| \xi_o \|^2 \, d\tau = 0,$$

whence $k = 0$, and therefore $\hat{y} = 0$.

5.   CONTINUATION METHODS

The following numerical approach to continuation is, as pointed out by Mehra and Carrol [22], to combine the methods of Lahaye [23] and Davidenko [24]. Consider the problem :

(5.1) $f(x,\lambda) = 0$

where x, $f \in \mathbb{R}^n$ and λ is the so-called continuation parameter. Beginning with a solution x_o at $\lambda = \lambda_o$, Lahaye uses $x(\lambda_{i-1})$ as the initial guess in Newton iterations at λ_i. Davidenko differentiates (5.1) with respect to λ to obtain :

(5.2) $f_x(x,\lambda) \dfrac{dx}{d\lambda} + f_\lambda(x,\lambda) = 0$

where f_x is the Jacobian $(\partial f_i / \partial x_j)$, $1 \le i$, $j \le n$, and f_λ is the vector $(\partial f_i / \partial \lambda)$, $1 \le i \le n$. The system of ordinary differential equations (5.2) is integrated from $x(\lambda_o) = x_o$. Kubicek's algorithm [13] uses Davidenko's method for prediction and Lahaye's method for correction. Parameterizing by arclenth s, Kubicek obtains the extended system :

$$(5.3) \quad \begin{cases} f_x \, \dot{x} + f_\lambda \, \dot{\lambda} = 0, \\[2mm] \| \dot{x} \|^2 + \dot{\lambda}^2 = 1, \\[2mm] x(o) = x_o \quad \text{and} \quad \lambda(o) = \lambda_o. \end{cases}$$

where an upper dot denotes d/ds.

Let $z(s)$ denote the $(n + 1)$ dimensional vector $(x(s), \lambda(s))$. Euler prediction for example consists in calculating $\dot{z}(s) = (\dot{x}(s), \dot{\lambda}(s))$ from (5.3) and defining :

(5.4) $\hat{z} = z(s) + h \, \dot{z}(s)$

as a first approximation to $z(s + h)$. In order to solve (5.3) for $\overset{\bullet}{x}$ and λ, Kubicek uses Gaussian elimination with complete pivoting applied to the $n \times (n + 1)$ matrix $[f_x \vdots f_\lambda]$. This procedure provides an "independent variable, say z_k, corresponding to the column which has been eliminated . Let Γ_k be the $n \times n$ submatrix of $[f_x \vdots f_\lambda]$ formed by eliminating column k. Gaussian elimination provides also the vector β such that :

$$(5.5) \quad \Gamma_k \, \beta \, + \, f_{z_k} \, = \, 0$$

Comparing (5.3) and (5.4) we see that, since Γ_k is nonsingular,

$$(5.6) \quad \overset{\bullet}{y} \, = \, \overset{\bullet}{z}_k \, \beta$$

where y is the n-dimensional vector formed by eliminating the kth component of z. Then $\overset{\bullet}{z}_k$ is given by

$$(5.7) \quad \overset{\bullet}{z}_k \, = \, \overset{+}{_-} \, (1 \, + \, \| \, \beta \|^{\, 2})^{- \, 1}$$

where the sign of $\overset{\bullet}{z}$ is + or - according to the direction for proceeding along the solution arc.
$\hat{z}$ is taken as the starting point for Newton corrections of a special type

$$(5.8) \quad \Gamma_{k_r} \, (z^r) \, \{z_i^{r+1} - z_i^r\}_{i \neq k_p} \, = \, -f(z^r), \quad z^\circ = \hat{z}.$$

Here k_r may change at each step. This feature enables in particular to pass past turning points.
Such methods of continuation can be extended to branches of periodic solutions. Parameterizing y, ρ and λ by arclength s, equations (4.2) and (4.6) give :

$$(5.9) \quad \begin{cases} \dfrac{d\overset{\bullet}{y}}{d\tau} + \rho \, f_y \, \overset{\bullet}{y} + \overset{\bullet}{\rho} \, f + \rho \, f_\lambda \, \overset{\bullet}{\lambda} = 0, \quad \overset{\bullet}{y}(o) = \overset{\bullet}{y}(2\pi) \\[2mm] \displaystyle\int_o^{2\pi} \, ((\overset{\bullet}{y}, \xi_o)) \, d\tau \\[2mm] \| \overset{\bullet}{y} \|^2 + \overset{\bullet}{\rho}^2 + \overset{\bullet}{\lambda}^2 \, = \, 1 \\[2mm] y(., s_o) \, = \, y_o(.), \quad \lambda(s_o) = \lambda_o, \, \rho(s_o) = \rho_o \end{cases}$$

where upper dot denotes d/ds and

$$(5.10) \quad \| \overset{\bullet}{y}(s) \|^2 \, = \, \int_o^{2\pi} \| \overset{\bullet}{y}(\tau, s) \|^2 \, d\tau.$$

For continuing an orbit $(y(\tau,s),\rho(s),\lambda(s))$ we have to calculate $\dot{y}$, $\dot{\rho}$, $\dot{\lambda}$, predict a new orbit, then correct by Newton iterations. It is what is done in AUTO [15].

Some numerical experiments done with AUTO have been shown on figures 2.1, 2.2 and 2.3. They correspond to the 0-dimensional case (2.2), (2.6) with $k = 0.1$, $s_o = 100$, $a_o = 500$ and $\alpha = 0.2$.

AUTO was also applied to the 1-dimensional case (3.7) with the reaction rate (2.6), the parameters being the same as above and the continuation parameter being σ. The system of O.D.E.s solved after discretization in space was 20-dimensional, and the Floquet multipliers were computed. The results where quite similar to those shown in Figure 2.1.

6.   POLARITY IN A TWO-CELL SYSTEM

Maybe one of the simplest dissipative structures is the one we are going to introduce now. Consider again the S-A system described by equations (2.2), (2.6), but with the parameter values

(6.1) $a_o = 79.2$, $k = 0.1$, $s_o = 102.5$, $\alpha = 1.45$

and $\rho = 13$.

Then there is only one steady state defined by equations (2.8), and it is a stable node. The behavior of system (2.2) is not very interesting : $s(t)$ and $a(t)$ tend towards $\tilde{s}$ and $\tilde{a}$ as $t \to \infty$.

The situation becomes much more interesting if the reactor vessel is separated into 2 compartments by a membrane imposing diffusional constraints on the transport of S and A from each compartment to the other. The state variables are now s_1, a_1 and s_2, a_2, concentrations of S and A in both compartments. s_1 and a_1, for example, are governed by :

(6.2)
$$\begin{cases} \dfrac{ds_1}{dt} = -\dfrac{1}{\Theta_R} a_1 F(s_1) + \dfrac{1}{\Theta_T} (s_o - s_1) + \dfrac{1}{\Theta_D} (s_2 - s_1) \\[4mm] \dfrac{da_1}{dt} = -\dfrac{1}{\Theta_R} a_1 F(s_1) + \dfrac{\alpha}{\Theta_T} (a_o - a_1) + \dfrac{\beta}{\Theta_D} (a_2 - a_1) \end{cases}$$

where Θ_R, Θ_T and Θ_D are characteristic times for reaction, transport and diffusion respectively , and we have analogous equations for s_2 and a_2. Here $F(s) = s / (1 + s + ks^2)$.

It is easy to check that $s_1 = s_2 = \tilde{s}$, $a_1 = a_2 = \tilde{a}$ is still an equilibrium solution that one could still think of as stable. However this is not true. The steady states are the solutions of :

$$(6.3) \quad \begin{cases} s_1 - s_2 + \lambda[\rho a_1 F(s_1) - (s_0 - s_1)] = 0, \\[2mm] \beta(a_1 - a_2) + \lambda[\rho \hat{a}_1 F(s_1) - \alpha(a_0 - a_1)] = 0, \\[2mm] -s_1 + s_2 + \lambda[\rho a_2 F(s_2) - (s_0 - s_2)] = 0, \\[2mm] \beta(-a_1 + a_2) + \lambda[\rho a_2 F(s_2) - \alpha(a_0 - a_2)] = 0 \end{cases}$$

where $\lambda = \Theta_D/\Theta_T$ and $\rho = \Theta_T/\Theta_R$.

The representation of s_1 for example as a function of λ for $\beta = 5$ looks like Figure 6.1, where full (resp. dashed) lines represent stable (resp. unstable) steady states. Thus when λ is small or large the trivial steady state (s,a) is stable, which can be easily understood since in the first case we are approaching the condition where there is no diffusional constraint $(\Theta_D = 0)$ and in the second we are approaching the condition where both compartments are separated by an impermeable wall $(\Theta_D = \infty)$. But there is an interval (λ', λ'') such that, for each value of λ between λ' and λ'', the trivial steady state is unstable and there exist two steady states which are stable and non-symetric (i.e. $s_1 \neq s_2$ and $a_1 \neq a_2$). Usually diffusion has a smoothing effect and tends to make the concentrations uniform. Here it is the contrary : diffusional constraints may cause a gradient of concentrations.

We must point out the analogy with polarity in biology. In the above model, diffusion constraints, interacting with a very common enzyme activity, may cause a differentiation between 2 compartments. In biology too, polarity phenomena (i.e. for example anterior-posterior differentiation) may be due to a similar cause.

7.   KAUFFMAN'S MODEL

Insect imaginal discs are assemblages of cells which metamorphose
into the different adult appendages (wing, leg, genital, haltere,
eye-antenna,...). During the development of a disc, say the Drosophila wing disc for example, there is a sequential formation of compartments : anterior-posterior, dorsal-ventral, wing-thorax,...
(Figure 7.1). Kauffman [25] observed that the compartment lines
resemble the nodal lines of the mode shapes :

$$
(7.1) \quad
\begin{cases}
-\Delta w = \mu w \quad \text{in } \Omega, \\
\dfrac{\partial w}{\partial \nu} = 0 \quad \text{on } \Gamma = \partial\Omega
\end{cases}
$$

the nodal lines being those points (x,y) such that $w(x,y) = 0$. Whence
the idea that diffusion of "morphogens" was playing a role, together
with some reaction. Kauffman's theory is that a reaction-diffusion
system :

$$
(7.2) \quad
\begin{cases}
\dfrac{\partial s}{\partial t} - \Delta s + \lambda f(s,a) = 0 \text{ in } \Omega, \\
\dfrac{\partial a}{\partial t} - \beta\Delta a + \lambda g(s,a) = 0, \\
+ \text{ no-flux B.C.s}
\end{cases}
$$

acts throughout development and generates a sequence of differently
shaped chemical patterns. More precisely the concentration field
passes, as λ varies, through a sequence of stable spatially non uniform steady states of (7.2), inducing one commitment (for example
anterior) in cells where s (or a) is above some threshold level, and
the alternate commitment (posterior) in cells below threshold. Here
the parameter λ represents the size of the disc and increases with
size.

8. STEADY STATES OF THE S-A SYSTEM

We focus hereafter on a generalization of the two-cell system of Section 6 to a system with infinitely many cells distributed in an active layer (Figure 8.1), separated from a bulk solution of substrates S and A by an unstirred layer. The substrates are transported by diffusion from this reservoir, where they are at fixed concentrations s_o and a_o, across the unstirred layer, to the active layer, which is assumed to be thin enough for the concentrations in this disc to be independent of the coordinate z in the transverse direction. The concentrations s and a of the diffusing and reacting substrates in this active disc Ω are governed by the following equations :

$$(8.1) \quad \begin{cases} \dfrac{\partial s}{\partial t} - \Delta s + \lambda[\rho a F(s) - (s_o - s)] = 0 \quad \text{in} \quad \Omega, \\[2mm] \dfrac{\partial a}{\partial t} - \beta \Delta a + \lambda[\rho a F(s) - \alpha(a_o - a)] = 0, \\[2mm] \text{with no-flux boundary conditions} \\[2mm] F(s) = s / (1 + s + ks^2). \end{cases}$$

Here Ω is a (wing) disc-shaped planar surface, λ is a parameter proportional to the actual disc size and in the first equation for example the terms $-\Delta s$, $\lambda \rho a F(s)$ and $\lambda(s_o - s)$ correspond respectively to diffusion within Ω, reaction within Ω and transport across the unstirred layer. In the second equation α (resp. β) is the ratio of diffusion coefficients in the unstirred layer (resp. Ω). The parameters λ and ρ are the ratios

$$(8.2) \qquad \lambda = \Theta_D/\Theta_T \quad \text{and} \quad \rho = \Theta_T/\Theta_R$$

of Θ_D, Θ_T and Θ_R, characteristic times respectively of diffusion within Ω, transport across the unstirred layer and reaction in Ω. The steady states of system (8.1), solutions to the system

$$(8.3) \quad \begin{cases} -\Delta s + \lambda[\rho a F(s) - (s_o - s)] = 0, \\[2mm] -\beta \Delta a + \lambda[\rho a F(s) - \alpha(a_o - a)] = 0, \\[2mm] \dfrac{\partial s}{\partial \nu} = 0, \qquad \dfrac{\partial a}{\partial \nu} = 0, \end{cases}$$

have been studied in [26]. For realistic values of the parameters,
for example

(8.4) a_0 = 79.2, k = 0.1, s_0 = 102.5, α = 1.45, β = 5,

             ρ = 13

corresponding to uric acid and oxygen, the enzyme being uricase,
(8.3) admits, in addition to a trivial, spatially uniform solution
$(\tilde{s}, \tilde{a})$, defined by the algebraic equations

(8.5)
$$\begin{cases} \tilde{s} - s_0 - \rho \tilde{a} F(\tilde{s}) = 0 \\ \alpha(\tilde{a} - a_0) - \rho \tilde{a} F(\tilde{s}) = 0, \end{cases}$$

others solutions which are patterned, and which are stable steady
states of the dynamical system (8.1).
Finite element approximations of solutions to (8.3) were calculated
with the mesh shown in Figure 8.2. By solving the evolution equations (8.1) until attaining a stable steady state, the patterns of
Figure 8.3 were obtained. They correspond, from left to right and
top to bottom, to increasing values of λ.

By applying Kubicek's method of continuation and Keller's method
of bifurcation to equations (8.3), the parameter values being

(8.6) a_0 = 92.8 , k = 0.1 , s_0 = 102.5, α = 1.2 ,

             β = 5   , ρ = 13

the diagram of Figure 8.4 was obtained. Here the concentration s at
a given point of Ω is plotted against λ. The straight line s = $\tilde{s}$ = 8
represents the trivial steady state, whereas the loops represent
patterned steady states. All the states are stable, excepted those
corresponding to the segments of the trivial line within the loops.
The patterns on the kth loop look like the kth eigenfunction of $-\Delta$;
this result, obtained by solving the nonlinear system (8.3), is in
agreement with Kauffman's prediction that the system undergoes sequential chemical patterns resembling the successive mode shapes.
Additional numerical experiments were performed with the parameter
values (8.4) in the one-dimensional case Ω = (0,1), Δ = $\partial^2/\partial x^2$,
thus yielding the bifurcation diagram of Figure 8.5. Here the inter-

val (0,1) was divided into 100 equal parts for a finite difference
approximation of equations (8.3), so that a problem with 2 x 99 = 198
degrees of freedom was solved.

On the diagram of Figure 8.5 the abscissa is λ and the ordinate is
the value of s at some point of Ω. Full (resp. dotted) lines correspond to stable (resp. unstable) solutions to (8.3). The straight
line A - I corresponds to the trivial steady-state $(\tilde{s},\tilde{a})$, and the
points A - I are bifurcation points from this branch. Points J - Q
are secondary bifurcation points. The path followed by system (8.3)
as λ increases (we assume the variation of λ slow enough for sequential steady states to settle, i.e. we make the quasi-steady-state
hypothesis) can be inferred from this bifurcation diagram. Before
attaining point A, the system follows the trivial branch. Then it
follows an arc AB of the first loop. Between B and C, $(\tilde{s},\tilde{a})$ again is
stable, but after C it becomes unstable, and the system passes smoothly to steady states which are structured in space, between C and
J, then jumps from J to one of the 2 branches of stable steady states
existing for $\lambda > \lambda_J$, say the upper one, until N, jumps again to, say,
the upper line and follows it until R,... . Of course, if λ was per-
mitted to decrease, the system would describe arc RP, jump from P
to arc NL, jump from L to arc JC, ..., so that an hysteresis phenomenon would be observed : for a given value of λ the system can
occupy different steady statesaccording to its past history.

Discussion : It is striking that an enzyme with a rather common activity (inhibited by exceeding S and activated by A), placed in a
frequent situation (immobilized within a membrane separated by a
boundary layer from an external bath), can exhibit pattern formation.
They precise geometry of the "disc" is unimportant : whatever the
geometry, if pattern formation occurs in the two-cell system of
Section 6, it occurs also in an array of N cells, in the one-dimensional case, in the two dimensional case for every shape of Ω, and
on non planar surfaces such as egg shaped surfaces, etc... . This
can be mathematically proved [26]. Moreover, whatever the geometrical domain, the first pattern to appear is always the onset of polarity.
Thus pattern formation, starting with polarity, occurs naturally as
the consequence of interacting diffusion and reaction, together with
transport of substrates from outside. In a situation such as shown
in Figure 8.4, it can be proved that the patterns which arise from
the trivial branch look like the sequential mode shapes [26].

REFERENCES

[1]   Aschoff, J.(Ed.) Circadian clocks (North Holland, Amsterdam, 1965.

[2]   Chance, B., Pye, E.K., Ghosh A.K. and Hess, B., Biological and biochemical oscillators (Academic Press, New York,1973).

[3]   Winfree, A.T., The geometry of biological time (Springer-Verlag New York, 1980).

[4]   Goldbeter, A. and Caplan, S.R., Oscillatory enzymes, Ann. Rev. Biophys. and Bioeng., vol. 5 (1976) 449 - 476.

[5]   Hess, B. and Boiteux, A., Oscillatory phenomena in biochemistry, Annu. Rev. Biochem. 40 (1971) 237 - 258.

[6]   Nicolis, G. and Portnow, J., Chemical oscillations, Chem. Rev. 73 (1973) 365 - 366.

[7]   Goldbeter, A. and Nicolis, G., an allosteric enzyme model with positive feedback applied to glycolytic oscillations, pp. 65-160 in : Rosen, R., ed., progress in theoretical biology, vol. 4 (Academic, New York, 1976).

[8]   Crandall, M.G. and Rabinowitz, P.H., the Hopf bifurcation theorem, MRC technical summary report   1604, University of Wisconsin, 1976.

[9]   Marsden J.E. and Mac Cracken M., the Hopf bifurcation and its applications, Applied Mathematical Sciences 19, Springer Verlag New York (1976).

[10]   Turing, A.M., the chemical basis of morphogenesis, Phil. Trans. Roy. Soc. London, vol. B 237 (1952) 37 - 72.

[11]   Gierer A. and Meinhardt H., Biological pattern formation involving lateral inhibition, pp. 163 - 183 in : Levin, S.A., (ed.) some mathematical questions in biology.6 (the American Mathematical Society, Providence, 1974).

[12]   Nicolis, G. and Prigogine, I., Self-organization in nonequilibrium systems, from dissipative structures to order through fluctuations, Wiley-Interscience, New York, 1977.

[13]   Kubicek M., Dependence of solution of nonlinear systems on a
       parameter ACM transactions on mathematical software, vol. 2,
        1, March 1976, p 98-107.

[14]   Keller, H.B., Numerical solution of bifurcation and nonlinear
       eigenvalue problems, pp. 359 - 384, in : Rabinowitz, P. H.
       (ed.), applications of bifurcation theory (Academic Press,
       New York, 1977).

[15]   Doedel, E., Auto : a program for the automatic bifurcation
       analysis of autonomous systems, Congressus Numerantium,
       vol. 30 (1981) 265 - 284.

[16]   Pettigrew, D.W. and Frieden, C., Rabbit Muscle Phosphofructo-
       kinase, a model for regulatory kinetic behavior, J. Biol.
       Chem. vol. 254, n° 6 (1979) 1896 - 1901.

[17]   Hervagault, J.F. et Duban, M.C., Oscillations de la phospho-
       fructokinase dans un système compartimenté,C.R.A.S.Paris, T.290,
       21, série D (1980) 1357 - 1360.

[18]   Hervagault, J.F., Friboulet, A., Kernevez, J.P. and Thomas, D.,
       Hysteresis, oscillations and pattern formation in immobilized
       enzyme systems, Ber. Bunsenges. Phys. Chem., 84, 358 (1980).

[19]   Hervagault, J.F., Friboulet, A., Kernevez, J.P. and Thomas, D.,
       Spatiotemporal behaviors in immobilized enzyme systems, Bio-
       chimie, 62 (1980) 367.

[20]   Hervagault, J.F. and Thomas D., Experimental evidence and
       theoretical discussion for an oscillatory behavior of phos-
       phofructokinase in a compartmentalized system, to appear in
       Eur. J. Biochem.

[21]   Cambou, B., Hervagault, J.F., Laurent, M. and Thomas, D., Eur.
       J. Biochem. (in press).

[22]   Mehra, R.K. and Carroll, J.V., Bifurcation analysis of air-
       craft high angle of attack flight dynamics, pp. 127 - 146
       in : Holmes, P.J., ed., New approaches to nonlinear problems
       in dynamics (Siam, Philadelphia, 1980).

[23]   Lahaye, E., une méthode de résolution d'une catégorie d'équa-
       tions transcendantes, C.R. ACAD. SCI. Paris, 198 (1934)
       pp. 1840 - 1842.

[24]   Davidenko,D., on a new method of numerically integrating a
        system of nonlinear equations, Dokl. Akad. Nauk. SSSR, 88
        (1953), pp. 601 - 604 (in Russian).

[25]   Kauffman, S.A., Shymko, R.M., and Trabert, K., Control of
        sequential compartment formation in Drosophila, a uniform
        mechanism may control the location of successive binary
        developmental commitments, Science, vol. 199, 1978.

[26]   Kernevez, J.P., Enzyme mathematics (North-Holland, Amsterdam,
        1980).

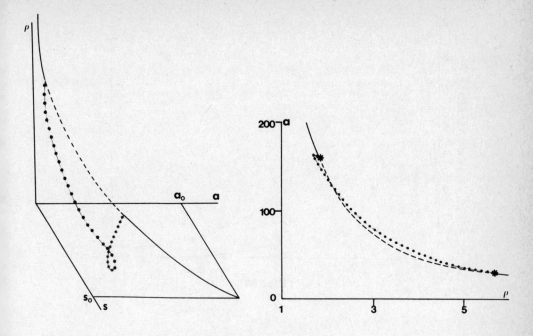

Figure 2.1   Figure 2.2

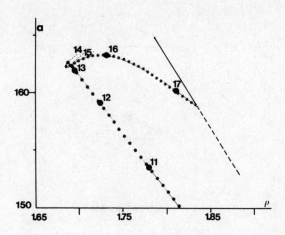

Figure 2.3

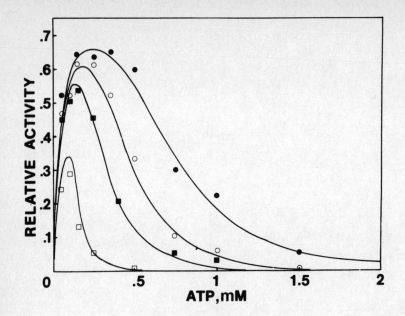

Figure 3.1

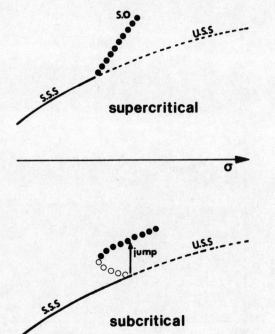

Figure 3.2

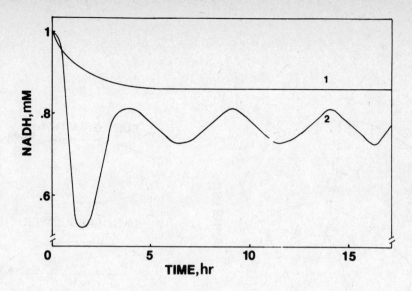

Figure 3.3

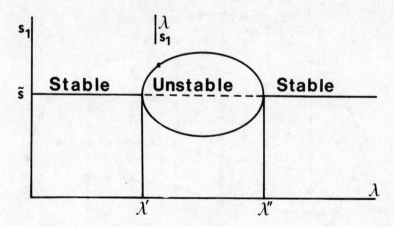

Figure 6.1

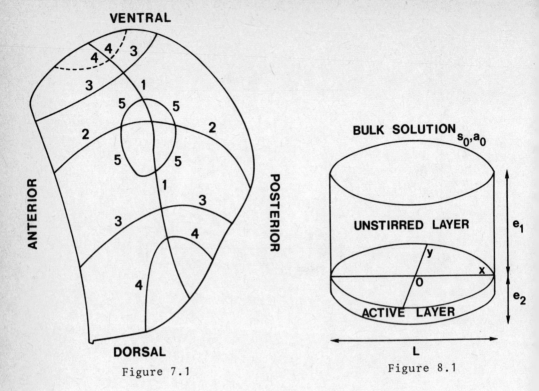

Figure 7.1

Figure 8.1

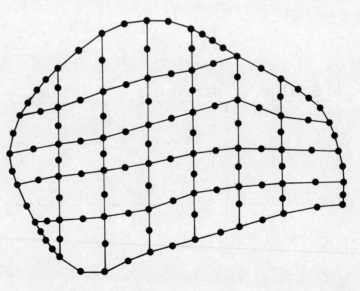

Figure 8.2

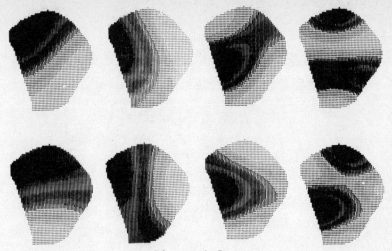

Figure 8.3

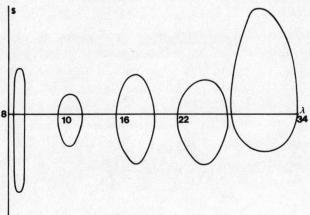

Figure 8.4

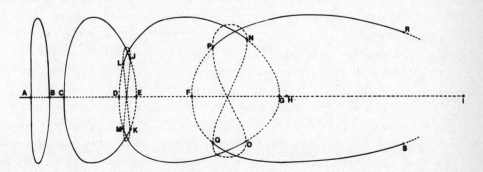

Figure 8.5

STEREOLOGICAL ANALYSIS OF CIRCADIAN RHYTHMS
IN NUCLEOLI OF RAT SYMPATHETIC NEURONS

M.J. PEBUSQUE and R. SEÏTE

Groupe de Neurocytobiologie

Faculté de Médecine

27, Boulevard Jean Moulin

13385 - MARSEILLE CEDEX 5

FRANCE

INTRODUCTION

While numerous chronobiological studies have been reported in the fields
of hormone activity, behavior and pharmacology (3, 12), only a few reports have been
devoted to rhythmic modifications at the structural or ultrastructural level of cells.

We recently focused our attention on nucleoli of rat sympathetic neurons.
The nucleolus represents a highly structured and specialized cell compartment having
for principal and perhaps only function the production of ribosomes. Electron microscopy has shown that the nucleoli contain different components i.e. fibrillar, granular and vacuolar components that can be considered constant and general and low
density electron zones which RECHER et al. (11) have called fibrillar centers regar-
ded as nucleolar organizer regions. In some cell types or during certain functional
events, fibrillar centers are very conspicuous as for example, in prophase nuclei or
in tumor cells, but it is generally claimed that they are difficult to identify in
interphase nuclei. The fibrillar centers contain proteins and DNA and the transcriptional activity of the nucleolus occurs at the level of the fibrillar centers and
more precisely at their periphery in the region of fibrillar RNP component (7).

By using both a stereological and ultrastructural analysis, we previously
showed that the size of nucleoli and of their fibrillar centers in sympathetic
neurons which are permanent interphasic cells, exhibits circadian changes with a
maximum value during the dark period (9). In order to determine whether such circadian variations follow an actual circadian rhythm or not, we have performed, observations on animals subjected to artificial synchronization. Such a purpose can be realized by stereological analysis. Stereology is the three-dimensional interpretation of
flat images, such as sections, by criteria of geometric probability. It is the rigou-
rous extrapolation from two - to three dimensional space and is practised by measuring
with different means, profiles in sections with aim to determine volume and volume
densities (2, 5, 14, 15).

MATERIALS AND METHODS

ANIMALS

Twenty-seven male Wistar rats weighing 300-350 g were used in this study. Three animals were randomly assigned to each cage. The animals were kept in a windowless, soundproof, vibration-free and temperature-controlled room. Access to food and water was allowed ad libitum. Artificial lighting was used and the light/dark cycle was 12 hours of light (0700-1900 h) and 12 hours of darkness (1900-0700 h).

After 3 weeks under these conditions of artifical synchronization, the animals were sacrificed three by three during a 24-hour period. Beginning at 1500 h the animals were sacrificed every 4 hours except from 2200 to 0700 h when sacrifice was performed every 2 hours. Thus 9 groups of 3 animals were used, the sacrifice of each group being obtained by an intracardiac perfusion not exceeding 1 hour. At the time of sacrifice all rats were anaesthetized by intraperitoneal sodium barbiturate (40 mg/kg) after which intracardiac perfusion was carried out with a solution of 1 % glutaraldehyde - 1 % paraformaldehyde in 0.12 M phosphate buffer, pH 7.4.

MICROSCOPY PREPARATIONS

The right superior cervical ganglion (SCG) of each animal was dissected out, fixed in the above solution for 1 hour at 4°C and postfixed for 1 hour in 2 % osmium tetroxide in the same phosphate buffer. After dehydration by acetone the blocks were embedded in Epon and sections were made on a Reichert Ultramicrotome as follow :
- 1 semi-thin section (1 μm thick) mounted on a glass slide and stained with a solution of 1 % toluidine blue.
- 1 thin-section (80 nm - thick) was picked up on a copper grid (200 mesh), contrasted by uranyl acetate and lead citrate and examined in a Siemens Elmiskop 101 electron microscope at 80 kv.
- 4 consecutive semi-thin sections (1 μm thick) were discarded (to avoid re-sectioning the same nucleolus) and then a semi-thin section and thin section were made as described above. The entire procedure (1 semi-thin, 1 thin, 4 discarded sections) was performed 5 times.

STEREOLOGICAL ANALYSIS

This study was performed in three consecutive steps.

1. Determination of mean volume of the nucleolus ($\bar{V}$nu) on semi-thin sections of neurons from the superior cervical ganglion.

The surface area of 150 sectionned nucleoli from each SCG was measured using a camera lucida (magnification : 800x) and a MOP-Kontron AM/01 analyzer. The apparent diameter of the sectionned nucleoli was calculated (the nucleoli being considered as spheres). A histogram of the frequency of the apparent

nucleolar diameters from each SCG (based on 150 nucleoli per SCG) was made
in order to verify that the distribution of these diameters followed a normal curve.
The χ^2 test showed that the observed distribution did not differ from the normal
distribution having the same mean and variance. After mathematical transformation of
the data as developed by WICKSELL (16) for spherical bodies, the mean nucleolar
diameter and mean nucleolar volume ($\bar{V}$nu) of each SCG were calculated. Calculations
were performed on a Hewlett-Packard HP 67 calculator.

The $\bar{V}$nu of the three animals belonging to the same group were compared
by the Student's t test, after verifying that variance was homogeneous. It was found
that the values of $\bar{V}$nu within each group of 3 animals were not significantly different (95 % confidence level). Accordingly, the $\bar{V}$nu of the sympathetic neurons of the
SCG, its standard deviation and standard error of the mean were calculated for each
group of 3 animals.

2. Determination of the volume density of nucleolar fibrillar centers
/Vvfc(nu)/ of SCG neurons on thin sections and calculation of mean volume of fibrillar centers /$\bar{V}$fc(nu)/.

For each SCG, the thin sections made 4 µm apart (to avoid resectioning
the same nucleolus) were picked up one by one on identical grids, using conditions
described by WEIBEL (14, 15). Twenty nucleoli were photographed (X 10 000). The
negatives developed using an automatic apparatus yielded a final magnification of
X 25 000. Calibration of the microscope magnification and that of the photographic
enlarger was checked using a negative displaying a linear grid (54,684 lines/inch,
Balzers Union) and its corresponding positive.

The surface section of each nucleolus (Snu) and that of its corresponding
fibrillar center /Sfc(nu)/ were measured using a MOP-Kontron apparatus. The volume
density of the fibrillar centers within the nucleoli was established according to
the principles of morphometry published by DELESSE (4) and developed by WEIBEL (14,
15). The volume density is given by the equation :

$$Vvfc(nu) = \frac{\bar{V}fc(nu)}{\bar{V}nu} = \frac{1}{n} \times \sum_{1}^{n} \frac{Sfc(nu)}{Snu}$$

(n = number of profiles).

The volume densities showed a normal distribution as confirmed by a χ^2
test comparing the observed distribution with a normal one having the same mean and
the same variance.

The volume densities of the fibrillar centers in the SCG nucleoli were
compared among the three animals in a given group, after verifying that variance
was homogeneous. Since volume densities were not significantly different (at the 5 %
level) within each group, the volume density of the fibrillar centers in the nucleoli
of SCG neurons, its standard deviation and standard error of the mean were calculated
for each group.

Finally, knowing the volume density of the fibrillar centers in the nucleoli and the $\bar{V}nu$ in each group of animals, the $\bar{V}fc(nu)$, its standard deviation and standard error of the mean were computed.

3. Determination of mean volume of the nucleolar components, i.e., fibrillar RNP, granular RNP and vacuolar components. It is rather difficult to precisely individualize and measure the dimensions of each of them from electron micrographs. Knowing for each group the $\bar{V}nu$ and the $\bar{V}fc(nu)$, the mean volume of fibrillar RNP, granular RNP and vacuolar components /$\bar{V}fgvac(nu)$/ was calculated.

RESULTS

All the parameters studied, in SCG neurons from each group are shown in figure 1. Results of the stereological analysis show that the $\bar{V}$nu, $\bar{V}$fc(nu) and $\bar{V}$fgvac(nu) varied according to the time of sacrifice, the variation following a normal curve with the maximum values occurring during the dark period (see Table I.)

TABLE I

RESULTS OF THE STEREOLOGICAL ANALYSIS

Time (hours)	$\bar{V}$nu n=450 μm^3	$\bar{V}$fgvac(nu) μm^3	$\bar{V}$fc(nu) n=60 μm^3
1500 h	6.451 ± 0.540	6.277 ± 0.517	0.174 ± 0.013
1900 h	5.961 ± 0.612	5.812 ± 0.596	0.149 ± 0.012
2300 h	10.532 ± 0.588	9.921 ± 0.533	0.611 ± 0.045
0100 h	13.443 ± 0.705	11.709 ± 0.599	1.734 ± 0.108
0300 h	11.122 ± 0.609	10.088 ± 0.556	1.034 ± 0.073
0500 h	7.337 ± 0.701	6.985 ± 0.669	0.352 ± 0.038
0700 h	7.794 ± 0.609	7.459 ± 0.573	0.335 ± 0.046
1100 h	7.601 ± 0.607	7.411 ± 0.598	0.190 ± 0.019
1500 h	6.202 ± 0.420	6.041 ± 0.400	0.161 ± 0.011

$\bar{V}$nu = mean volume of nucleolus

$\bar{V}$fgvac(nu) = mean volume of fibrillar RNP granular RNP and vacuolar components of the nucleolus

$\bar{V}$fc(nu) = mean volume of fibrillar centers

n = number of profiles

Results are means ± SEM for three animals

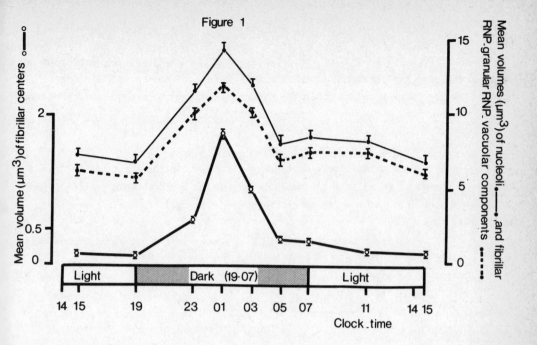

Circadian rhythms of mean volumes of nucleoli and their different components in
sympathetic neurons. The data are the average ± SEM of three animals.
- ●——● Represents the curve of the mean nucleolar volume
- ○——○ Represents the curve of the mean volume of fibrillar centers and,
- ●----● That of fibrillar RNP, granular RNP and vacuolar components of the
  nucleoli.

MEAN VOLUME OF NUCLEOLI

Figure 1 demonstrates that the peak $\bar{V}nu$ occurred in the dark period when
sacrifice is performed at 0100 h. The $\bar{V}nu$ (± SEM) which was low at 1500 h (6.451 ±
0.540 μm^3), began to rise at the onset of the dark period, reaching a zenith of
13.443 ± 0.705 μm^3 at 0100 h. The $\bar{V}nu$ then progressively decreased to a minimum
value of 6.202 ± 0.420 μm^3 at 1500 h on the following day, the lowest value being
5.961 ± 0.612 μm^3 at 1900 h. It shoud be noted that when the $\bar{V}nu$ of rats sacrificed

at 1500 h was compared to that of rats sacrificed at 1900 h no statistically significant difference was found (P $<$ 0.05). Likewise, comparison of the $\bar{V}$nu of animals
sacrificed at 0500 h with that of rats sacrificed at 0700 h showed no significant
difference. These results thus demonstrate that the $\bar{V}$nu of the rat SCG increases twofold during the dark period and that the variations of $\bar{V}$nu correspond to a circadian
rhythm.

MEAN VOLUME OF NUCLEOLAR FIBRILLAR CENTERS

For these data, it was necessary to examine, in the light period, as
well as in the dark period, all the nucleoli present on a single thin section picked
up on one copper grid. All nucleolus sections were 4 μm apart to avoid resectioning
of the same nucleolus.

Figure 1 shows that $\bar{V}$fc(nu) exhibits a peak in the dark period when animals are sacrificed at 0100 h. It was found that $\bar{V}$fc(nu) ($\pm$ SEM), which is 0.174 $\pm$
0.013 μm^3 at 1500 h, starts to increase at the beginning of the dark period, reaching
a maximum value of 1.734 $\pm$ 0.108 μm^3 at 0100 h. It then progressively decreases,
reaching 0.161 $\pm$ 0.011 μm^3 the next day at 1500 h. The lowest value 0.149 $\pm$ 0.012 μm^3
was detected at 1900 h.

A statistical analysis of this parameter with Student's t test between
the two groups of rats sacrificed at 1500 h and 1900 h did not prove any significant
difference (P $<$ 0.05). Similarly, no statistically significant difference was observed between the values obtained in groups of animals sacrificed at 0500 h and 0700 h
(P $<$ 0.05).

The results obtained show that $\bar{V}$fc(nu) increases ten-fold during the
1500-0100 h interval. The considerable dimensional changes in fibrillar centers
correspond to a diurnal rhythm.

MEAN VOLUME OF FIBRILLAR RNP, GRANULAR RNP AND VACUOLAR COMPONENTS OF THE NUCLEOLUS

In this case also, a single thin section of SCG was picked up on one
copper grid and all nucleoli encountered were measured. Figure 1 shows that
$\bar{V}$fgvac(nu) exhibit a peak in the dark period when rats are sacrificed at 0100 h.
$\bar{V}$fgvac(nu) ($\pm$ SEM) increases from 6.277 $\pm$ 0.517 μm^3 at 1500 h to a maximum of
11.709 $\pm$ 0.599 μm^3 at 0100 h and then decreases to 6.041 $\pm$ 0.400 μm^3 at 1500 h on
the following day, reaching a minimum of 5.812 $\pm$ 0.596 μm^3 at 1900 h.

A statistical analysis of this parameter with Student's t test was performed between the two groups of rats sacrificed at 1500 h and 1900 h and also between
those sacrificed at 0500 h and 0700 h. No statistically significant difference was
observed in both cases (P $<$ 0.05).

Thus, $\bar{V}$fgvac(nu) undergoes a 1.8 fold during the dark period and it
must be pointed out that these parameter changes follow a circadian rhythm.

DISCUSSION AND CONCLUSIONS

A very few studies have reported rhythmic variations of nucleolar size under physiological conditions. To our knowledge only observations reported by QUAY (10) and BENSON et al. (1) showed that the nucleoli size in the pinealocytes of rodents displays a circadian rhythm.

In the present study we demonstrate that in sympathetic neurons, the nucleolar volume displays a diurnal rhythm and that such a circadian rhythm concerns nucleolar components at the ultrastructural level. Indeed, the nucleolar volume increases 2 fold during the dark period (0100 h) and, at the same time, mean volume of fibrillar centers and fibrillar RNP, granular RNP and vacuolar components reach their zenith.

Moreover this study clearly shows : 1) that fibrillar centers are not responsible for the overall increase of the nucleolar volume and 2) that the modifications triggered by darkness firstly concern fibrillar RNP, granular RNP and vacuolar components. It is well known that rhythmic variations of nucleolar volume are related to the functional activity of the cell (8, 12, 13). An increase of nucleoli size is generally interpreted as reflecting increased transcriptional activity (6).

However, on the basis of our results, we cannot define whether the rhythmic variations observed are correlated to the level of transcriptional activity of the nucleolus of rat sympathetic neurons or not. Experiments are in progress to answer this important question.

ACKNOWLEDGEMENTS

All the members of our laboratory are acknowledged for their taking part in this work.

The authors are grateful to Prof. I. ASSENMACHER and Dr. A. SZAFARCZYK for their interest to this work and for the use of the specialized animal laboratory to achieve artificial synchronization of the animals.

They are also indebted to Prof. P. BOUYARD and Dr. B. BRUGUEROLLE for helpful suggestions.

This work was supported by grant from DGRST (N° 81.E.0538).

REFERENCES

1. BENSON B. and KRASOVICH M., 1977, Circadian rhythm in the number of granulated vesicles in the pinealocytes of mice, Cell Tissue Res., 184, 499-506, "Chemical Abstracts"

2. BOLENDER R.P., 1979, Surface area ratios. II. A stereological method for estimating changes in average cell volume and frequency, The Anat. Rec., 195, 257-264, "Chemical Abstracts"

3. BUNNING E., 1973, "The physiological clock", Springer Verlag, Berlin and New York "Chemical Abstracts"

4. DELESSE M.A., 1847, Procédé mécanique pour déterminer la composition des roches C.R. Acad. Sci., 25, 544. "Chemical Abstracts"

5. ELIAS H. and HYDE D.M., 1980, An elementary introduction to stereology (quantitative microscopy), Amer. J. Anat., 159, 411-446. "Chemical Abstracts"

6. GIMENEZ-MARTIN G., DE LA TORRE C., LOPEZ-SAEZ J.F. and ESPONA P., 1977, Plant nucleolus : structure and physiology, Cytobiol., Eur. J. Cell Biol., 14, 421-462 "Chemical Abstracts"

7. GOESSENS G. and LEPOINT A., 1979, The nucleolus-organizing regions (NOR'S) : recent data and hypotheses, Biol. Cell., 35, 211-220 "Chemical Abstracts"

8. LEPOINT A., 1978, Analyse stéréologique au niveau ultrastructural des nucléoles et des ribosomes cytoplasmiques de cellules tumorales d'Ehrlich au cours de la préparation à la mitose, Arch. Biol., 89, 129-137, "Chemical Abstracts"

9. PEBUSQUE M.J. and SEÏTE R., 1980, Circadian change of fibrillar centers in nucleolus of sympathetic neurons : an ultrastructural and stereological analysis, Biol. Cell., 37, 219-222, "Chemical Abstracts"

10. QUAY W.B., 1974, Pineal chemistry in cellular and physiological mechanisms, Springfield, III, Charles C. Thomas, 63-329, "Chemical Abstracts"

11. RECHER L., WHITESCARVER J. and BRIGGS L., 1969, The fine structure of a nucleolar constituent, J. Ultrastruct. Res., 29, 1-14, "Chemical Abstracts"

12. SCHEVING L.E., MAYERSBACH H. and PAULY J.E., 1974, An overview of chronopharmacology, J. Europ. Toxicol., 7, 203-227, "Chemical Abstracts"

13. SMETANA K. and BUSCH H., 1974, The nucleolus and nucleolar DNA, "The Cell Nucleus" (ed. H. Busch), Academic Press, New York, 73-147, "Chemical Abstracts"

14. WEIBEL E.R., 1969, Stereological principles for morphometry in electron microscopic cytology, Int. Rev. Cytol., 26, 235-302, "Chemical Abstracts"

15. WEIBEL E.R., 1979, Stereological methods. I. Practical methods for biological morphometry. Academic Press Inc. London LTD, "Chemical Abstracts"

16. WICKSELL S.D., 1925, The corpuscule problem. A mathematical study of a biometric problem. Biometrika, 17, 84-99, "Mathematical Reviews".

FORMALIZATION OF ADRENAL-POSTPITUITARY CIRCADIAN RHYTHMS BY THE MODEL FOR THE REGULATION OF AGONISTIC-ANTAGONISTIC COUPLES. PARAMETER IDENTIFICATION.

F. SANTI, A. GUILLEZ, Y. CHERRUAULT & E. BERNARD-WEIL

I. THE MODEL FOR THE REGULATION OF AGONISTIC-ANTAGONISTIC COUPLES (MRCAA).

The MRCAA may be considered as a function model, i.e. a general model that could be common to several concrete systems in so far as it would allow us to simulate a function belonging to all these systems.

Nevertheless, the MRCAA was conceived from a specified biological system, the system formed by the adrenals and the neuropostpituitary. Such a system has already been considered in an empirical manner, seing the particular type of endocrine actions and their interelationships.

This model could be built as a knowledge model, in the usual sense of the term, which would have accumulated a great number of equations and variables in order to take into account all the data about secretion, transport, clearance, molecular actions... In fact, we prefered a simpler model, with only two variables (in its basic version), the one assembling the two principal adrenocortical hormones (cortisol and aldosterone)/(ACH), the other corresponding to the vasopressin (VP), and with parameters without physical meaning, i.e. phenomenological parameters. But this model cannot be considered as a "black box", because it tries to express two series of facts with which the physician or the physiologist are familiar : on one hand, the fact that these hormones have some <u>antagonistic</u> actions on some receptors, and on the other hand some <u>agonistic</u> actions on some other receptors.

Antagonistic actions concern, among others, water diuresis, cell hydration, mitosis... Agonistic actions concern volemia and stress.
The regulations that ensue are very complicated, because an imbalance, according as it concerns antagonistic or agonistic actions, will elicit either variations of the two hormonal secretions in opposite senses, or variations in the same sense.

Without going into all the details of the elaboration and justification of the model, it is given now in its present version, under the form of a set of non linear differential equations. One can see a kind of "series expansion" of two expressions, the one antagonistic ($u = x(t) - y(t)$), the other agonistic ($x(t) + y(t) - m$) (m = constant parameter or variable) (x = ACH, y = VP).

$$(1) \quad \begin{aligned} \dot{x} &= k_1 u + k_2 u^2 + k_3 u^3 + c_1 v + c_2 v^2 + c_3 v^3 \\ \dot{y} &= k_1' u + k_2' u^2 + k_3' u^3 + c_1' v + c_2' v^2 + c_3' v^3 \end{aligned}$$

k_i, c_i, k'_i, c'_i = constant parameters

The end of this model,if it suitably acts,is to reestablish u = v = 0 (or x = y = m/2) after a perturbation.The singular point (u,v) = (0,0) may be asymptotically stable, but we will consider only its limit-cycle form.

Complements (2,3,4):

a) other expressions for v (logarithmic) and u (allosteric),taking into account some data of the molecular biology.

b) variable parameters : $-$ k_i ,c_i : we do not consider periodic coefficients,but the possibility that these parameters could change in relation to stress or other pertur-bations;

$-$ m can be variable in relation to u and v (in order to make a constraint of positivity for x and y).

c) optimal control: it consists here in the addition of two new differential control equations.

$$\dot{X} = k_5(u+r) + k_6(u+r)^2 + k_7(u+r)^3 + c_5(v+s) + c_6(v+s)^2 + c_7(v+s)^3$$
$$\dot{Y} = k'_5(u+r) + k'_6(u+r)^2 + k'_7(u+r)^3 + c'_5(v+s) + c'_6(v+s)^2 + c'_7(v+s)^3$$

with r = X(t) $-$ Y(t) and s = X(t) + Y(t) (in eqs. (1),u is substituted with (u + r) and v with (v + s)).

d) supermodel combining several MRCAA.

II. APPLICATIONS

In spite of $-$ or owing to $-$ its relative simplicity and its basic conveiving,this mo-del allowed us to qualitatively simulate nearly the whole of the phenomena concerning the endocrine system,at least at a certain level of description (macroscopic changes)
$-$ circadian rhythms with their characteristic phase-shift (acrophase of VP towards, midnight,of ACH towards 7 h. A.M.)
$-$ synchronization of these endogenous rhythms by an external periodic stimulus such as the alternance day-night (represented by q(t) in the agonistic expression v = x+y-m+q)
$-$effects of a change in osmolarity,volemia,stress action
$-$effects of ACH suppression on VP,of VP suppression on ACH
$-$simulation of the pathological facts:according to the parametric field,we can obtain a bistable model with a physiological stable limit-cycle and a pathological attractor ((x,y) $\neq$ (0,0)) or a pathological monostable model
$-$the optimal control simulations allowed us to propose some efficient therapeutics in certain cases of adrenal postpituitary imbalances (cerebral edema,cerebral collapse, grade II recurrent astrocytomas)
$-$the supermodel may account for the possible relationships between several internal os cillators acting upon the same receptor.

III. PARAMETER IDENTIFICATION

-A- "Qualitative" identification: it proceeded from considerations about the model
stability (because one imagined that the concrete system never diverged) and also from
considerations about the clinico-experimental data.

As it has been demonstrated elsewhere (4),the parametric conditions to obtain a physiological limit-cycle are:

a) by linearization:the point $(x,y) = (m/2,m/2)$ is an instable focus if

(3)
$$k_1 - k_1' + c_1 + c_1' > 0$$
$$(k_1-k_1'+c_1+c_1')^2 - 4\left[(k_1-k_1')(c_1+c_1') - (k_1+k_1')(c_1-c_1' \right] < 0$$

b) by the second Lyapounov method and the method of the asymptotic lines of the trajectories at the infinite: a divergence will be avoided if a global stability is performed
with:

(4)
$$k_3 \text{ and } c_3' < 0 \qquad k_3'c_3 < 0 \qquad (\text{ with } |k_3'c_3| < |k_3c_3'|)$$
$$k_2, k_2' , c_2, c_2' \quad \text{of weak value}$$
$$k_1' + c_1 = 0$$

If we take into account the clinical and experimental data, i.e if we adopt the hypothesis according which some continuous variations of the parametric field are able to
provoke the catastrophic changes in the phase-portrait (cf. supra),a supplementary condition will be established:

(5) k_1 , k_1' and $c_1' < 0$ and $c_1 > 0$ (or conversely)

-B- "Quantitative" identification: let us denote the system (1) as

(11)
$$\dot{u}(t) = a_1 u(t) + a_2 u^2(t) + a_3 u^3(t) + a_4 v(t) + a_5 v^2(t) + a_6 v^3(t)$$
$$\dot{v}(t) = a_1' u(t) + a_2' u^2(t) + a_3' u^3(t) + a_4' v(t) + a_5' v^2(t) + a_6' v^3(t)$$

where
$$a_i = k_i - k_i' \quad , \quad a_i' = k_i + k_i' \quad , \quad i = 1,2,3$$
$$a_i = c_i - c_i' \quad , \quad a_i' = c_i + c_i' \quad , \quad i = 4,5,6$$
$$u = x - y \quad , \quad v = x + y - m$$

The problem we now consider is to find the parameters (a_i) and (a_i') (i=1 to 6) so
that the solution curves $x_c(t)$ and $y_c(t)$ tend to the experimental curves $x(t)$ and $y(t)$.
Generally we get only noisy experimental data points and it is rather unlikely that this
data could be simulated by a possible parametric field for our model.
Therefore we used to smooth the data points.

a)smooth curves : we will smooth the data with analytical functions to facilitate the
analytical expressions of the derived functions.To determinate the analytical functions
of the smooth curves is a very critical problem,especially if the data points are scarce
and if the errors on the data are correlated.Our investigations started using "exact"
data and "noisy" data for which the errors are not correlated and with zero-average.
Thus we built a method to resolve our identification problem.This method is then used
to find the model for the experimental data of the literature.

We have studied two different analytical smooth functions:

-splines functions

-Fourier series functions: this kind of function is natural to approximate periodic functions.The present work deals with the circadian rhythms of the variables x and y. Generally a simpler sinusoidal function is too regular to approximate this kind of rhythm.A Fourier series function allows a better approximation.We tried different numerical methods to calculate the coefficients of the series:linear least squares methods,an integration method ...

b)matrix systems: assuming that we have analytical smooth functions for x(t) and y(t) then the expressions for their derivatives $\dot{x}(t)$ and $\dot{y}(t)$ immediately follow.This allows us to calculate the values of this functions for any time during a period.Let us write the equation system (11) for a time sequence (t_i) (i=1 to M) which yields two equation systems,each with M equations and six unknown parameters.

Let us denote A,A' the 6-vectors $A_i = a_i$, $A_i' = a_i'$ i = 1 to 6

B,D the M-vectors $B_i = \dot{u}(t_i)$, $D_i = \dot{v}(t_i)$ i = 1 to M

M the Mx6-matrix $M_{ij} = u^j(t_i)$ (j = 1 to 3) and $v^{j-3}(t_i)$ (j = 4 to 6)

Thus the systems are MA = B and MA' = D .

c)resolution: we have to resolve this two linear systems by numerical methods.We have studied a few methods of linear algebra and least squares methods.The systems are ill-conditionned so it is necesserary to choose a well-adapted method.The numerical method for solving linear least squares problems due to G. GOLUB (6) with the extension for very ill-conditionned systems dues to RIBIERE (7) was found to be relatively successfu On this case the numerical and experimental errors can not be disregarded and are such that the calculated curves are only approximations of the "true" curves.To obtain a better approximation we proceed to use an iterative optimization from the algebric solution.The optimization we studied is an iterative minimization of a quadratic criteria with local variation methods or gradient techniques and Newtons methods.

d) results: we first work with the data points which we obtain through the solution of the simulated curves were found to be very acceptable in the sense that the deviation from the "true" curves was almost negligible; The approximation of the parameters is rather satisfying; However the deviation on each parameters seems generally depend on its influence on the varation of the curves (its sensibility).

example 1

The given parameters for the system (1) :

$$P_v \quad \begin{array}{cccccc} -0.062 & -0.250 & -0.600 & 0.162 & 0.100 & -0.500 \\ -0.162 & 0.550 & 0.500 & -0.062 & -0.300 & -0.600 \end{array}$$

The solution of matrix resolution is :

$$P_f \quad \begin{array}{cccccc} -0.082 & -0.161 & -0.377 & 0.144 & 0.030 & -0.325 \\ -0.156 & 0.531 & 0.491 & -0.084 & -0.314 & -0.360 \end{array}$$

The solution of the optimisation is :

$$P_f \quad \begin{matrix} -0.050 & -0.267 & -0.641 & 0.160 & 0.102 & -0.485 \\ -0.161 & 0.545 & 0.496 & -0.062 & -0.296 & -0.598 \end{matrix}$$

the residual error on the curves = 0.0012

the residual error on the 12 parameters = 0.027

···· curve : simulated curve with the parametric point P_0

—— curve : simulated curve with the parametric point P_f

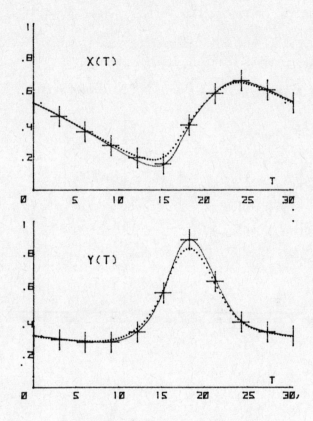

The experimental points gave rise to a lot of difficulties. First of all, the data for the vasopressin are almost absent. We only find a few data in (5) but each point has a large standart deviation. Then it is not easy to find the smooth curves of these data points which could be represented by the model. But in spite of this we tried and we got a solution which turne out not to be "too bad": The signs of the parameters agreed with the conditions that the qualitative study of the model established; The values of the quadratic parameters are not really weak but we got the global stability, we can observe this fact in the phase-portrait.

example 2

The experimental points are very inaccurate. They did not allow a "proper" resolution of the matrix system. A (x-y) data analysishas determined the significant points. The approximative functions of these points allowed us to solve the matrix system and gave the solution P_0:

$$P_0 \quad \begin{matrix} -0.155 & 0.170 & -0.127 & 0.118 & 0.070 & -0.153 \\ -0.368 & -0.755 & 1.505 & -0.065 & -0.128 & -0.697 \end{matrix}$$

The minimization is used to fit the experimental points which are represented with thei: standart deviation on the figure. The solution of the optimization is

$$P_f \quad \begin{matrix} -0.223 & 0.148 & -0.133 & 0.093 & 0.097 & -0.182 \\ -0.331 & -0.735 & 1.512 & -0.061 & -0.149 & -0.699 \end{matrix}$$

···· curve : simulated curve with the parametric point P_0

—— curve : simulated curve with the parametric point P_f

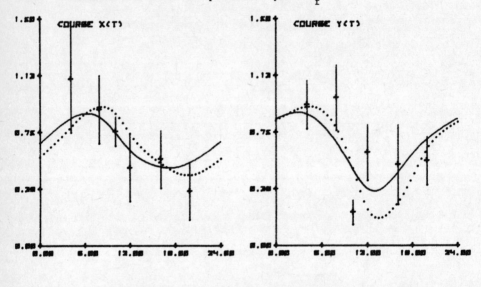

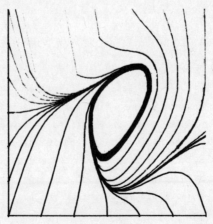

Phase-portrait

IV. CONCLUSIONS

A- We note for the signs of the parameters the similarity of the results between the qualitative and the quantitative studies.

B- The MRCAA can represent a new type of method for the simulation of biological rhythms (however degenerated MRCAA can be considered as a differential equation of the second order) : it allows us to reproduce simultaneously two circadian rhythms if they belong to an ago-antagonistic system,with their characteristic phase-shift. While,if the rhythms are taken separately,they benefit a more complet representation than with just one simple sinusoidal function.

C-It seems that the model is still valid to simulate one rhythmic function if we consider a standard sinusoidal function as second variable.

D- Any improvement of the model must seem to depend on
a) the expansion of the MRCAA itself (u and v expansions)
b) added experimental data which are still rare for the VP and totally absent for the simultaneous dosage of VP and ACH.

REFERENCES

(1) BERNARD-WEIL E. L'endocrinologie sous l'angle de la theorie des systemes.Rev. Franc.Endocrin.Cli. 1975,16,335-406

(2) BERNARD-WEIL E.,DUVELLEROY M. and MULLETIN J. Etude analytique et analogique d'un modele de la fonction surreno-posthypophysaire. Ann.Endocrinol. 1976,27,1

(3) BERNARD-WEIL E.,CHERRUAULT Y. Separate or combined agonistic-antagonistic models. A new approach to the optimal control.Medical implications. In 32nd Congress of Applied Systems and Cybernetics (Acapulco,1980),Pergamon,1981

(4) BERNARD-WEIL E. Formalisation d'un systeme endocrinien surreno-posthypophysaire par le modele mathematique de la regulation des couples ago-antagonistes. These de Doctorat ès-Sciences.Universite Paris VI,1979

(5) GEORGE C.P.L. and al.   Diurnal variation of plasmatic vasopressin in man. J.Cli.Endocrin. 1974,41,332-338

(6) GOLUB G. Numerical Methods for Solving Linear Least Squares Problems. Num.Math. 7,1965

(7) RIBIERE G. Amelioration du residu dans la resolution de systemes lineaires au sens des moindres carres. Mathematiques à l'usage du calculateur. 20,CNRS,Fev. 1967

CHAPTER 2

THEORETICAL STUDY OF BIOLOGICAL MODELS

THE SPRUCE BUDWORM-FOREST AND OTHER ECOSYSTEMS

Luis L. BONILLA and Manuel G. VELARDE,
Departamento de Física Fundamental,UNED,
Apartado Correos 50 487, Madrid-3(Spain)

1.INTRODUCTION

In the past decade quite a number of publications have appeared describing properties of time- and/or space-dependent phenomena and *dissipative structures* in nonlinear systems. Reactor kinetics /1/, non-equilibrium thermodynamics /2/, synergetics
/3/, ecology /4,5/ and other disciplines have strongly benefited from the detailed
mathematical analysis of model problems. Nearly all the publications refer, however,
to processes with instantaneous responses and it is only very recently /6-18/ that
phenomena with time- or space-delays have received some attention. Time-delay problems
arise in many areas of physics, physical chemistry, chemical engineering, biochemistry, ecology, economy, etc.

We have studied a model problem where time-delay, diffusion and advection compete
We have shown that dissipation can play a *dual* role in the stability of a limit cycle
and that slowly modulated variations of its amplitude obey a Landau-Ginzburg equation.
Our model is

$$\partial N/\partial t - rN(1 - BN/K) + bN^2/(H^2 + N^2) =$$

$$= \partial/\partial X \, [D(N)\partial N/\partial X] - \partial/\partial X \, [V(N)N] \tag{1.1}$$

where N is the unknown. N may represent some population density. BN accounts for
a time-delay . This is either
i) discrete or punctual(with time-delay, T)

$$BN \equiv N(x,t-T) \tag{1.2 a}$$

or ii) continuous, although peaked around t = T

$$BN \equiv \int_0^\infty (\sigma/T^2) \exp (-\sigma/T)N(x,t-\sigma)d\sigma \tag{1.2 b}$$

D and V   denote diffusion and velocity coefficients which are taken density dependent.

Specific examples exist in the literature to which the model could apply. One
case is the spruce budworm-forest ecosystem /9-16/ where the time-delay, T , corresponds to the seven to ten year time interval that balsam fir trees take to complete

their refoliage. Worms, however, reproduce yearly with a birth rate r. K is the carrying capacity of the ecosystem. Another example has been recently suggested by E.Parisi to account for some features in the development of sea-urchin eggs.

The depletion term in (1.1) is called Holling's S-shaped functional law, and it accounts for predation of the worms by birds. H determines the scale of budworm densities at which saturation begins to take place. b is the rate of worms consumption by the birds. H and K are quantities usually taken proportional to the available branch surface in the forest, say. Holling's law is the Michaelis-Menten law in enzyme catalyzed reactions and the Langmuir-Hinshelwood law in heterogeneous catalytic reactors /1/.

For certain values of the parameters in (1.1) the time-delay equation has two homogeneous steady states: $N = 0$ (extinction) and $N = N_0$ where N_0 is some constant whose actual value dependes on the given values of the parameters of the problem. In the absence of time-delay and dispersion (no spatial effects) N_0 can be a *stable* steady state of (1.1) whereas $N = 0$ becomes *unstable*. On the other hand, provided the time-delay, T, is large enough, N_0 can be unstable to time-periodic oscillatory disturbances /4,7/.

We call $\tilde{D} \equiv D(N_0) \neq 0$, $\tilde{V} = V(N_0)$, and define

$$u = N/H, \quad \tau = t/T, \quad x = X/(\tilde{D}T)^{1/2}, \quad \beta = rT, \quad R = rH/b,$$

$$Q = K/H, \quad c = V(T/\tilde{D})^{1/2}, \quad \tilde{V}c(u) = V(N), \quad \tilde{D}d(u) = D(N).$$

With the new scales the equation (1.1) becomes in dimensionless form

$$\frac{\partial u}{\partial \tau} - \beta u \left[1 - \frac{Bu}{Q} - u/R(1 + u^2) \right] = \frac{\partial}{\partial x} [d(u) \, \partial u/\partial x] - c \frac{\partial}{\partial x} [c(u)u] \quad (1.3)$$

where

$$d(u_0) = c(u_0) = 1, \quad u_0 = N_0/H \quad (1.4)$$

and

$$Bu = u(x, \tau-1) \quad (1.5 \text{ a})$$

or

$$Bu = \int_0^\infty \sigma \exp(-\sigma) u(x, \tau-\sigma) d\sigma \quad (1.5 \text{ b})$$

2. LINEAR STABILITY ANALYSIS

2.1. Dispersion-free case,

In the absence of space-dependent phenomena linearization of eq.(1.3) around the homogeneous steady state u_0 (which is stable in the absence of delay)leads to the following equation

$$du/dt = -\{a_{10}(\alpha)u + \alpha Bu\} \tag{2.1.a}$$

with

$$a_{10} = -\beta u_0(u_0^2 - 1)/R(u_0^2 + 1)^2 \equiv -\alpha Q(u_0^2 - 1)/R(u_0^2 + 1)^2 \tag{2.1.b}$$

and

$$\alpha = \beta u_0/Q \tag{2.1.c}$$

The characteristic equation for the eigenvalues λ is

$$\lambda + a_{10}(\alpha) + \alpha \tilde{B}(\lambda) = 0 \tag{2.2.a}$$

where

$$\tilde{B}(\lambda) = \exp(-\lambda) \tag{2.2.b}$$

for discrete delay, and

$$\tilde{B}(\lambda) = (1 + \lambda)^{-2} \tag{2.2.c}$$

for continuous delay.

It happens that for $\alpha < \alpha_0$ all roots of (2.2) have negative real parts ,with

$$\nu_0 \cot \nu_0 = -a_{10}, \text{ with } \quad 0 < \nu_0 \leqslant \pi , \tag{2.3.a}$$

$$\nu_0 \text{cosec } \nu_0 = \alpha_0 \tag{2.3.b}$$

$$a_{10} + \alpha_0 > 0 \tag{2.3.c}$$

for discrete time delay /5/, and

$$\alpha_0 = 2(1 + a_{10})^2 \tag{2.4.a}$$

$$\nu_0 = (1 + 2a_{10})^{1/2} \qquad\qquad\qquad\qquad (2.4.b)$$

for continuous time delay (Routh-Hurwitz criterion).

At $\alpha = \alpha_0$ there are two purely imaginary roots $\pm i\nu_0$ that cross the axis with positive speed, $\mathrm{Re}\,\lambda_1 > 0$, where

$$\lambda_1 = \lambda'(\alpha_0) = - [a_{10}'(\alpha_0) + B(i\nu_0)]/[1 + \alpha_0 B'(i\nu_0)]$$

Here prime denotes derivative with respect to the argument. Thus, we have a Hopf bifurcation to a limit cycle whose stability is exchanged with the trivial solution /7,8,13/.

2.2. Purely diffusive dispersion (no advection).

If we set $a = a_{10} + b$, $b > 0$ (not depending of α by assumption) instead of a_{10} in (2.1.a) and again perform the stability analysis, it turns out that b is always a stabilizing parameter for the homogeneous steady state. Therefore, when adding diffusion here restricted to dimension one, $\partial^2 u/\partial x^2$, we obtain the following results:
(i) In unbounded media or in bounded media with Neumann zero-flux b.c. there is bifurcation to homogeneous limit cycle. The most unstable Fourier mode in (2.1) has zero wavenumber.
(ii) In bounded media (length, L) with Dirichlet zero-data conditions there is bifurcation to a space modulated limit cycle with wavelength $L/2$. Thus in dimensional units time-delay and length act destabilizing and diffusion stabilizing the trivial state.

2.3. General dispersion with Dirichlet zero-data b.c. (diffusion and advection).
Here

$$b = \pi^2/L^2 + c^2/4$$

or

$$b = \pi^2 DT/L^2 + v^2 T/4D$$

in dimensional units. Diffusion plays a dual role:
(i) If the dimensionless number

$$\mathrm{Re} \equiv VL/D$$

is less than 2π , diffusion tends to stabilize the trivial (homogeneous) solution.
(ii) If $\mathrm{Re} > 2\pi$ diffusion can play a destabilizing role of that solution.

The critical value $\mathrm{Re}^c = 2\pi$ comes from the geometry and b.c. of the problem. Here Re is the Reynolds or Péclet number of fluid dynamics /29/.

3. NONLINEAR ANALYSIS

Search for direction of bifurcating solutions is carried out by taking into account the specific nonlinearity of the model. We have used a multiscale method/13, 19,20/to derive from (1.1) the following Landau-Ginzburg equation for the slowly varying complex nonlinear amplitude of the limit cycle:

$$\frac{\partial a}{\partial \tau} = \delta \frac{\partial^2 a}{\partial \xi^2} + (\alpha_2 \lambda_1 + \mu |a|^2)a$$

where $\alpha = \alpha_0 + \alpha_2 \epsilon^2 + \theta(\epsilon^3); \lambda_1, \delta, \mu$ are complex quantities, ξ, τ are rescaled space and time variables. Homogeneous time periodic solutions of (3.1) represent those of (1.1)which are stable to homogeneous disturbances if and only if Re $\mu < 0$.

3.1. Dispersion-free case. Here $\delta = 0$ in (3.1) and there is a Hopf bifurcation/21/ which is supercritical (stable) if Re $\mu < 0$ and subcritical (unstable) if Re $\mu > 0$.

3.2. Bounded media. The b.c. impose an exponential decay to all Fourier modes except one whose complex amplitude verifies (3.1) with $\delta = 0$. As μ depends on the nonlinear dispersion, thus an appropriate density-dependent diffusion can change the direction of bifurcation and the stability of the limit cycle/13/.

3.3. Purely diffusive dispersion in unbounded media. We have eq.(3.1) with $\delta \neq 0$. Even limit cycles which are stable to homogeneous disturbances can be destabilized by diffusion, if a number,κ,(essentially the nonlinear frequency correction ν_1), is negative /13.See also 24,25/.
According to the sign of

$$\kappa = \text{Re } \delta \left(1 + \frac{\text{Im } \delta}{\text{Re } \delta} \frac{\text{Im } \mu}{\text{Re } \mu}\right)$$

either local spatial oscillators can be sinchronized through diffusion if $\kappa > 0$ /22-23/, or if $\kappa < 0$ a stationary turbulent state (chemical turbulence)appears/26-28/.

4. APPLICATIONS

4.1. Budworm-forest ecosystem.

In this particular case, relevant ecological data are/12,13/:r = 1.52/year, and T ~ 7-10 years,R = 0.994,Q = 302 and u_0 = 300.991.Then Re $\mu < 0$ and $\nu_1 < 0$ thus,in the dispersion-free case there is bifurcation to a stable limit cycle, whereas a turbulent state is expected in the purely diffusive case if the space is unbounded.

In the dispersion-free case, at larger supercritical values ($\beta > \beta c$) the limit cycle appears like a relaxation oscillation. Figure 1 corresponds to the case $\beta = 14$. For about 2/3 of the period(4T ~ 37 years) there are few worms (endemic state) whereas in the later third of the period there is the outbreak which is expected to repeat periodically some forty years later. The population ratio between the densities at the two states is about 25×10^5.Such predicted values (period and ratio) agree satisfactorily with data given in the literature /14/. We have numericaly tested

the stability of the limit cycle to various illustrative disturbances: $u \approx u_0$
$u = 5 \, u_0, u = u_0 + e^{\tau+1} - 1 \, (-1 \leqslant \tau \leqslant 0)$. It takes about $\tau \sim 120$ for such initial
conditions to decay into the stable limit cycle within less than one per cent error
bar.

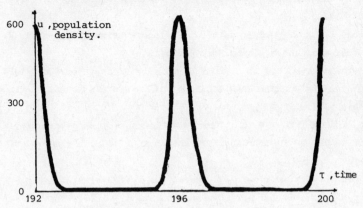

Figure 1. Stable limit cycle of Eq.(1,3) for $\beta = 14$, and $u(\tau) = 300.991$,
$-1 \leqslant \tau \leqslant 0$. Note that the minimum value of u is 2×10^{-4}, and it is not zero. The
ratio u_{max}/u_{min} is about 25×10^5. The period is $4T \sim 37$ years.

4.2. Time-delay in an ionic pump of sea-urchin eggs.

The equation
$$du/d\tau = 1 - \alpha u[\beta + \gamma \, u^n(\tau-1)] \qquad (4.1)$$
is a model recently proposed by E.Parisi /30/ to account for an ionic pump in the
sea-urchin eggs. As for (1.1), here (4.1) has a unique physically observable steady
state $u_0 > 0 (\alpha, \beta, \gamma$ positive numbers) and there is a Hopf bifurcation for suitable
values of the parameters if $n > 1$. For $n = 1$ the steady state can only be destabilized for $\alpha\gamma = \infty$, $u_0 = 0$, $\nu_0 = \pi$.

As an illustration, for $\beta = 0$, $n = 2$, $u_0 = \Gamma^{-1/3}$ with $\Gamma = \alpha\gamma$ there is a supercritical Hopf bifurcation for $\Gamma > \Gamma_0 \equiv (2\pi\sqrt{3}/9)^3$. The nonlinear correction to the linear
frequency $\nu_0 = 2\pi/3$ is $\nu_1 > 0$ (the period is slightly less than 3 minutes). If diffusion is added to the model, this homogeneous limit cycle is stable to inhomogeneous
spatial disturbances.

ACKNOWLEDGMENTS

Our thanks to A. Fernandez-Cancio fur useful discussions and to Dr.Elio Parisi
for suggesting the sea-urchin model. This work has been sponsored by the Stiftung
Volkswagenwerk.

REFERENCES

1. R. Aris, THE MATHEMATICAL THEORY OF DIFFUSION AND REACTION IN PERMEABLE CATALYSTS, (Two volumes),Clarendon Press, Oxford, 1975.

2. G.Nicolis and I. Prigogine. SELF-ORGANIZATION IN NON-EQUILIBRIUM SYSTEMS,Wiley, New York,1977.

3. H. Haken, SYNERGETICS,2nd. edition, Springer-Verlag, New York,1977.

4. G.E.Hutchinson, Ann.N.Y.Acad.Sci.50,221(1948).

5. J.Maynard-Smith,MODELS IN ECOLOGY,University Press, Cambridge, 1974.

6. J.M.Cushing, INTEGRODIFFERENTIAL EQUATIONS AND DELAY MODELS, Springer-Verlag, New York, 1977.

7. J.Hale, in NONLINEAR OSCILLATIONS IN BIOLOGY, Lect. Appl.Math.17,157(1978).

8. J.Hale, THEORY OF FUNCTIONAL DIFFERENTIAL EQUATIONS, Springer-Verlag,New York, 1977.

9. D.S.Cohen,E.Coutsias and J.C.Neu,Math.Biosci.44,255(1979).

10. D.S.Cohen,P.S.Hagan and H.C.Simpson,Math.Biosci.44,167(1979).

11. L.L.Bonilla and M.G.Velarde, J.interdiscipl.Cycle Res.,in the press.

12. L.L.Bonilla,A.Fernández-Cancio and M.G.Velarde,J.interdiscipl.Cycle Res. , in the press.

13. L.L.Bonilla and M.G.Velarde,J.Math.Phys.(submitted).

14. W.C.Clark,D.D.Jones and C.S.Holling, in SPATIAL PATTERNS IN PLANKTON COMMUNITIES, edited by J.H.Steele,Plenum Press,New York, 1978,p.385.

15. D.Ludwig ,D.P.Jones and C.S.Holling,J.Animal Ecol.47,315(1978).

16. D.Ludwig ,D.G.Aronson and H.F.Weinberger,J.Math.Biol.,8,217(1979).

17. G.S.Jones,J.Math.Anal.Appl.4,440(1962).

18. J.L.Kaplan and J.A.Yorke,SIAM J.Math.Anal.6,268(1975).

19. L.L.Bonilla and M.G.Velarde,J.Math.Phys.20,2692(1979).

20. A.H.Nayfeh,PERTURBATION METHODS,Wiley,1973;chapter 6.

21. S.N.Chow and J.Mallet-Paret,J.Diff.Eqs.26,112(1977).

22. Y.Kuramoto and T.Tsuzuki,Prog.Theor.Phys.55,356(1976).

23. Y.Kuramoto, in SYNERGETICS, edited by H.Haken, Springer-Verlag,New York, 1977,p.164.

24. G.B.Whitham, LINEAR AND NONLINEAR WAVES, Wiley, New Yor,1974.

25. D.Cope,SIAM J.Appl.Math.38,457(1980).

26. H.Fujisaka and T.Yamada, Prog.Theor.Phys.57,734(1977).

27. Y.Kuramoto and T.Yamada, Progr.Theor.Phys.56,679(1976).

28. T.Yamada and Y.Kuramoto, Prog.Theor.Phys.56,681(1976).

29. Ch. Normand, Y.Pomeau and M.G.Velarde, Rev.Mod. Phys.49 ,581(1977).

30. E. Parisi(private communication) and report in preparation.

ON THE CONSERVATION OF PHYSIOLOGICAL FUNCTION IN A POPULATION OF INTERACTIVE AND SELF REPLICATIVE UNITS

G. CHAUVET   D. GIROU
Laboratoire de Biologie Mathématique
U.E.R   ANGERS

Abstract :

The purpose of this study is the research of conditions which lead to the conservation of a given physiological function in a given population. In particular it is shown that a new hierarchical organization of different units in the population is obtained. The stability of non linear phenomenological systems is studied for a known relationship between two levels of organization.

The first objective is the validity of the following fundamental hypothesis : the substitution of a unit by an association is the consequence of a micromutation which breaks a biochemical pathway and stops the synthesis of a given product in any population unit. From an example of a $(\mathcal{M} - \mathcal{R})$ system where $\mathcal{M}$ is a Goodwin metabolic network and $\mathcal{R}$ is a particular Eigen sytem, this possibility of association is confirmed by a mathematical study. Indeed the areas of stability increase when association occurs.

The second objective is the influence of a coupling parameter between the two levels of organization on the behaviour of populations. It is shown that these coupling parameters are necessary for studying the selection of species.

INTRODUCTION

The problem discussed in this paper is the conservation of a
given physiological function in a population of selfreplicative and metabolic units. This basic property of living organisms was called elsewhere
[1] <u>vital coherence</u>. It means that during their evolution, there exists
a fundamental condition between elements of a population in order that a
given physiological function which is neccessary to their existence, be
conserved. This concept, which was much discussed in the evolutionary framework with regard to both species and tissular specialization, is based,
as will be shown, on the hierarchized system and on the relationship between organization levels. In particular with an example of the general metabolic system, we show how the extension of the study of the evolution of
a dynamic sytem to a larger system permits the observation of a new functionnal order.

This includes of course the mathematical study of a larger system from an
analysis of its subsystems, which is a very important problem in biology.
In a more general way the study of the evolution of a dynamic sytem of progressively increasing size, is in progress. In effect, two aspects have
to be considered : on the one hand, the extension or the reduction from one
organization level to another, i.e. the transcription of the language of
description at a given level into another different one; on the other hand
the description of the evolution of systems at each level.

Therefore it is a question here of functionnal self organization and we
show how, with an example of a ($\mathcal{M} - \mathcal{R}$) general system, it is possible to
formulate and develop this problem. Another direction in the laboratory
concerns structural self organization of hierarchized physical system [2].
We recall the following definitions [1] of levels of organization : The
first level concerns chemical reactions $\mathcal{C}$: the second, metabolic networks
$\mathcal{M}$ and the third, self replicative unit $\mathcal{U}$.

For each level there exist several populations of elements whose organiza-
tion is different, say $\mathcal{C}_1 \ldots \mathcal{C}_p$, $\mathcal{M}_1 \ldots \mathcal{M}_q$, $\mathcal{U}_1 \ldots \mathcal{U}_r$. By supposing these
populations arranged in ascending organizational order for a given defini-
tion of organization according to the given problem, we say that the degree
of organization of ($\mathcal{M} - \mathcal{R}$) systems increases with association of units
which belong to populations which are different from a functionnal point
of view for an identical organization level. With these definitions the
complexity of a system is related not only to the level but also to the
degree of organization.

While it is possible to describe more or less correctly the extension to
level $\mathcal{C}$ from the molecular level, with a principle of optimization of
potential energy during the association of molecules called chemical reaction, it is much more different to create a network $\mathcal{M}_0$ and then a selfreplicative unit according to a global principle.

The principle we have used is the one here called the vital coherence of living
organisms : a physiological function could be suppressed in a unit belonging to $\mathcal{U}$ if the product which is necessary to its life was provided
by other units. So it is the association of elements with the same properties, which increases the degree of organization influenced by external or
internal conditions.

DESCRIPTION OF THE ELEMENTARY MODEL : elements u and groups $\mathcal{U}$.

Let $\mathcal{U}$ be a population of selfreplicative and metabolic units which have
two basic properties :
(i) it is a very general metabolic system as described by Goodwin [3]
and which constitutes two control loops, one is an inhibition with a feedback at a point of the metabolic pathway (I-loop), the other is a repression of structural genes (R-loop). Figure 1 gives an example of this network. The essential difference between these two mechanisms resides on the
one hand in the localization of the point of impact of product P_n which
acts on the I-loop on the enzyme E at the point of the metabolic pathway
and on the R-loop on the structural gene G; on the other hand, in response
time because inhibition is fast and repression is slow. The connections
between passages of this type, say $\mathcal{C}$, constitute a metabolic pathway $\mathcal{M}_0$.
In a first study we simplify the above problem by considering figure 2,
where the regulation of the biochemical system is only that of an epigenetic system.

In other words there is a feedback of the end product P_2 on m RNA whose
concentration is X. This inhibiting interaction is cooperative and P_2 limits the transcription rate of the genetic message according to the formula :

$$\frac{dX}{dt} = f(P_2,\rho) = \frac{\alpha}{\beta+\gamma P_2^\rho} = \frac{\alpha_0}{1+KP_2^\rho} \quad \text{with } \alpha_0 = \frac{\alpha}{\beta}, \quad K = \frac{\gamma}{\beta}$$

and ρ is the molecularity of interaction. This signifies that ρ molecules of P_2 are binding with the aporepressor.

The dynamical evolution of the chemical reactions of an epigenetic system (figure 2) is described by :

I-1
$$\begin{cases} \dfrac{dX}{dt} = -\alpha_1 X + f(P_2,\rho) \\[2mm] \dfrac{dY}{dt} = -\alpha_2 Y + \alpha_1 X \\[2mm] \dfrac{dP_1}{dt} = -\alpha_3 P_1 + \alpha_2 Y \\[2mm] \dfrac{dP_2}{dt} = -\alpha_4 P_2 + \alpha_3 P_1 \end{cases}$$

where α_1 is the constant for the degradation of mRNA, α_1 the constant which expresses biosynthesis of protein Y, and α_2 its degradation. P_1 and P_2 are two intermediate products in the metabolic chain.

Such a system has been studied by several authors. For example Rapp [4] has shown that the stability of this system implies a relation between the molecularity ρ and the number of steps in the metabolic pathway. In the following lines, u denotes a unit belonging to $\mathcal{U}$ whose evolution satisfies the dynamic system (I-1).

(ii) It is also a selfreplicative unit which can reproduce itself by the following neodarwinian criteria, that is to say the basic equations first given by Eigen [5] . If we suppose that there exist several unit types, say u_i, in a certain sense which will appear in following lines, then $\mathcal{U} = \bigcup_i \mathcal{U}_i$ must satisfy a constant overall organizational constraint. Eigen had also studied the case of a constant overall flux constraint but this is not the objective here. Therefore we require the conservation of species, i.e $\sum_i u_i$ = constant.

The evolution of population $\mathcal{U}$ is given by the system :

II-1
$$\begin{cases} \dfrac{du_i}{dt} = (a_i - \dfrac{1}{c}\lambda(u_1 \ldots u_r)) u_i \\[2mm] \sum_{i=1}^{r} u_i = c \end{cases}$$

Now we are in a position to signify the type of organization for $\mathcal{U}$ and each $\mathcal{U}_1$. Let r- $\mathcal{U}$ be this group (which is not a mathematical group) of elements $\mathcal{U}_i$, i = 1 to r. It is the postulate of vital coherence which imposes system organization. Thus let u_1^* be a unit element of $\mathcal{U}1$ affected by a micromutation, occuring in a certain step of the metabolic pathway, defined by the biochemical reaction : $S_o \longrightarrow P_2$, and blocking the whole reaction.

For example, biosynthesis of protein Y is stopped as a consequence of a mutation of gene G. The survival of u_1^* is therefore completely dependent upon whether product P_1 (synthetized by other units of u_1-type) is used by u_1^* or not. This is the postulate of vital coherence which is well developped in other papers [1] . Other hypotheses like the transport process from one unit to another are not necessary in this first study. The final result is the functionnal association of both u_1 and u_1^* to generate another type of unit, say $u_2 = (u_1, u_1^*)$. A more detailed discussion and its consequences will be found in [1] .

Thus a new group (2-$\mathcal{U}$) is obtained from unit u_1. It is the set which is formed by elements like u_2. More explicitly the epigenetic regulation of u_2, represented in figure 3 is described by the dynamic system :

$$(\text{I-2}) \quad \begin{cases} \dfrac{dX}{dt} = -\alpha_1 X + f(P_2, \rho) + f(P_2^*, \rho) \\[2mm] \dfrac{dY}{dt} = -\alpha_2 Y + \alpha_1 X \\[2mm] \dfrac{dP_1}{dt} = -\alpha_3 P_1 - \alpha_5 P_1 + \alpha_2 Y \\[2mm] \dfrac{dP_2}{dt} = -\alpha_4 P_2 + \alpha_3 P_1 \\[2mm] \dfrac{dP_2^*}{dt} = -\alpha_4 P_2^* + \alpha_5 P_1 \end{cases}$$

and this functionning of metabolic units at organization level denoted by $\mathcal{M}$ is well known. At the highest level $\mathcal{U}$, system II can be written :

$$(\text{II-2}) \quad \begin{cases} \dfrac{du_1}{dt} = (a_1 - \dfrac{1}{c} \lambda (u_1, u_2)) u_1 \\[2mm] \dfrac{du_2}{dt} = (a_2 - \dfrac{1}{c} \lambda (u_1, u_2)) u_2 + ku_1^2 \\[2mm] u_1 + 2u_2 = c \end{cases}$$

where we have defined a constant overall organization by requiring that
the total number of u_1-units be equal to c.
The fundamental term in this new system is ku_1^2 which expresses the generation of new units like u_2 from u_1. As k is a function of P_2 which controls
the association between u_1-units, we say that it is a coupling parameter
between the two levels of organization $\mathscr{M}$ and $\mathscr{U}$ or a functionnal self organization parameter. Here we have used the chemical formalism for bimolecular
reactions. The association of two units u_1 and u_1^* occured at the rate k . The phenomenological significance of the constant k derives from the principle of
vital coherence because a unit of u_1^* type must associate with a unit of u_1
type. If not u_1 dies. There are certainly some possibilities of such association and a tissue is the best example. In a population whose degree of
organization equals three, there would be a third equation in u_3 with a term
which expresses the generation of new units such as u_3 from u_2 and u_1, and
a second coupling parameter k' :

$$\frac{du_3}{dt} = (a_3 - \frac{1}{c} (u_1,u_2,u_3)) u_3 + k' u_1 u_2$$

and $u_1 + 2u_2 + 3u_3 = c$ is the relation of constant overall organization.

Such a hierarchically organized system is a realistic example deduced from
known theories (Goodwin [3],Eigen [5]) and can lead simultaneously to a
rational explanation of both species evolution and tissular specialization
[1] . But it is also possible in this framework to give a formalized meaning to several concepts such as the self organization parameter, and the
degree of organization and specialization.

In this paper we have limited ourselves to the study of mathematical stability of systems (I-2) and (II-2) which are deduced from (I-1) and (II-1) by
adding an equation of the same type.

STABILITY OF SYSTEMS (I-1) and (I-2)

1. Coordinate transformation $(X,Y,P) \longrightarrow (x_i)$

The study of these non-linear systems is easier when the following transformation due to Rapp, [4] is used :

$$a_o = (K^{\frac{1}{\rho}} \alpha_0 \alpha_1 \alpha_2 \alpha_3)^{\frac{1}{4}}$$

$$a_i = K^{\frac{1}{\rho}} \prod_{j=i}^{3} b_j \qquad i = 1 \text{ to } 3$$

with

$$a_4 = K^{\frac{1}{\rho}}$$

$$b_j = \frac{\alpha_j}{a_o} \qquad j = 1 \text{ to } 4$$

and

$$f(P,\rho) = \frac{\alpha_o}{1 + KP^\rho}$$

in the first case (system I), we have by putting $t^* = a_o t$:

$$x_1(t^*) = a_1 X(t)$$

$$x_2(t^*) = a_2 Y(t)$$

$$x_3(t^*) = a_3 P_1(t)$$

$$x_4(t^*) = a_4 P_2(t)$$

and the system (I-1) may be written in the new coordinates (x_1, x_2, x_3, x_4) :

$$(I-3) \quad \begin{cases} \dot{x}_1 = -b_1 x_1 + \dfrac{1}{1+x_4^\rho} \\[2ex] \dot{x}_2 = -b_2 x_2 + x_1 \\[2ex] \dot{x}_3 = -b_3 x_3 + x_2 \\[2ex] \dot{x}_4 = -b_4 x_4 + x_3 \end{cases}$$

In the second case (system I-2), the same coordinate transformation with a complementary relation :

$$x_5(t^*) = a_5 P_2^*(t)$$

and
$$a_5 = \frac{\alpha_3}{\alpha_5} a_4 \quad , \quad b_5 = \frac{\alpha_5}{a_0}$$

leads to system (I-4)

$$(I-4) \quad \begin{cases} \dot{x}_1 = -b_1 x_1 + \dfrac{1}{1+x_4^\rho} + \dfrac{1}{1+(\frac{b_5}{b_3} x_5)^\rho} \\[2ex] \dot{x}_2 = -b_2 x_2 + x_1 \\[2ex] \dot{x}_3 = -(b_3+b_5) x_3 + x_2 \\[2ex] \dot{x}_4 = -b_4 x_4 + x_3 \\[2ex] \dot{x}_5 = -b_4 x_5 + x_3 \end{cases}$$

It is now possible to study the (I-4) system dependance on the (I-3) system. In particular the immediate problem to be solved is the study of the stability of the (I-2) system when α_3, α_4 and α_5 vary from values which satisfy the stability of (I-1) system. Another problem is the influence of the epigenetic system represented by coefficients (α_1, α_2, ρ) on the stability of the system.

2. Linear stability analysis :

The (I-3) system (non equivalent to (I-1), but studied for its compatible numerical values of parameters) is linearized around the steady-stade $(x_1^o, x_2^o, x_3^o, x_4^o)$ given by :

x_4^o which is a solution of : $x_4^{\rho+1} + x_4 \dfrac{1}{\prod\limits_{i=1}^{4} b_i} = 0$

$x_i^o = x_4^o \prod\limits_{j=i+1}^{4} b_j$ for i = 1 to 3

The Routh-Hurwitz criteria applied to the linear system :

$$\frac{dU}{dt} = LU \quad \text{with } U = \begin{pmatrix} \delta x_1 \\ \delta x_2 \\ \delta x_3 \\ \delta x_4 \end{pmatrix} \quad, \quad L = \begin{pmatrix} -b_1 & 0 & 0 & -\gamma \\ 1 & -b_2 & 0 & 0 \\ 0 & 1 & -b_3 & 0 \\ 0 & 0 & 1 & -b_4 \end{pmatrix}$$

and $\qquad \gamma = \dfrac{\rho (x_4^o)^{\rho-1}}{(1+(x^o)^{\rho})^2_4}$

give the condition of stability :

$$\mu^2 T \delta_1 \delta_2 + (\mu + \rho(\mu - x_4^o))T^2 + \mu^2 \delta_2^2 \leqslant 0$$

with $\qquad \mu = \dfrac{1}{\prod\limits_{i=1}^{4} b_i}$, $T = -\sum\limits_{i=1}^{4} b_i$, $\delta_i = \sum\limits_{1 \leqslant i < j \leqslant 4} b_i b_j$, $\delta_2 = \sum\limits_{1 \leqslant i < j < k \leqslant 4} b_i b_j b_k$

The case of the (I-4) system is more complicated but it is possible to follow the same calculations. We also have a unique steady state, denoted $(\tilde{x}_i^o)$ for i = 1 to 5, given by the equations : $\tilde{x}_4^o$ solution of the algebraic equation :

$$A x_4^{2\rho+1} + (1+A) x_4^{\rho+1} - \tilde{\mu}(1+A) x_4^{\rho} + x_4 - 2\tilde{\mu} = 0$$

with
$$A = (\frac{\alpha_5}{\alpha_3})\rho = (\frac{b_5}{b_3})\rho \quad \text{and} \quad \tilde{\mu} = (b_1 b_2 b_4 (b_3 + b_5))^{-1}$$

$$\tilde{x}_1^o = b_2 (b_3 + b_5) b_4 \, \tilde{x}_4^o$$

$$\tilde{x}_2^o = (b_3 + b_5) b_4 \, \tilde{x}_4^o$$

$$\tilde{x}_3^o = b_4 \, \tilde{x}_4^o$$

$$\tilde{x}_5^o = \tilde{x}_4^o$$

The linearized equation around this steady state is :

$$\frac{dU}{dt} = LU \quad \text{with} \quad U = \begin{pmatrix} \delta x_1 \\ \cdot \\ \cdot \\ \delta x_5 \end{pmatrix} \quad \text{and}$$

$$L = \begin{pmatrix} -b_1 & 0 & 0 & -\gamma_1 & -\gamma_2 \\ 1 & -b_2 & 0 & 0 & 0 \\ 0 & 1 & -(b_3+b_5) & 0 & 0 \\ 0 & 0 & 1 & -b_4 & 0 \\ 0 & 0 & 1 & 0 & -b_4 \end{pmatrix}$$

with
$$\gamma_1 = \frac{\rho(\tilde{x}_4^o)^{\rho-1}}{(1+(\tilde{x}_4^o)^{\rho})^2} \quad \text{and} \quad \gamma_2 = \frac{A\rho(\tilde{x}_4^o)^{\rho-1}}{(1+A(\tilde{x}_4^o)^{\rho})^2}$$

The Routh-Hurwitz criteria give the following condition of stability :

$$\tilde{T}\delta_1\delta_2 + \delta_2^2 + \Delta\tilde{T}^2 \leqslant 0$$

with
$$\tilde{T} = -\prod_{i=1}^{5} b_i = T - b_5$$

$$\delta_1 = b_1 b_2 + b_1 b_4 + b_2 b_4 + (b_1 + b_2 + b_4)(b_3 + b_5) = \delta_1 + (b_1 + b_2 + b_4) b_5$$

$$\delta_2 = b_1 b_2 b_4 + (b_1 b_2 + b_1 b_4 + b_2 b_4)(b_3 + b_5) = \delta_2 + (b_1 b_2 + b_1 b_4 + b_2 b_4) b_5$$

$$\Delta = b_1 b_2 (b_3 + b_5) b_4 + \gamma_1 + \gamma_2$$

For the values of α_i as given by Walter [6] in the original publication
we have determined the regions of stability. The results are shown in fi-
gure (4) when α_1, α_2, α_0, K and ρ are fixed. The diagram (α_3, α_4) gives
closed lines for several values of α_5 and we see that the inside area which
represents the instability condition decreases.

The first simulations we have undertaken thus give an interesting conclusion : $u_2 = (u_1, u_1^*)$ unit is more stable than u_1 in the level of organization $\mathcal{M}$. The second problem is also fundamental. What is the behaviour
of the $\mathcal{U}$-population when the self organization parameter varies versus
the concentration of P ?

STABILITY OF SYSTEMS (II-2)

The (II-2) system is now written for simplicity :

(II-3)
$$
\begin{cases}
\dot{x} = (\alpha - f)x \\[2mm]
\dot{y} = (\beta - f)y + kx^2 \\[2mm]
x + 2y = c
\end{cases}
$$

It is easy to show that the conservation relation $x+2y=c$ implies the
form of f :

$$f(x,y) = \frac{\alpha}{c}x + \frac{2\beta}{c}y + \frac{2k}{c}x^2$$

The calculation gives four steady states :

$$X_1 = (0,0)$$

$$X_2 = (0, \frac{c}{2})$$

$$X_3 = (a_1, \frac{1}{2}(c-a_1)) \qquad \text{with} \quad a_1 = \frac{\beta - \alpha + \sqrt{\Delta}}{4k}$$

$$X_4 = (a_2, \frac{1}{2}(c-a_2)) \qquad \text{and} \quad a_2 = \frac{\beta - \alpha - \sqrt{\Delta}}{4k}$$

We have put $\Delta = (\beta - \alpha)^2 - 8kc(\beta - \alpha)$ which is the discriminant of the
second order steady-stade equation :

$$2kx^2 - (\beta - \chi)x + (\beta - \alpha)c = 0$$

The problem is now the analysis of the stability around X_i, $i = 1$ to 4, and the determination of conditions concerning α, β, and k. The full calculations are long and fastidious. So here we only give the principal results.

c is always stricly positive. So the trivial case X_1 is not possible. It is the same for X_4 which is negative with these conditions.

Study of the X_2-state : It is easy to find Jacobian J and its eigenvalues $\lambda_1 = -\beta$ and $\lambda_2 = \alpha - \beta$. If $\alpha < \beta$, both λ_1 and λ_2 are real negative. If $\alpha < \beta$, one root is real positive and the other is real negative. In the first case X_2 is a stable state. Evidently it is unstable in the second case.

Study of the X_3-state : After long calculations the linearized system deduced from (II-3) is written :

$$\begin{pmatrix} \delta \dot{x} \\ \delta \dot{y} \end{pmatrix} = \begin{pmatrix} 2r_1 - \alpha & -2r_2 \\ -r_1 & r_2 - \alpha \end{pmatrix} \begin{pmatrix} \delta x \\ \delta y \end{pmatrix}$$

which gives two eigenvalues :

$$\lambda_1 = 3r_1 + r_2 - \alpha$$

$$\lambda_2 = -\alpha$$

where $r_1 = (\beta - \frac{\alpha}{2})(1 - \frac{a_1}{c})$ and $r_2 = \frac{\beta}{c} a_1$

It is possible to show that both λ_1 and λ_2 have negative real parts because $\lambda_1 = (\beta - \alpha) \gamma$ where γ is positive.

Finally two stable areas are found for the X_2 and X_3 states respectively. Evidently in this simple case the interpretation of results shown in figure 5 is easy : the evolution of units u_1 and u_2 depends on the coupling parameter $k(P)$ as well as on coefficients α, β and k which results in the selection of species. Such calculations could usefully be extended to more complex systems.

DISCUSSION :

         The results which are obtained from the analysis of linear
stability confirm the possibility of association of units with different properties. This self organization leads to selection of species
which have the "best" set of parameters including the coupling parameter between two levels of organization. Indeed it is possible to study
a more complex system than (II-3) by adding another equation which represents the association of u_1 and u_2 units. The behaviour of this new
system depends on two coupling parameters denoted by k and k'. First
results are shown on figure 6 for several values of k and k'.

         Evidently this is a preliminary study of the effect of cou-
pling between several levels of organization on the association of units
with given properties. Though the mechanisms which lead to the association of units have to be studied further a fundamental result has been
obtained : it is shown that the selective value as defined by several
authors [5]   needs to be completed by a new parameter called the self
organizational parameter. This parameter is a function of the concentration of product P_2 formed at the metabolic level. Thus although we
have not taken account of the effect of the spatial diffusion in the units
in this preliminary study, we have obtained two results : (i) the stable
zone of the type u_2 composite unit is greater than that of a type u_1 simple unit, such an organization is therefore favorable for a given set of
parameters (α_3, α_4, α_5) (figure 4) ; (ii) If the self organization parameter $k(P_2)$ is the same for the association (u_1, u_1^*) u_2 or (u_2, u_1^*) u_3,
which is justified in the absence of the spatial effect, in other words if
k' = k , the population of u_3 units becomes preponderant (figure 7).

REFERENCES

1- G.CHAUVET. Functionnal self organization: Consequences on the evolu-
         tion of species and tissular specialization (tc appear)

2- P.AUGER. Coupling between N levels of observation of a system (biolo-
         gical or physical) resulting in creation of structures.
         Int. J. General systems 6, 83 (1980)

3-B.C. GOODWIN. Analytical cell physiology (1978) - Academic Press -
         and Temporal organization in cell (1963)Academic Press(LONDON)

4-P.RAPP. Analysis biochemical phase shift oscillators by a harmonic
         balancing technique -J.Math.Biol. 3, 203 (1976)

5-M.EIGEN. Self organization of matter and the evolution of biological
         molecules- Naturwissenschaften 58, 465 (1971)

6-C.F. WALTER. The occurence and the significance of limit cycle behavior
         in controlled biochemical systems.-J.Theor.Biol. 27, 259
         (1970)

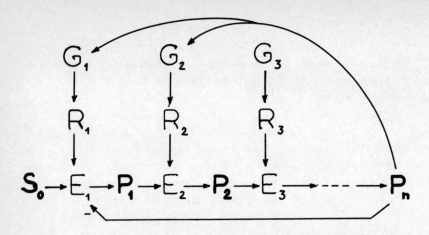

Figure 1 (After Goodwin, modified)

S_i = substrate; G_i, R_i, E_i are respectively structural genes, polysomes and synthetized enzymes.

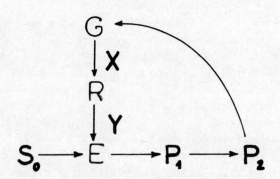

Figure 2

Epigenetic model obtained from figure 1

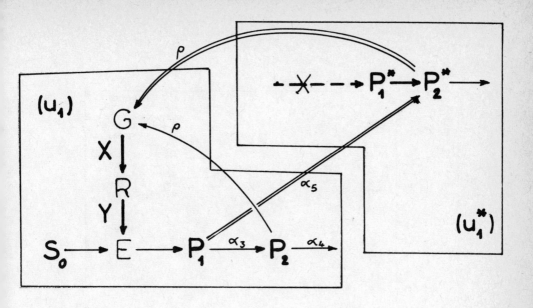

Figure 3
$u_2 = (u_1, u_1^*)$ unit obtained from an increase in degree of
organizational

116

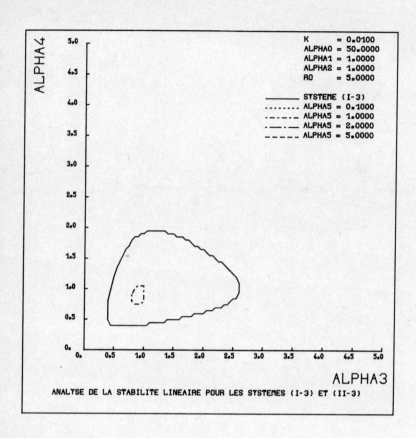

ANALYSE DE LA STABILITE LINEAIRE POUR LES SYSTEMES (I-3) ET (II-3)

Figure 4

Linear stability analysis for systems (I-3) and (I-4) with
two different values of k.

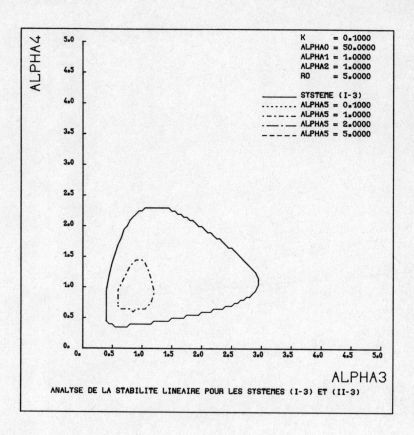

ANALYSE DE LA STABILITE LINEAIRE POUR LES SYSTEMES (I-3) ET (II-3)

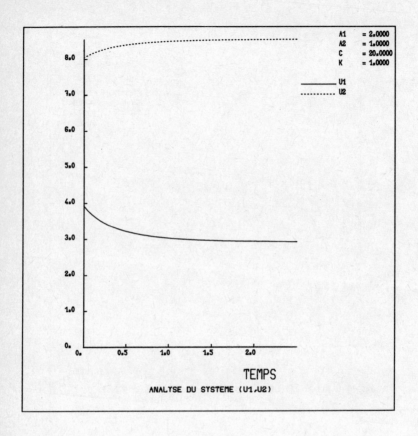

Figure 5

Analysis of system II-3 (u_1, u_2) around the X_3-steady state- (concentration vs time)

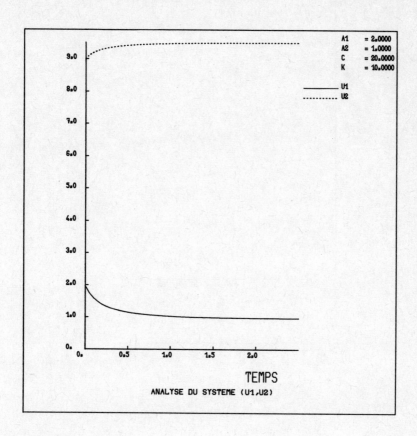

ANALYSE DU SYSTEME (U1,U2)

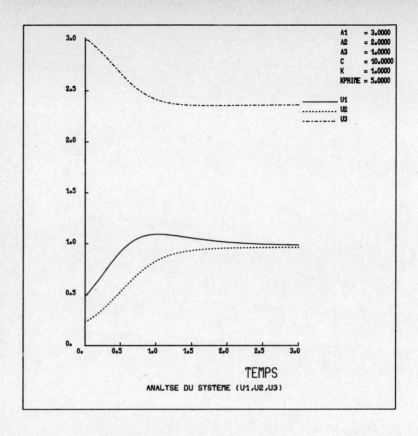

Figure 6

Analysis of a system like II-3 (u_1, u_2, $u_3 = (u_1^*, u_2)$) for different values of the coupling parameters k and k'.

(concentration vs time)

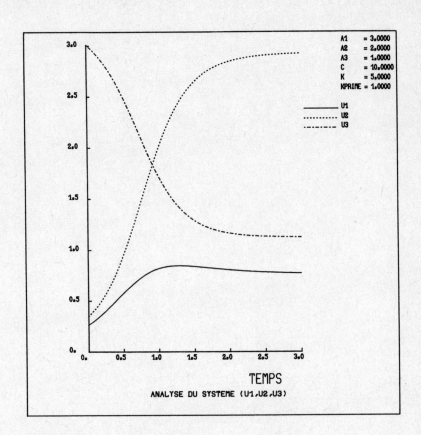

ANALYSE DU SYSTEME (U1,U2,U3)

122

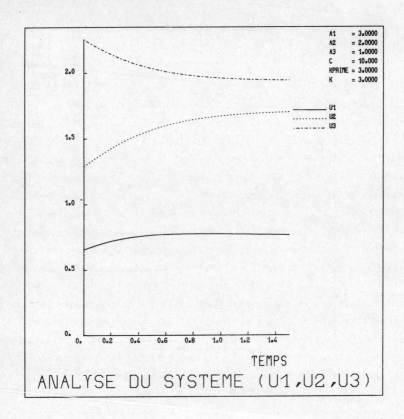

Figure 7

Analysis of system $(u_1,\ u_2,\ u_3 = (u_1^*,\ u_2))$ for $k = k'$.

DYNAMICS AND STABILITY OF INDUCTION OF
THE LACTOSE OPERON OF ESCHERISCHIA COLI

Florence CORPET, Claude CHEVALET, Michel GILLOIS(*)
and Artibano MICALI(**)

ABSTRACT.   The genetical and biochemical mechanisms of the induction process of
lactose operon are modeled by a set of nine differential equations, with delayed
arguments. A preliminary numerical investigation has shown that the dimension
of the system could be reduced to four or even two, so as to allow for an analytical study of stability. When the external concentrations in lactose and glucose
are kept fixed, the main results are :
(i)   There is a unique fixed point ; necessary conditions for existence of multiple steady states involve parameters values far beyond any biological meaning.
(ii) Parameters values describing known wild and mutant genotypes are within the
domain of stability of the unique fixed point, whichever external concentrations
may be.
(iii) Sets of parameters values involving at least two mutations may be found, for
which the stability depends on the external lactose concentration, and such that
intracellular concentrations can undergo sustained oscillations ; however the
periods are quite large and the delays seem to stabilize the system, so that such
periodic behaviour has not yet any clear biological meaning.

CONTENTS

4.   Stability analysis

    4.1 Two dimensional stability of the fixed point

    4.2 Stability of the critical point in the four-dimensional system

    4.3 Sensitivity of the system with respect to delays

5.   Conclusion

    References

1.   <u>Introduction</u>

       Life is rythm. Circadian, monthly and annual changes may be related
to astronomical periodicities, but specific biological mechanisms must be invoked
to account for autonomous oscillations like cell divisions and precise timing in
morphogenesis and development. The search for subcellular and supercellular mechanisms that could be responsible for stable sustained oscillations has been undertaken along two epistemological lines, and has been focused on two main systems :
metabolic pathways, and genetic control circuits. The first trend is the finding
of mathematical metaphors, which can mimic some biological behaviours [1,2,3].
These models are not dependent on specific biological systems, nor on peculiar
biochemical substrates, and they derive by some inductive process, from general
concepts such as gradients of effectors among cells [2], inhibition and activation
of enzymatic catalysis [4], genetic regulation [5], genetic coupling of enzymatic
reactions [6]. The second trend is the developing of ad-hoc models for systems
which can be submitted to experiments. Best studied systems are the phosphofructokinase enzyme [7,8,9], and the lactose operon control circuit. The latter system
embodies both kinds of biological systems, as it is a metabolic pathway controlled
by a genetic system of regulation.

       As soon as the main phenomena involved in the functioning of operon
lactose were discovered, Monod stated that it might be the source of some self
sustained oscillations. As it is a system that works as a response to environmen-
tal changes, it is not expected to be any basic element in a biological clock ;
however it may be an archetype for a biological dissipative structure that
exhibits some periodical behaviour, in addition to its main and evident feeding
role. In fact, several authors [10,11,12] have found that models of its functioning might possess several stationary states and periodical solutions for some values
of the parameters. However some new biological results have been obtained, that
need some of these models to be re-written. Specially, the predicted self sustained oscillations, irrespective of the fact that they occur with parameter values
outside the range of any biological meaning, are basically dependent on the way

catabolic repression was taken into account [13].

We have undertaken a new modeling of the lactose operon system, yet restricted to the induction process. At present we have included catabolic repression in the adjusting of some unknown parameters, but have not yet entered into the analysis of conditions in which the phenomenon does have dynamical importance, such as diauxic growth.

We have another aim in developing this work, that is the synthetic modeling of a whole polygenic system. Presently, only poor mathematical models of the joint effects of genes on some quantitative trait are available, which are mainly derived from the early Fisher's one [14]. In quantitative genetics, genes are mostly considered as independent factors, contributing small and additive amounts to any metric trait. This view has had, and still has, considerable impact on the statistical methods of crop and animal improvement. Nevertheless, the general discoveries in molecular biology, as well as the experimental ability to study the genetical basis of compound characters in cultured cells, should make it possible and useful to build up specific models for such traits. At present we think it is necessary to work with a few well known systems, and to build some substrate dependent models that could be contrasted with experimental evidence, before proposing any general set of metaphors as mathematical descriptions of inherited complex characters.

2. Statement of the model and numerical results

The present study is only concerned with the mechanism of induction, so that amounts of molecular species involved in catabolic repression are kept constant. The specific elements of the model (figure 1) are the states of the control region, and the head of the metabolic pathway of lactose. The linkage between them is due to the control region state dependence on inducer's concentration, and to the dependence of enzymes synthesis rate on the control region state.

The control region may be in different states, according to the macromolecules bound to DNA. Modeling of that part has been performed by several authors [16, 17], we use Mandecki's model modified to take account of the antipolar effect of CAP (figure 2). Rate equations for probabilities $x_i(t)$ of the six possible states are :

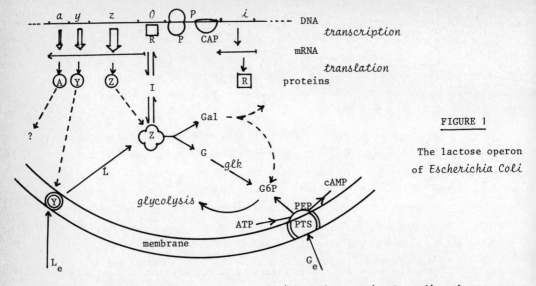

FIGURE 1

The lactose operon
of *Escherichia Coli*

When the bacterium is grown on glucose and without lactose in the medium, the repressor R encoded by gene i binds to the operator of the operon and allows for a very small synthesis of the proteins Z, Y and A. If lactose is present in the medium, it first enters the cell at a very low rate, but the few Z proteins convert it partially into an isomer, allolactose, which can bind to the repressor and weaken its affinity with the operator. The latter gene is then "open" and allows the transcription of lac-mRNA and its translation into greater amounts of proteins Z and Y. This autocatalytic process enables the cell to use lactose as a carbone source. However, as long as glucose is present in the medium, the rate of transcription remains low and the cell grows with glucose as its carbon source. If glucose is removed, the PEP used in the permeation system of glucose (PTS) may be used to activate the adenylate cyclase enzyme which converts ATP into cAMP, which in turn activates the CAP protein. The binding of the latter to the promoter region increases the rate of transcription and thus allows the operon to be fully induced. Conversely, adding of glucose in the medium lowers the intracellular concentration of cAMP and resumes the lac operon expression to its repressed level (catabolic repression).

FIGURE 2 : States of the control region

(i) The inducer I (allolactose) may bind to the free repressor ($R + I \rightleftharpoons RI$) and to the repressor bound to operator ($OR + I \rightleftharpoons ORI$) with equilibrium constants $1_1/1_1'$ and $1_2/1_2'$; the kinetic association constants of R and RI to the operator are known to be equal (k_1), but the kinetic dissociation constant of complex ORI is much larger than that of complex OR. (ii) The kinetic constants of the binding of the CAP protein to the

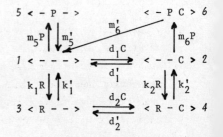

promoter region are unknown. (iii) The binding of polymerase P to the promoter is inhibited when the repressor is bound to operator, its efficiency is dependent upon the presence or absence of protein CAP, which tightens the binding of P so as to enhance the transcription rate ($m_6' < m_5'$) , and allows for longer messengers RNAs.

Abbreviations used: DNA:deoxyribonucleic acids. mRNA:messenger ribonucleic acids. A:thiogalactoside transacetylase. Y:lactose permease. Z:β-galactosidase. R:repressor. L:intracellular lactose. L_e:extracellular lactose. I:allolactose, the natural inducer. G:intracellular glucose. G_e:extracellular glucose. Gal:intracellular galactose. G6P:glucose-6-phosphate. ATP:adenosine triphosphate. cAMP:cyclic adenosine monophosphate. PEP:phosphoenol-pyruvate. C:the CAP protein activated by cAMP. *glk*:glucokinase enzyme.

$$\frac{dx_1}{dt} = - (d_1 C + k_1 R + m_5 P) \, x_1 + d_1' \, x_2 + k_1' \, x_3 + m_5' \, x_5 + m_6' \, x_6$$

$$\frac{dx_2}{dt} = d_1 C \, x_1 - (d_1' + k_2 R + m_6 P) \, x_2 + k_2' \, x_4$$

$$(1.1) \quad \frac{dx_3}{dt} = k_1 R \, x_1 - (k_1' + d_2 C) \, x_3 + d_2' \, x_4$$

$$\frac{dx_4}{dt} = k_2 R \, x_2 + d_2 C \, x_3 - (k_2' + d_2') \, x_4$$

$$\frac{dx_5}{dt} = m_5 P \, x_1 - m_5' \, x_5$$

$$\frac{dx_6}{dt} = m_6 P \, x_2 - m_6' \, x_6$$

Parameters are defined in figure 2, as differential transition rates.

The intracellular inducer concentration I commands the rate at which the repressor-operator complex may be dissociated. We assume a rapid diffusion of allolactose within the bacterium, so that the kinetic dissocation coefficients of repressor from the operator are

$$(1.2) \qquad k_i' = k_{i1}' \, (1 + K_i \, \ell_2 \, I/\ell_2') \, / \, (1 + \ell_2 \, I/\ell_2') \qquad i = 1,2$$

according to the hyperbolic relationship given by in vitro experiments [23].

The general hypotheses used in the derivation of (1) are :
(i)   mass action law is valid for any uni- or bi-molecular reaction ;
(ii)   when the equilibrium constant of two interacting molecules is affected by the binding of an effector to one of them, the change is only due to some modification in the kinetic dissociation constant, whereas the association kinetic constant is assumed to be unaffected;
(iii) known kinetic hierarchies are used to replace differential equations by algebraic ones (such a simplification is implicit in figure 2, where it was taken advantage of the higher magnitude of kinetic parameters $\ell_2 I$ and ℓ_2', compared to k_1' and k_2').

The operon system controls the metabolism of lactose by means of enzymes Y and Z. Associated equations are the Michaelis equation for permease Y [18] and the complete rate equation for β-galactosidase Z [19]. Taking account of passive permeation, rate equations for intracellular lactose L, allolactose I and glucose G are

$$\frac{dL}{dt} = k_s \ (L_e - L) + V_M \ \frac{L_e}{L_e + K_M} \ Y - Z \ \frac{(a+b) \ L}{L + \alpha I + \beta} \ ,$$

(2)

$$\frac{dI}{dt} = Z \ \frac{bL - \alpha c \ I}{L + \alpha I + \beta} \ , \quad \frac{dG}{dt} = Z \ \frac{aL + \alpha c \ I}{L + \alpha I + \beta} \ .$$

Two kinds of important hypothesis are made in writing down these equations :

(iv)   numbers of substrates molecules are large as compared to numbers of enzymatic sites (it is a necessary condition for applying the pseudo steady state hypothesis [20, 21, 22]);

(v)   some enzymatic activites are irreversible, so that lactose cannot leave the cell through the permease system, and intracellular galactose and glucose do not alter the rate of hydrolysis of lactose.

Synthesis of enzymes Y and Z is a stochastic process, the main steps of which are : initiation of messenger RNA transcription, at a rate proportional to $x_5(t) + x_6(t)$ at time t, possible early termination of transcription when it starts from state $< 5 >$, translation of RNA transcripts into proteins, rapid decay of messenger RNA molecules (with a half life of about one minute), maturation of enzymes. All these steps are summed up in the following equations for the expected values of Y and Z amounts :

$$\frac{dY}{dt}(t) = K_y \ (\alpha_y \ x_5(t-\tau_y) + x_6(t-\tau_y)) - K_y' \ Y(t)$$

(3)

$$\frac{dZ}{dt}(t) = K_z \ (\alpha_z x_5(t-\tau_z) + x_6 \ (t-\tau_z)) - K_z' \ Z(t)$$

Parameters α_y and α_z, $\alpha_y \le \alpha_z \le 1$, express polarity effects ; τ_z and τ_z are delays between transcription initiation and beginning of enzymatic activities ; K_y and K_z express the efficiency of the whole process ; K_y' and K_z' give the rates at which enzymes are lysed. Most restrictive in these equations is the deterministic formulation that may make the model questionable when dealing with states involving few enzymes and rare transcriptional events.

Equations (1.1, 1.2), (2) and (3) make up the full system. The model embodies many parameters whose actual values have important bearing on the qualitative nature of the trajectories. A thorough numerical investigation

was carried out that allowed firstly to estimate some unknown parameters by
contrasting model predictions with experiments, secondly to propose some simple
analytical expressions of some sub-systems that seemed to keep the main qualitative
features of the original model, thirdly to state a few conjectures about the
reduction of the differential system to fewer   dimensions, which allowed further
analytical studies. The numerical integration was performed on a IBM 3031 computer
with a Runge-Kutta program given to us by Pr. I. Gumowski (Université Paul Sabatier,
Toulouse). Details and main biological consequences will be reported elsewhere
[24]. The set of parameters values given in table 1 is representative of the wild
type bacterium, but known mutations may be reflected by changes in the parameters.
Conversely, the stability analysis carried out in the following section involves
bifurcation values of the parameters and we shall discuss whether they may be trans-
gressed in some mutant strains.

   Setting to zero the derivatives dx_i/dt in (1) yields the dependence
of the control region state on a constant inducer concentration I :

$$x_i(u) = Q_i(u) / Q(u) \qquad i = 1,2,\ldots,6$$

where $\qquad u = \ell_2 I / \ell_2' \quad , \quad Q = \sum_{i=1}^{6} Q_i \text{ and}$

$$Q_1 = k_{11}'(1 + K_1 u) k_{21}' (1 + K_2 u) (d_1' + m_6 P) +$$
$$+ (1 + u) (k_{11}'(1 + K_1 u) d_2'(d_1' + k_2 R + m_6 P) + k_{21}'(1 + K_2 u) d_2 C(d_1' + m_6 P)),$$

$$Q_2 = k_{11}'(1 + K_1 u) k_{21}'(1 + K_2 u) d_1 C +$$
$$+ (1 + u)(k_{11}'(1 + K_1 u) d_2' d_1 C + k_{21}'(1 + K_2 u) d_2 C(d_1 C + k_1 R)),$$

$$Q_3 = (1 + u)((1 + u) d_2'(k_2 R d_1 C + k_1 R(d_1' + k_2 R + m_6 P)) +$$
$$+ k_{21}' (1 + K_2 u) k_1 R (d_1' + m_6 P)) ,$$

$$Q_4 = (1 + u)((1+u) d_2 C(k_2 R d_1 C + k_1 R(d_1' + k_2 R + m_6 P)) + k_{11}'(1+K_1 u) k_2 R d_1 C),$$

$$Q_5 = \frac{m_5 P}{m_5'} Q_1 ,$$

$$Q_6 = \frac{m_6 P}{m_6'} Q_2 .$$

Parameters known from direct in vitro experiments

Symbol	Value	Unit
R	0.2	mol
k_1	6	$mol^{-1}s^{-1}$
k'_{11}	$6\ 10^{-4}$	s^{-1}
K_1	500	-
ℓ_2/ℓ'_2	$5\ 10^{-6}$	mol^{-1}
τ_z	240	s
τ_y	300	s
K'_z	$1.1\ 10^{-3}$	s^{-1}
a	64	s^{-1}
b	56.5	s^{-1}
c	97.5	s^{-1}
β	$2.5\ 10^6$	mol
α	2.1	-
K_M	10^{-4}	M

Parameters derived from indirect experimental evidence

Symbol	Value	Unit
k_2	6	$mol^{-1}s^{-1}$
V_M	55	s^{-1}
k_s	10^{-3}	s^{-1}
K_z	50	$mol\ s^{-1}$
K_y	25	$mol\ s^{-1}$
K'_y	$5.5\ 10^{-4}$	s^{-1}
α_y/α_z	0.2	-

Unknown parameters, estimated from the model

Symbol	Value	Unit
k'_{21}	$6\ 10^{-4}$	s^{-1}
K_2	5000	-
m'_6	1	s^{-1}
$m_5 P = m_6 P$	0.75	s^{-1}
$d_1 C = d_2 C$	2	s^{-1}
d'_1	0.2	s^{-1}
d'_2	0.2	s^{-1}
$\begin{pmatrix}\alpha_z\\ m'_5\end{pmatrix}$	$\begin{pmatrix}1\\ 25\end{pmatrix}$ or $\begin{pmatrix}0.04\\ 1\end{pmatrix}$	- s^{-1}

Table 1

Numerical values of the parameters for the wild type operon.

Concentrations are expressed as numbers of molecules (or active sites for polymeric enzymes) per cell. With a cell volume of about 1.5 μm^3, one molar concentration involves 10^9 molecules per cell. "mol" stands for molecules per cell. Symbols refer to those in the text.

The full system effective dimension might be reduced if some variables undergo rapid variations, relative to other ones, towards some local pseudo-equilibrium [25]. Sub-system (1) is a natural candidate for such a reduction, since it is linear with a stable equilibrium state for any I concentration. Exhibiting a small parameter multiplying x_i's derivatives for every i is possible when the full system is considered around its equilibrium state (§ 3), but is not possible for state values involving few enzymes or few intracellular substrates. Numerical integration of the system provides strong evidence that reducing the dimension of the system does not alter its quantitative nor its qualitative properties. Replacing the x_i values by their equilibrium values depending on present I value is shown to be valid in every condition, including the early steps of the induction process : this reduces the system dimension from nine to four (§4.2). Numerical results suggest a further reduction, but restricted to near-equilibrium states : it turns out that substrates concentrations I and L . remain close to the equilibrium values of sub-system (2), where Z and Y are taken constant . With both simplifications, the reduced system is two dimensional in Y and Z ; although it is an oversimplified version of the model, it is an easy and efficient tool to enter into the bifurcation analysis of the full system (§ 4.1). It may be noted here that the reduction of the system does not follow the same rationale as in [12] where the control region is set at equilibrium with substrates, as we do, but where it is assumed that enzymes concentrations Y and Z are adjusted to substrates concentrations, in sharp opposition with our numerical results.

The four dimensional system studied is :

$$\frac{dY}{dt} = K_y \, P_y \, (u(t-\tau_y)) - K'_y \, Y$$

$$\frac{dZ}{dt} = K_z \, P_z \, (u(t-\tau_z)) - K'_z \, Z$$

(4)

$$\frac{dL}{dt} = V_M \frac{L_e}{L_e + K_M} Y + k_s \, (L_e - L) - Z \frac{(a+b)L}{L + \alpha I + \beta}$$

$$\frac{dI}{dt} = Z \frac{bL - \alpha c I}{L + \alpha I + \beta}$$

where
$$P_y(u) = (\alpha_y \, Q_5(u) + Q_6(u)) \, / \, Q(u)$$
$$P_z(u) = (\alpha_z \, Q_5(u) + Q_6(u)) \, / \, Q(u) \ .$$

P_y and P_z are thus ratios of second degree polynomials in $u = \ell_2 I / \ell'_2$. Numerical results indicate that P_y and P_z are increasing functions of u that can be approximated by homographic functions. More precisely we shall make use of the following inequalities :

$$(5) \qquad 0 \le \frac{P'_y(u)}{P_y(u)} \le \frac{1}{u} \quad \text{and} \quad 0 \le \frac{P'_z(u)}{P_z(u)} \le \frac{1}{u}$$

3. Existence and uniqueness of an equilibrium point

When there is no lactose in the medium $(L_e = 0)$, system (4) has only one constant steady state

$$Y_o = K_y P_y(0)/K'_y \quad , \quad Z_o = K_z P_z(0)/K'_z \quad , \quad L_o = I_o = 0.$$

The Jacobian around this point has negative real eigenvalues, $- K'_y$, $- K'_z$, $- (k_s + Z_o(a+b)/\beta^2)$, and $-Z_o \, \alpha \, c/\beta$, so that the constant steady state is a stable node. Very low values of Y_o and Z_o describe a repressed bacterium, this state will be the initial point for simulating the induction process.

When there is lactose in the medium, system (4), with the preceding point as initial condition, has a unique solution that describes the induction of the bacterium and tends to some stable steady state. In the following, we show that, for parameters values of biological meaning, system (4) has only one constant steady state.

At any fixed point, values of Y, Z, L, I are such that

$$Y = K_y P_y(u)/K'_y \quad , \quad Z = K_z P_z(u)/K'_z \quad , \quad L = \frac{\alpha c}{b} \frac{\ell'_2}{\ell_2} u \quad , \quad I = \frac{\ell'_2}{\ell_2} u \quad ,$$

where u is a positive zero of function F defined by

$$F(u) = k_s \, L_e + h \, P_y(u) - \varphi u - g \, u \, P_z(u)/(1 + \epsilon u)$$

with

$$h = V_M \frac{L_e}{L_e + K_M} \frac{K_y}{K'_y} \quad , \quad \varphi = k_s \frac{\alpha c}{b} \frac{\ell'_2}{\ell_2} \quad , \quad g' = \frac{a+b}{\beta} \frac{\alpha c}{b} \frac{\ell'_2}{\ell_2} \quad , \quad g = g' \frac{K_z}{K'_z} \quad ,$$

$$\epsilon = \frac{\alpha}{\beta} \left(1 + \frac{c}{b} \right) \frac{\ell'_2}{\ell_2} \; .$$

3.1. A sufficient condition for uniqueness. We define the fourth degree polynomial G as $G(u) = F(u) (1 + \epsilon u) Q(u)$, where Q is the second degree polynomial with positive coefficients defined in the previous section. As u goes to infinity, G is infinite negative , G(0) is positive, so G has one or three positive roots. We now state sufficient conditions for the existence of a unique positive root :

Theorem 3.1.1. With the following conditions, G has one positive root and only one :

(1.1) $K_2 \geq K_1 \geq 1$; (1.2) $m_5/m'_5 \leq m_6/m'_6$; (1.3) $\alpha_y \leq 1$ and $\alpha_z \leq 1$;

(1.4) $\dfrac{K_2 k'_{21}}{K_1 k'_{11}} \geq \mathrm{Sup}\ (\dfrac{k_2 R + d_1 C + d'_1 + m_6 P}{k_1 R + d_1 C + d'_1 + m_6 P}\ ,\ \dfrac{d'_2 d_1}{d_2(d'_1 + m_6 P)}\ \dfrac{k_2}{k_1})$; (1.5) $\epsilon \leq 1$

Proof. Let X_1 and Y_1 (resp. X_2 and Y_2) be the roots of Q_1 (resp. Q_2), with : $-1 \leq X_i \leq -\dfrac{1}{K_1} \leq Y_i \leq -\dfrac{1}{K_2}$ $(i = 1,2)$. Roots of $Q_3 + Q_4$ are -1 and X_3 with : $-1 \leq X_3 \leq -1/K_2$. So $Q(u)$, $P_y(u)$ and $P_z(u)$ are positive for $u \leq -1$ or $u \geq -1/K_2$. From condition (1.5), $G(-1/\epsilon)$, $G(-1)$ and $G(-1/K_2)$ are positive, so there is at least one root of G in $]-\infty, -1/\epsilon[$ and one in $[0, +\infty[$. We show now that the other two roots are in $[-1, -1/K_2]$.

If $X_3 \geq -1/K_1$, then $Q(-1/K_1) < 0$, $P_y(-1/K_1) \geq 0$, and $P_z(-1/K_1) \geq 0$. So $F(-1/K_1) \geq 0$ and $G(-1/K_1) \leq 0$; there is one root in $[-1, -1/K_1]$ and the fourth one in $[-1/K_1, -1/K_2]$.

If $X_3 < -1/K_1$, it follows from condition (1.4) that $(Q_1+Q_2)(X_3)$ is negative and that $Q_1(X_2)$ is positive, so that $(Q_1+Q_2)(X_2)$ is positive too ;

Q_1+Q_2 is a second degree polynomial, positive in X_2, negative in X_3 and in $-1/K_1$, then $X_2 \leq X_3 < -1/K_1$ and $Q_2(X_3) \leq 0$. As Q_1+Q_2 and Q_2 are negative at X_3 , we have

$$\forall \gamma, \quad 0 \leq \gamma \leq 1 , \quad (\gamma Q_1 + Q_2)(X_3) \leq 0.$$

Using condition (1.2) we then derive $Q(X_3) \leq 0$, and using condition (1.3) yields $Q(X_3) P_y(X_3) \leq 0$ and $Q(X_3) P_z(X_3) \leq 0$. We have $P_y(X_3) \geq 0$, $P_z(X_3) \geq 0$, $F(X_3) \geq 0$ and $G(X_3) \leq 0$, so there is one root in $[-1, X_3]$ and the fourth one in $[X_3, -1/K_2]$.

In either case, $X_3 + 1/K_1$ positive or negative, G has four real roots, three are negative, and a single one is positive.

Conditions (1.1) to (1.4) are filled by the model, since they express
the known effects of active cAMP-CAP complex on transcription rates and on polarity. Condition (1.5) is filled by the values describing the wild type strain
(ϵ = .46), but mutants of the i gene are known that transgress the condition.
This condition is in fact much too strong, as shown by numerical investigation of
the following necessary and sufficient condition for uniqueness.

3.2. <u>The necessary and sufficient condition for uniqueness.</u> Let ' denote
the derivation with respect to u and R be defined as
$$R(u) = u \left(\frac{P'_y(u)}{P_y(u)} - \frac{P'_z(u)}{P_z(u)} \right). \quad \text{We have :}$$
<u>Theorem 3.2.1.</u> A necessary and sufficient condition for F to have three
positive zeros is that there exists some u, u > 0, such that

(2.1) $R(u) > 0$,   (2.2) $\epsilon > \frac{1}{u} \left(\frac{1}{R(u)} - 1 \right)$,

(2.3) $\frac{\varphi}{g} < \frac{P_z(u)}{1+\epsilon u} \frac{R(u) - \sqrt{(1+\epsilon u)}}{1 - u\, P'_y(u)/P_y(u)}$, and

(2.4) $\bar{h} = V_M \frac{K_y}{K'_y} > \frac{s'(u)}{P'_y(u)} \left(1 + k_s K_M/(s(u) - s'(u) P_y(u)/P'_y(u)) \right)$

where
$$s(u) = \varphi u + \frac{gu}{1 + \epsilon u} P_z(u).$$

<u>Proof</u>. For G to have three positive roots, it is necessary and sufficient
that there exists a positive root where the derivative G' is positive. For a root
of G, F' and G' have the same sign, so the condition may be written as
$$\exists\, u > 0 , \quad F(u) = 0 \quad \text{and} \quad F'(u) > 0, \text{ that is :}$$

(6) $\begin{cases} k_s L_e + \bar{h} \dfrac{L_e}{L_e + K_M} P_y(u) - s(u) = 0 \\[3mm] \bar{h} \dfrac{L_e}{L_e + K_M} P'_y(u) - s'(u) > 0 \end{cases}$

Making use of inequalities (5), (6) and the following four statements are
equivalent :
$$(7)\; \begin{cases} 1 > L_e/(L_e + K_M) > s'(u) / (\bar{h}\, P'_y(u)) \\[3mm] \left(1 - \dfrac{L_e}{L_e + K_M}\right) \left(\bar{h} \dfrac{L_e}{L_e + K_M} P_y(u) - s(u)\right) + k_s K_M \dfrac{L_e}{L_e + K_M} = 0 \end{cases}$$

$$(8) \quad \begin{cases} s'(u) < \bar{h}\, P'_y(u) \\ P_y(u)(s'(u))^2 - P'_y(u)s'(u)(k_s K_M + \bar{h}P_y(u) + s(u)) + \bar{h}(P'_y(u))^2 s(u) > 0 \end{cases}$$

$$(9) \quad \begin{cases} \bar{h} > s'(u) \,/\, P'_y(u) \\ \bar{h}\, P'_y(u)\, S(u) - s'(u)\,(S(u) + P'_y(u)\, k_s K_M) > 0 \\ \text{with } S(u) = P'_y(u)\, s(u) - P_y(u)\, s'(u). \end{cases}$$

$$(10) \quad \begin{cases} P'_y(u)/P_y(u) > s'(u)/s(u) \\ \bar{h} > \dfrac{s'(u)}{P'_y(u)}\,(1 + k_s K_M\, P'_y(u)/S(u)) \end{cases}$$

Second condition in (10) is condition (2.4), and the first one is condition (2.3). As φ/g is positive, $R(u) - 1/(1+\varepsilon u)$ must be positive, so that conditions (2.1) and (2.2) must be true.

With the wild type parameters values, we find that $\frac{1}{u}\left(\frac{1}{R(u)} - 1\right)$ remains very large, greater than $4.7\ 10^6$, whichever u may be. A necessary condition for F to have three positive zeros is thus that ε be at least 10^7 times greater than in the wild type ; also, φ/g must be taken 10^7 times smaller than in the wild type. Recalling the expressions for these parameters,

$$\frac{1}{\varepsilon} = \frac{\beta}{\alpha}\,\frac{b}{b+c}\,\frac{\ell_2}{\ell'_2} \quad \text{and} \quad \frac{\varphi}{g} = \frac{k_s\,\beta}{(a+b)K_z/K'_z}\ ,$$

we see that the extreme reduction in both quantities, needed to obtain multiple steady states, cannot be achieved. Specially, any decrease in φ/g would imply a more efficient β-galactosidase than in the wild type (lower Michaelis constant and higher maximum velocity for the total enzyme content in a cell), on the other hand I^s mutants are known that could increase ε by a factor of 10^2 to 10^3. Figure 3 shows the equilibrium values of u and Z as functions of the external lactose concentration, L_e, for the wild type strain.

4. Stability analysis.

Stability of the equilibrium point of system (4) is difficult to study because of its fourth order. As outlined in section 2, the system may be approxima-ted by reducing the equations in L and in I to algebraic equations. The stabi-lity of the equilibrium point is first considered in this reduced system, which

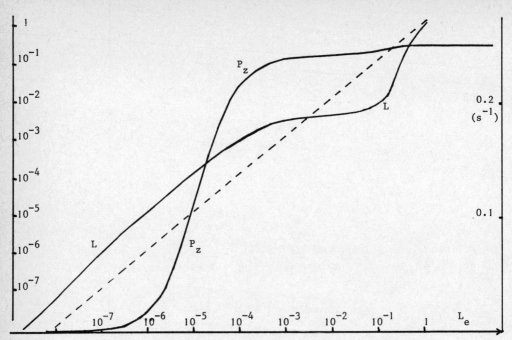

FIGURE 3 : Molar concentration of intracellular lactose (L and left ordinates),and transcription rate (P_z and right ordinates), as functions of external molar concentration of lactose (L_e) in the wild type bacterium.

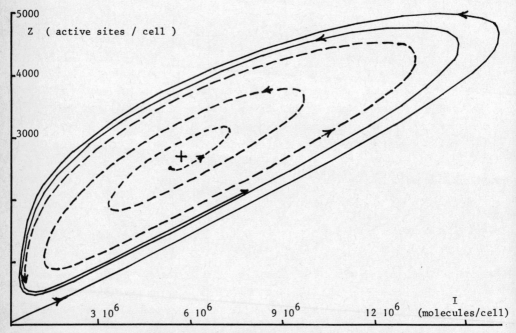

FIGURE 4 : Projection on the plane (I,Z) of two approaches to a periodic solution , from the repressed state (solid curve trajectory), and from a state in the neighborhood of the critical point (dashed curve trajectory). Modified parameters are : $1_2/1_2'=10^{-8}mol^{-1}$, $K_y'=.0022s^{-1}$ and $V_M=330s^{-1}$; with $L_e= 2\ 10^{-3}$ M.

gives some preliminary ideas for the stability of full system (4).

4.1. <u>Two dimensional stability of the equilibrium point</u>. We choose to express any variable as function of Z and u. Then

(11) $Y = (\varphi u + Zg'u/(1+eu) - k_e)/\delta$, $\quad L = \dfrac{\alpha c}{b} \dfrac{\ell_2'}{\ell_2} u$, $\quad I = \dfrac{\ell_2'}{\ell_2} u$,

where $\quad k_e = k_s L_e$ and $\delta = V_M \dfrac{L_e}{L_e + K_M}$ are constant if the external lactose concentration is kept fixed. Differentiating (11), we get the partial derivatives $\partial u/\partial Y$ and $\partial u/\partial Z$, from which we may write the system in Z and u as follows :

(12)
$$\frac{dZ}{dt} = K_z P_z(u) - K_z' Z$$
$$\frac{du}{dt} = (K_y' F(u) + (K_y'-K_z') \frac{g'u}{1+eu} \frac{K_z}{K_z'} (\frac{K_z}{K_z'} P_z(u)-Z))/(\varphi+Z \frac{g}{(1+eu)^2})$$

Equilibrium points of systems (4) and (12) are the same, so (12) has one critical point :
$$\bar{u} > 0,\ F(\bar{u}) = 0 \ ,\ \bar{Z} = \frac{K_z}{K_z'} P_z(\bar{u}) \ .$$

Denoting by z and v the disturbances of variables Z and u around the equilibrium point, the linearized operator associated to the system (12) is :

(13)
$$\frac{dz}{dt} = -K_z' z + K_z P_z(\bar{u}) v$$
$$\frac{dv}{dt} = (\frac{g'\bar{u}(K_z'-K_y')}{1+e\bar{u}} z + (K_y'F'(\bar{u}) + \frac{g\bar{u}(K_y'-K_z')}{1+e\bar{u}} P_z'(\bar{u})v)/(\varphi+P_z(\bar{u})\frac{g}{(1+e\bar{u})^2})$$

From Lyapunov's theory, the critical point is stable if the Jacobian given by (13) has two eigenvalues with negative real parts. The sum, $\lambda_1+\lambda_2$, and the product $\lambda_1\lambda_2$ of the roots of the characteristic polynomial are :

$$\lambda_1+\lambda_2 = -K_z' + (K_y' F'(\bar{u}) + \frac{g\bar{u}(K_y'-K_z')}{1+e\bar{u}} P_z'(\bar{u}))/(\varphi+P_z(\bar{u}) \frac{g}{(1+e\bar{u})^2})$$

$$\lambda_1 \lambda_2 = -K_y' K_z' F'(\bar{u})/(\varphi + P_z(\bar{u}) \frac{g}{(1+e\bar{u})^2})$$

Since $F'(\bar{u}) < 0$, the product is positive, and we have :

<u>Proposition 4.1.1</u>.   A sufficient condition for stability is $\quad K_z' > K_y'$.

<u>Proof</u>.   The condition implies, with $F'(\bar{u}) < 0$, that both roots have a negative real part.

Although there is no direct evidence that the condition holds for the wild type, its fulfilment in our parameters values is a consequence of the natural polar effect between genes for Z and for Y $(K_y \leq K_z)$, and of the observation that Y and Z amounts are equal under full induction $(K_y/K_y' \simeq K_z/K_z')$.

More generally, a necessary and sufficient condition for stability is that the sum $\lambda_1 + \lambda_2$ is negative, since the product is positive. Replacing F' by its expression, we get

$$(\varphi + P_z(\bar{u}) \frac{g}{(1+\epsilon\bar{u})^2})(K_y'+K_z') + K_z \frac{g'\,\bar{u}}{1+\epsilon\bar{u}} P_z'(\bar{u}) - K_y \, \delta \, P_y'(\bar{u}) > 0 \ ,$$

and we have :

Theorem 4.1.2. A necessary and sufficient condition for the equilibrium point of the two-dimensional system (12) to be unstable is that there exists $\bar{u}$, with $F'(\bar{u}) < 0$, and such that

$$(3.1) \quad T(\bar{u}) = \bar{u} \, (\frac{P_y'(\bar{u})}{P_y(\bar{u})} - \frac{K_z'}{K_y'} \frac{P_z'(\bar{u})}{P_z(\bar{u})}) > 0 \ ,$$

$$(3.2) \quad \epsilon > \frac{1}{u} \, ((1 + \frac{K_z'}{K_y'})/T(\bar{u}) - 1) \ ,$$

$$(3.3) \quad \frac{\varphi}{g} < \frac{P_z(\bar{u})}{1+\epsilon\bar{u}} \frac{T(\bar{u}) - (1+K_z'/K_y')/(1+\epsilon\bar{u})}{1 - \bar{u}P_y'(\bar{u})/P_y(\bar{u})+K_z'/K_y'} \ ,$$

$$(3.4) \quad \bar{h} > \frac{r(\bar{u})}{P_y'(\bar{u})} \, (1+k_s K_M P_y'(\bar{u})/(P_y'(\bar{u}) \, s(\bar{u}) - P_y(\bar{u}) \, r(\bar{u}))) \ ,$$

where $s(u)$ is defined in Theorem 3.2.1 and $r(\bar{u}) = (1 + \frac{K_z'}{K_y'})s'(\bar{u}) - \frac{g\,\bar{u}}{1+\epsilon\bar{u}} P_z'(\bar{u})$.

The proof follows the same lines as that of Theorem 3.2.1. Conditions here are easier to fill, and may be achieved in keeping the same orders of magnitude as in the wild type set of parameters. Denoting by subscript w the wild strain values, we get an unstable point with the following changes :

$$V_M = 6 \, V_{Mw} \ , \ K_y' = 4 \, K_{yw}' \ \text{ and } \ \frac{\ell_2'}{\ell_2} = 500 \ (\frac{\ell_2'}{\ell_2})_w \ .$$

With such a "genotype", we find that the equilibrium point is stable for low or high external lactose concentration $(L_e < 3 \ 10^{-4} \text{ M, or } L_e > 3.5 \ 10^{-2} \text{ M})$, and is unstable for intermediate concentrations.

4.2. Stability of the critical point in the four-dimensional system.

4.2. <u>Stability of the critical point in the four-dimensional system</u>. The Jacobian of system (4) around the equilibrium point is

$$
\begin{vmatrix}
- K'_y & 0 & 0 & K_y P'_y(\bar{u}) \dfrac{\ell_2}{\ell'_2} \\[2em]
0 & - K'_z & 0 & K_z P'_z(\bar{u}) \dfrac{\ell_2}{\ell'_2} \\[2em]
\delta & \dfrac{g'\,\bar{u}}{1+\epsilon\,\bar{u}} & -(\varphi + \dfrac{g P_z(\bar{u})(1+\eta\bar{u})}{(1+\epsilon\,\bar{u})^2}) \dfrac{b}{\alpha c} \dfrac{\ell_2}{\ell'_2} & \dfrac{\ell_2}{\ell'_2} \dfrac{g\,P_z(\bar{u})\,\eta\,\bar{u}}{(1+\epsilon\,\bar{u})^2} \\[2em]
0 & 0 & (\dfrac{b}{\alpha c})^2 \dfrac{\ell_2}{\ell'_2} \dfrac{j\,P_z(\bar{u})}{1+\epsilon\,\bar{u}} & - \dfrac{b}{\alpha c} \dfrac{\ell_2}{\ell'_2} \dfrac{j\,P_z(\bar{u})}{1+\epsilon\,\bar{u}}
\end{vmatrix}
$$

where $\eta = \dfrac{\alpha}{\beta} \dfrac{\ell'_2}{\ell_2}$ and $j = \dfrac{K_z}{K'_z} \dfrac{\alpha c}{b} \dfrac{\ell'_2}{\ell_2} \dfrac{\alpha c}{\beta}$.

Writing the characteristic polynomial as $\lambda^4 + a_1 \lambda^3 + a_2 \lambda^2 + a_3 \lambda + a_4$, it is easily verified that a_1 and a_2 are positive ; we get also :

$$
a_4 = - K'_y K'_z (\dfrac{b}{\alpha c} \dfrac{\ell_2}{\ell'_2})^2 \, j\,P_z(\bar{u})\,F'(\bar{u}) \,/\, (1 + \epsilon\bar{u}) > 0
$$

Using a Liennard-Chipard theorem [26], we can express the condition for the roots to have negative real parts, in terms of Hurwitz's determinants. The necessary and sufficient condition for stability becomes : $a_3(a_1 a_2 - a_3) - a_1^2 a_4 > 0$. This condition is very complicated, and can only be used for numerical results. A necessary condition for the equilibrium point to be stable is $a_3 > 0$, so we can give sufficient conditions for it to be unstable :

<u>Theorem 4.2.1.</u> A sufficient condition for the equilibrium point of system (4) to be unstable is that there exists some $\bar{u}$, $\bar{u} > 0$, such that

(4.1) $\qquad T(\bar{u}) > 0 \quad$ (same condition as (3.1)) ,

(4.2) $\qquad \dfrac{\beta}{\alpha c} < K_z P_z(\bar{u})\,T(\bar{u})\,/\,(K'_z)^2$,

(4.3) $\qquad \dfrac{\ell'_2}{\ell_2} \dfrac{1}{c} < \dfrac{1}{\bar{u}}\,(K_z P_z(\bar{u})\,T(\bar{u})/(K'_z)^2 - \beta/\alpha c\,)$,

(4.4) $\qquad 1 + \dfrac{c}{b} > \dfrac{1}{\eta\bar{u}}\,(\,(1+\dfrac{K'_z}{K'_y})/(T(\bar{u}) - \dfrac{(K'_z)^2\,\beta(1+\eta\bar{u})}{K_z\,\alpha c\,P_z(\bar{u})}) - 1\,)$,

$$(4.5) \qquad \frac{\alpha c}{a+b} < \frac{K_z}{(K_z')^2} \quad \frac{\alpha c}{\beta} \quad \frac{P_z(\bar{u})}{1+\epsilon\ \bar{u}} \quad (T(\bar{u}) - \frac{1+K_z'/K_y'}{1+\epsilon\bar{u}}) - \frac{1+\eta\bar{u}}{1+\epsilon\bar{u}} \ ,$$

$$(4.6) \quad \frac{\varphi}{g} < \frac{\dfrac{P_z(\bar{u})}{1+\epsilon\bar{u}} \ (T(\bar{u}) - \dfrac{1+K_z'/K_y'}{1+\epsilon\bar{u}}) - \dfrac{(K_z')^2}{K_z} \ \dfrac{\beta}{\alpha c} \ (\dfrac{1+\eta\bar{u}}{1+\epsilon\bar{u}} + \dfrac{\alpha c}{a+b})}{1 - \dfrac{P_y'(\bar{u})}{P_y(\bar{u})} \ \dfrac{\bar{u}}{} + \dfrac{K_z'}{K_y'} + \dfrac{(K_z')^2}{K_z} \ \dfrac{\beta}{\alpha c} \ \dfrac{1+\epsilon\bar{u}}{P_z(\bar{u})}} \ ,$$

$$(4.7) \qquad h > \frac{q(\bar{u})}{P_y'(\bar{u})} \ (1 + k_s \ K_M \ P_y'(\bar{u})/(s(\bar{u}) \ P_y'(\bar{u}) - q(\bar{u}) \ P_y(\bar{u}))),$$

where

$$q(\bar{u}) = r(\bar{u}) + \frac{(K_z')^2}{K_z} \ \frac{\beta}{\alpha c} \ \frac{1+\epsilon\bar{u}}{P_z(\bar{u})} \ (\varphi + P_z(\bar{u}) \ g \ \frac{1+\eta\bar{u}}{(1+\epsilon\bar{u})^2} + P_z(\bar{u}) \ \frac{j}{1+\epsilon\bar{u}}) \ .$$

This theorem can be demonstrated as theorems 3.2.1 and 4.1.2.

If we consider the same mutant genotype as in section 4.1, the equilibrium point is now found to be unstable in a narrower range of lactose concentration, for :
$$5.25 \ 10^{-4} \ M < L_e < 5.75 \ 10^{-3} \ M$$

In this case, there is a limit cycle around the critical point, all variables are periodic functions of time. For $L_e = 2 \ 10^{-3}$ M, the period is about 175 minutes, figure 4 shows the projection of the cycle on the plane (Z, I).

4.3. <u>Sensitivity of the system with respect to delays</u>. Until now we have studied stability of the equilibrium point of (4) without taking account of the delays τ_y and τ_z. With them, the characteristic equation of (4) is transcendental, it may be written as :

$$(\lambda + K_y')(\lambda + K_z')(\lambda^2 + \frac{b}{\alpha c} \ \frac{\ell_2}{\ell_2'} \ (\varphi + g \ P_z(\bar{u}) \ \frac{1+\eta\bar{u}}{(1+\epsilon\bar{u})^2} + P_z(\bar{u}) \ \frac{j}{1+\epsilon\bar{u}}) \ \lambda +$$

$$+ (\frac{b}{\alpha c} \ \frac{\ell_2}{\ell_2'})^2 \ \frac{j \ P_z(\bar{u})}{1+\epsilon\bar{u}} \ (\varphi + \frac{g \ P_z(\bar{u})}{(1+\epsilon\bar{u})^2})) +$$

$$+ (\frac{b}{\alpha c} \ \frac{\ell_2}{\ell_2'})^2 \ \frac{j \ P_z(\bar{u})}{1+\epsilon\ \bar{u}} \ (K_z' \ P_z'(\bar{u}) \ \frac{g\ \bar{u}}{1+\epsilon\bar{u}} \ (\lambda + K_y') \ e^{-\tau_z \lambda} - K_y' \ P_y'(\bar{u})h \ (\lambda+K_z')e^{-\tau_y \lambda})=0$$

A necessary and sufficient condition for stability is that every zero of this equation has a negative real part. As there are two delays, it is difficult to find the limits of the stability domain, that are sets of parameters values for which the equation has pure imaginary zeros. We only did numerical studies and found that the delays had a stabilizing effect. For instance, introduction of delays (τ_y = 5 min., τ_z = 4 min.) cancelled the periodic solution found above and yielded a stable focus.

5. Conclusion

Lactose operon has been the subject of many theoretical works. The most complete of them is by Sanglier and Nicolis [12]. These authors translate intracellular glucose and lactose variations as two differential equations of rational fraction shape. Their model, in addition to sustained oscillations and multiple steady states, may present multiple limit cycles and associated threshold phenomena, for certain ranges of parameters values. These results, however, depend on the way they have modeled the mechanism of catabolic repression, assuming a direct binding of glucose to repressor. Although the equations so obtained may be accepted as a heuristic description, the hypothesis is at variance with experimental evidence. Also, the equations do not allow for any flux of glucose out of the system. We think that experimental data are not yet sufficient to build up a quantitative model of the dynamical aspects of catabolic repression. For that reason, there is no attempt in our model to take account of them, so that its mathematical properties cannot be validly compared with those found by Sanglier and Nicolis.

We have shown that, in the range of values of the parameters describing known genotypes, our model had only one constant steady state for any extracellular concentration. Every (but one) sufficient conditions are evident as they translate the operon polarity and CAP's role. Necessary and sufficient conditions can be broken only in extreme biological situation where β-galactosidase is infinitely more efficient than the wild type one.

We have shown that this steady state was stable. The biological translation of the conditions that lead to stability, when the dimension is two, is the following : firstly, the sum of permeases activities must be less than β-galactosidases' one ; secondly, the permease mean life must be longer than that of β-galactosidase ; thirdly, the repressor must be sufficiently sensitive to the inducer. All these properties are owned by bacteria of known wild or mutant genotype, such as I^-, I^q, I^{sq}, I^s, PI, PII, PIII. The stability in dimension four is got for wider ranges of values of the parameters. Introduction of delayed arguments in the equations seems to widen these ranges too. So, for wide ranges of parameters values, the topological situation is always the same in our model of the lactose operon : there is an only stable constant steady state. This situation is very well known by experimentators, who give it the name of homeostasis.

We have looked for genotype and medium properties that would break unicity and stability conditions. Biological conditions could not be found that led to multiple steady states. On the contrary, some ones were found that led to destabilizing the constant steady state and arising of a stable periodic steady state (limit cycle). The genotype must own at least two mutations, one in the i gene, and one in the structural y and z genes whose effect would be to bring the sum of permeases activities bigger than galactosidases', and their mean lives shorter. For such a genotype, that could involve an inversion of genes y and z, there is a range of values of extracellular lactose concentration that leads to destabilization. Simulations of these conditions with our model give birth to sustained oscillations of enzymes and substrates internal concentrations with large periods (about three hours). Perhaps some "leaky" mutants, that have been abandonned by experimentators because they failed to give repeatable responses, were of this kind. Now, we are studying the influence of delays on these sustained oscillations : they seem to decrease the amplitude of the oscillations, and even to make them damped. A question remains open : can mutants of the lactose operon be conceived and realized that present sustained oscillations for some range of values of extracellular lactose concentration ?

REFERENCES

[1] Rashevsky N., 1961, Mathematical Biophysics, Dover, New-York, (3rd edition).

[2] Turing A.M., 1952, Phil. Trans. Roy. Soc., B 237, 5-72.

[3] Rosen R., 1970, Dynamical system theory in Biology, Vol.1, Wiley-Interscience, New-York.

[4] Higgins J., 1967, Industrial and Engineering Chemistry, 59, 18-62.

[5] Goodwin B., 1963, Temporal organization in cells, Academic Press, London.

[6] Zeeman E.C., 1972, in : Towards a Theoretical Biology, 4 : Essays, Waddington C.H. (ed.), Edinburgh University Press, 63-66.

[7] Higgins J., 1964, Proc. Nat., Acad. Sci. U.S.A., 51, 989-993.

[8] Sel'kov E.E., 1968, European J. Biochem., 4, 79-86.

[9] Demongeot J., 1981, in : Modèles Mathématiques en Biologie, Chevalet C. et Micali A., (ed.), Lecture Notes in Biomathematics, 41, Springer-Verlag, Berlin, 40-62.

[10] Knorre W.A., 1968, Biochem. Biophys. Res. Commun., 31, 812-817 ; 1973, in :
     Biological and Biochemical Oscillators, Chance B. et al (ed.), Acade-
     mic Press, New-York, 449-457.

[11] Babloyantz A., Sanglier M., 1972, FEBS Letters, 23, 364-366.

[12] Sanglier M., Nicolis G., 1976, Biophysical Chemistry, 4, 113-121.

[13] Gillois M. et al. 1981, in : Modèles Mathématiques en Biologie, Chevalet C.,
     Micali A. (ed.), Lecture Notes in Biomathematics, 41, Springer-Verlag,
     Berlin, 3-13.

[14] Fisher R.A., 1918, Trans. Roy. Soc. Edinburgh, 52, 399-433.

[15] Watson J.D., 1976, Molecular Biology of the Gene, (3rd ed.), Benjamin,
     Menlo-Park, California.

[16] Mandecki W., 1979, J. Theor. Biol., 81, 105-122.

[17] Manabe, T., 1981, J. Theor. Biol., 89, 271-302.

[18] Kepes, A., 1978, Aspects moléculaires des fonctions membranaires, Masson,
     Paris, 114-150.

[19] Huber et al., 1975, Can. J. Biochem. 53, 1035-1038 ; 1976, Biochemistry, 15,
     1994-2001.

[20] Heineken F.G. et al., 1967, Math. Biosci., 1, 95-113.

[21] Chevalet C. et al., 1978, C.R. Acad. Sci. Paris, D , 287, 169-172 ; 1979,
     Tôhoku Math. J., 31 127-138.

[22] Göbber F., and Seelig F.F., 1975, J. Math. Biology, 2, 79-86.

[23] Barkley M.D., Bourgeois S., 1978, in : The Operon, Miller J.H. and
     Reznikoff W.S. (ed.), Cold Spring Harbor Laboratory, Cold Spring Harbor,
     New-York, 177-220.

[24] Chevalet C. et al., Second World Conference on Mathematics at the Service
     of Man, Las Palmas, Spain, June 28 - July 3, 1982. In press.

[25] Tikhonov A.N., 1952, Math. Sb., 31, 575-586.

[26] Philippov, A., 1976, Recueil de problèmes d'équations différentielles
     (trad. française : G. Petrossov), Editions Mir, Moscou, 79-81.

(*) Laboratoire de Génétique Cellulaire   (**) UER de Mathématiques
     Centre de Recherches INRA de Toulouse   Université Montpellier II
     B.P. 12   Place Eugène Bataillon

     31320 CASTANET-TOLOSAN   34060 MONTPELLIER CEDEX

AUTOMATA NETWORKS AS MODELS FOR BIOLOGICAL SYSTEMS : (A SURVEY)

F. FOGELMAN-SOULIE, M. MILGRAM, G. WEISBUCH

I - INTRODUCTION

Biological systems are usually made of many interacting components :

in molecular biology : molecules or macromolecules ;
in genetics : genes, proteines or enzymes ;
in immunology : lymphocytes and antigens ;
in embryology : cells or groups of cells ;
in the nervous system : neurons ;
in ecology : living beings or species.

To study such systems, one first has to define at which level
they will be viewed : from molecular to microscopic and macroscopic. Then
the description of the elements and their interaction rules at one level
would allow to understand better the behavior of the system at a more global
level.

The formalisms used at integrated levels are generally continuous :
typically they include systems of differential or partial differential
equations in variables describing the global behavior of the system (concentration, level of activity for example). These formalisms make possible
precise quantitative and qualitative analysis of many basic biological phenomena.

But in some cases, it appears necessary to go more deeply into the
details of the elementary levels. This may happen because of the very large
number of interacting components, the high complexity of their interactions
(which may determine in a basic fashion the over_all behavior) or simply
because the equations describing the system at a superior level are not
easily solved (too many equations or variables, high non-linearities).

Then discrete models may be useful : they include important simplifications which may still allow for a sufficiently accurate description
of the different possible behaviors of the system.

Among discrete models, automata networks have long been used in
biology. They seem to be particularly well adapted to describe the logics
of interactions and feedbacks between large number of functionnally different
elements.

In addition, recent developments in computers allow the simulation of
networks of thousands of elements, which is a size still insufficient in
biological contexts- for example, the brain is made up from about 10^{10}
neurons- but may yet ỹield some information upon the behavior of "natural"
networks.

II - THE PIONEERS

Automata theory was first used in the late 40's by John von Neumann
after his studies on computers. After world war II, he   became involved
in large projects for the realization of high-speed electronic computers
(ENIAC at Pennsylvania and, later, JONIAC at Princeton). He wanted to design
the logical organization of these machines independently of the technical
realization of the circuits and thus based his construction on the use of
idealized switch delays which had some similarities with neurons.

After these studies, he got into the more theoretical problem of
comparing computers to the brain, artificial automata to natural automata,and
concluded   that a new theory - Automata theory - was needed to improve our
understanding of both natural and artificial complex systems.

As an example of how such a theory could be useful, he discussed
the questions of reliability and self-reproduction. We will not describe
in details these problems that the reader could eventually find in von
Neumann's work ([24] and [25]). We just want to state some characteristics of the methods he used.

One of the most evident features of natural systems is their ability
of maintaining an organized behavior even when faced with important perturbations or partial destructions. It is a well known property of the brain
that thousands of its components - the neurons - die each day without being
replaced and that this does not imply a functional degeneracy of the brain.
Nobody knows of a computer which would allow for such amputations. Nevertheless
von Neumann has proved [24] that it was possible to design a network of non
reliable automata which could be reliable. His solution was to increase the
number of components and connections, in his words, to achieve a sufficient
"complexity" of the structure.

In the same fashion, he produced a system of finite-state automata which
was a universal constructor (able to reproduce itself or any other configuration)
and a universal calculator (able to simulate any Turing machine). He emphasized
the necessity of a critical level of complexity below which "the process of
synthesis is degenerative,but above which ... syntheses of automata can
proceed in such a manner that each automaton will produce other automata which
are more complex and of higher potentialities than itself"[25]. Further work
has been devoted to this important problem of biological organization and
complexity (Atlan[3]).

Along with von Neumann's pioneer work, many authors have used the
automata model to study the brain (see for example Ashby[2], Wiener [27],
Simon [18] and von Foerster [23]). But the work by Mac Culloch and Pitts [15] seems
to have been one of the most stimulating.

III - NEURAL NETWORKS

In 1943, they proposed to modelize the nervous system by networks
made of many interconnected components : the so-called "formal neurons".
They focused mainly on the logical power of their model : they proved that
such networks were able to simulate any Turing machine or any finite-state
automaton - Hence, any function performed by a computer may also be performed
by a Mac Culloch - Pitts network. The dynamical behavior of such networks thus
appears quite relevant to understand how the brain works, but this point was
not investigated by Mac Culloch and Pitts.

Formally, a Mac Culloch-Pitts network is made of formal neurons :
those are "all or none" devices which may be represented in the following way.

Each formal neuron has two internal states : o or 1 (inactive or
firing) and changes its state at each time of a discrete time scale according to a
"threshold" function. For example, formal neuron i will be, at time t, in
state $\phi_i(y) = \begin{cases} 0 & \text{if } \sum\limits_{j=1}^{n} \alpha_{ij} y_j < \theta_i \\ 1 & \text{otherwise} \end{cases}$

if $y_1 \ldots y_n$ were the internal states at time t-1 of the n neurons of the
network (including neuron i). The dynamical behavior of the network may then
be represented by an equation : $y^t = \phi(y^{t-1})$

where $y^t = (y_1^t, \ldots, y_n^t)$ is the state-vector of the neurons at time t and ϕ is a mapping from $\{0,1\}^n$ to $\{0,1\}^n$ whose components are $\phi_1, \ldots, \phi_n$.

$\theta_1, \ldots, \theta_n$ are called the thresholds of neurons $1, \ldots, n$. $\alpha_{ij} \in \mathbb{R}$ corresponds to a synapse between neurons i and j,which is inhibitory if $\alpha_{ij} < 0$.

Goles [11] proved that,if the matrix (α_{ij}) was symmetrical (i.e. $\alpha_{ij} = \alpha_{ji}$, $\forall$ i,j $\in$ (1,...,n) ,then all trajectories of solutions of the equation $y^t = \phi(y^{t-1})$ were periodic of period at most 2.Hence the behavior of such networks is very poor. But the symmetry assumption,which may be quite relevant in some sociological contexts (Goles [10]),must be rejected in modelling the nervous system.Unfortunately,no general result is known when the symmetry assumption is released.The network must always assume ,after some transient time,a periodic behavior - because the state-space is finite- but the possible periods have not been characterized yet (see Goles [10] for numerical examples showing periods > 2).Further work is needed on this point.

IV - GENE CONTROL SYSTEMS

Other models of automata networks have been used to model biological systems, mainly since the work by Kauffman [12] .

Kauffman wanted a theory for the "integrated gene control system" or "system of controls concerning DNA replication, transcription of particular genes, translation of particular mRNA, and enzymes activity" [13] . Such a theory would have to account for the following features :

1) - Restriction in gene activity : a metazoan cell may have up to 100 000 genes. Hence, assuming a gene is capable only of being active or inactive, the cell has $2^{100\,000}$ different patterns of gene activity. But changes in gene activity are relatively slow and, thus, the cell during its life time, is restricted to a small subset of these possibilities.

2) - Restricted number of cell types : any organism has a small number of cell types, which is certainly correlated to the number of distinct genes in the organism or DNA content of the cell.

3) - Restricted local accessibility : along the process of differentiation, the initial blastula cells differentiate into
   intermediate cell types which will further differentiate
   themselves. No cell differentiates directly into all possible
   different cells, but rather into a small number of other cell
   types.

Kauffman proposed to model a gene by an automaton with 2 internal
states (0 and 1 : inactive or active). A "model gene control system" is
then a set of N such binary genes connected together in such a way that each
gene receives as inputs the outputs of k genes. He assumes that, for each
gene, its output at time t is its internal state at time t, and that its
internal state at time t+1 is a boolean function of its k inputs at time t.

The dynamical behavior of the whole network can then be represented
by an equation : $x^t = F(x^{t-1})$ where $F : \{0,1\}^N \rightarrow \{0,1\}^N$

The state space being finite, all trajectories will be periodic.
For any initial condition, after some transient time, the network will enter
a limit cycle which it will never leave, unless perturbed.

The characterization of periods and limit cycles depends heavily
on k : for networks using functions distributed randomly among all possible
boolean functions, the k=2 case leads to behaviors qualitatively different
from the k > 2 cases. Kauffman argues that macromolecules - genes and
proteins - are specific and thus, that they are affected by only a few other
molecules [13] . Hence, only networks with low values of k are relevant
for modelling gene control systems.

In the k=2 case, a network of N binary genes may be characterized
by :

- its incidence matrix. A, which has N lines and N columns.
   $$A_{ij} = \begin{cases} 1 & \text{if gene i has gene j as one of its inputs.} \\ 0 & \text{otherwise} \end{cases}$$

Hence matrix A has two 1's per line and per column..

- its boolean function matrix F, which has N lines.

Element F_i specifies the number of the function used by gene i

149

to compute its state (see table 1).

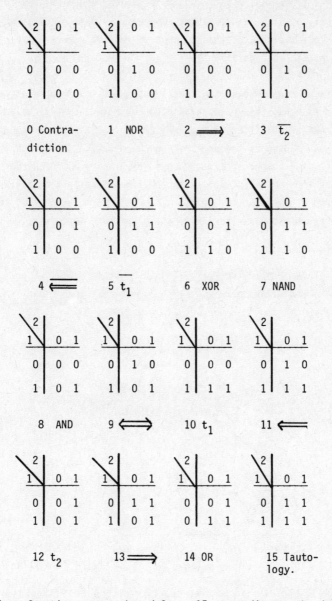

Table 1. Boolean functions are numbered 0 ... 15 according to the decimal representation of their table of values. Table $\begin{vmatrix} d & b \\ c & a \end{vmatrix}$ is numbered : $a.2^3 + b.2^2 + c.2 + d.$

It has been shown (see Kauffman [12]) that random networks (where matrices A and F are set at random) with connectance k = 2,are very stable: the mean period of limit cycles is $\sqrt{N}$ (which is very small when compared to 2^N,the number of initially possible states).Furthermore,the number of different limit cycles (for all possible initial conditions) is also restricted:there are only about $\sqrt{N}$ such asymptotic configurations.

Kauffman compares each limit cycle of the network to one type of cell in the organism which has this network as gene control system.He shows that the law relating the number of different types of cells to the number of genes or DNA content of the organism is the same as the law relating the number of different limit cycles to the number of binary genes (see figure 1).The period of each limit cycle is then to be related to the cell replication time.Biological data support this hypothesis:the law relating the cell replication time to the number of genes is the same as the law relating the mean period to the number of binary genes.

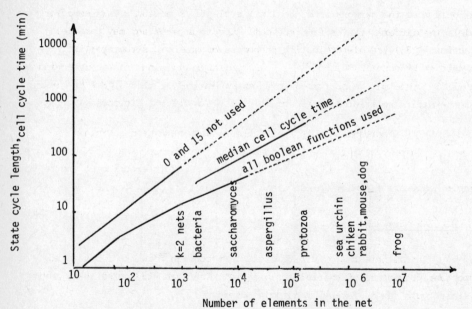

Figure 1: correlation between quantity of DNA per cell and cell cycle time.Also figured is state cycle length as a function of the number of elements N in a k=2 net,either using all 16 boolean mappings or excluding mappings 0 and 15 (constant mappings).   (Figure from Kauffman [12])

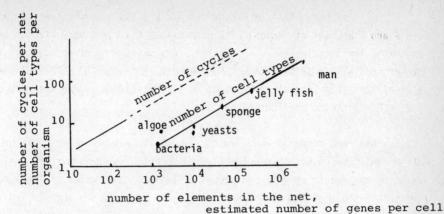

Figure 1:number of cell types against number of genes and number of
state cycles against number of elements (from Kauffman [12])

We have only described so far the behavior of autonomous networks :
what happens if they are perturbed ? The effect of perturbations on some gene
may only move the network from one limit cycle to an another. This behavior
models the differentiation from one cell type to another and may parallel
(Kauffman [13]) transdetermination phenomena of anatomic structures (for
example in Drosophila Melanogaster). As in differentiation or transdetermination
one limit cycle may be perturbed to a few others only : the network of binary
genes exhibits restricted local accessibility (as defined previously).

It is important to note that these results have been obtained on
networks randomly connected which means that it is not necessary to assume
that evolution has selected very specific patterns of interaction to ensure these
stable behaviors : random interactions would do.

V - BOOLEAN NETWORKS

Random networks of binary elements ("boolean networks") have also
important properties of spatial organization. Kauffman [13] noted that, during
a limit cycle, most elements remained constant.

We think that this fact may explain for many properties of boolean
networks.

We call subnet (see Atlan et al [2]), Fogelman et al [7]) an aggregate
of connected elements which oscillate during the limit cycle. A limit cycle
is then characterized by subnets of oscillating elements separated by elements
which remain constant (see figure 2 - figure 3).

152

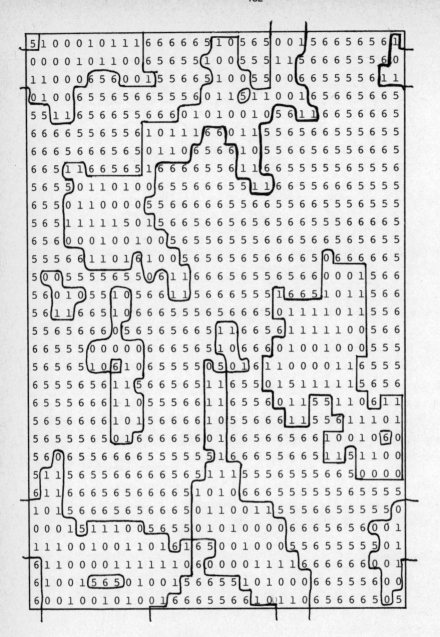

FIGURE 2

The figure represents the state of a random boolean network, with regular connections, at a given time of the limit cycle.

O and 1 correspond to oscillating elements 5 and 6 to modules which remain in a constant state (0 or 1) during the limit cycle.

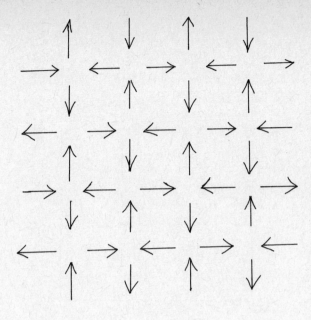

FIGURE 3 - REGULAR CONNECTIONS

Each element takes its input and output among its neighbours. The structure is completed at the boundaries by connecting symmetrical ñodes (the network can be viewed as drawn on a torus).

This connection structure allow for an easy representation of subnets because neighbour elements are also connected elements. Of course, subnet organization exists also for random connections.

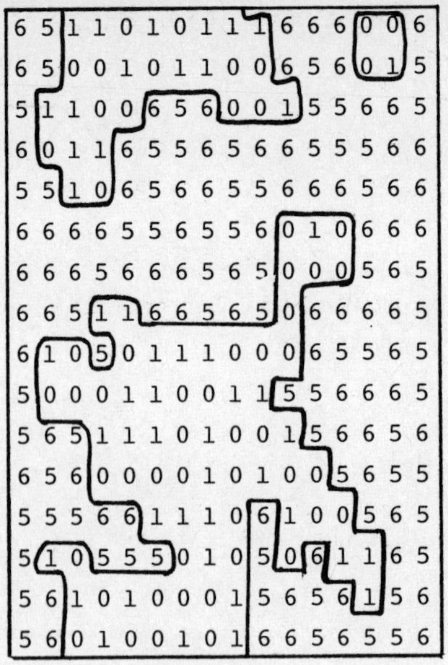

```
6 5 1 1 0 1 0 1 1 1 6 6 6 0 0 6
6 5 0 0 1 0 1 1 0 0 6 5 6 0 1 5
5 1 1 0 0 6 5 6 0 0 1 5 5 6 6 5
6 0 1 1 6 5 5 6 5 6 6 5 5 5 6 6
5 5 1 0 6 5 6 6 5 5 6 6 6 5 6 6
6 6 6 6 5 5 6 5 5 6 0 1 0 6 6 6
6 6 6 5 6 6 6 5 6 5 0 0 0 5 6 5
6 6 5 1 1 6 6 5 6 5 0 6 6 6 6 5
6 1 0 5 0 1 1 1 0 0 0 6 5 5 6 5
5 0 0 0 1 1 0 0 1 1 5 5 6 6 6 5
5 6 5 1 1 1 0 1 0 0 1 5 6 6 6 5
6 5 6 0 0 0 0 1 0 1 0 0 5 6 5 5
5 5 5 6 6 1 1 1 0 6 1 0 0 5 6 5
5 1 0 5 5 5 0 1 0 5 0 6 1 1 6 5
5 6 1 0 1 0 0 0 1 5 6 5 6 1 5 6
5 6 0 1 0 0 1 0 1 6 6 5 6 5 5 6
```

FIGURE 4

This is the subnet structure of a 16x16 network, with regular connections which corresponds to the left most quarter of the network shown on figure 2 (⌐).

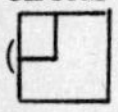

Subnets are very similar, especially in the interior part of the network, far from the cut.

This organization into subnets is very stable against perturbation :
if one cuts a hole in a network (the elements are held constant, irrespective of
their inputs) or a whole part of a network (for example 3/4 of it, see figure 4),
then the remaining network enters a limit cycle where the geometrical structure of the subnets is very similar to the initial network (in their common
part).

Roughly speaking, subnets oscillate independently, perturbations do
not propagate much through the stable parts.

This behavior is to be related to the question of reliability we
introduced previously : as for the brain, boolean networks accept important
disparition of their elements without significative perturbation of their
overall behavior (as characterized by their structuration in subnets).

Subnets seem then to be the active parts of the network. To understand
the behavior of random boolean network, it is thus necessary to have a theory
for the formation of subnets. Until now, the results come mainly from simulations on computers, some formal results exist, but only in particular cases (homogeneous networks where all elements perform the same boolean function) :
see Fogelman and al [7].

One important feature, which appeared from simulation (see Kauffman
[13] and Weisbuch [26]), is that all subnets have a common part : among the
N elements of the network, some are oscillating in all limit cycles, some
never (see figure 5). The sensitive part of the network is thus made of those
"doomed to live" elements which, whatever the initial conditions, will oscillate
forever.

```
80 80 80 80 80 80 56 74 79 80 80  0 80 80 80  0
80 80 80 80 80 80 80 80 79 80 80 80 80 80  0  0
80 80 80 80  0 80 80 80 80 76 80 80 80 80  0  0
 0  0 80  0  0  0 80 80 40 80 80 80 80  0  0  0
 0  0  0  0  0  0 80 80 80 80 80 80 80  0  0  0
80 80 80 80  0  0 80 80 80 80 80 80 79  0  0  0
80 80 80  0  0  0  0  0  0 80 80 79 79 79  0  0
 0  0 80 80  0  0  0  0 80 80 80 79 79 79 79 79
 0  0  0  0  0  0  0  0 80 80 78 77 78 76 79 79
 0  0  0  0 77 77 77 77 76 76 76 77 79 79 79 79
 0  0 53 53 77 77 77 77 77 76 76 79 79 69 59 69
69 69 63 53 77  0 56 56  0  0 79 79  0 69 69 69
69 63 69 53 53  0 56 56 56 56 56  0  0 69 69 69
 0 63 63  0 30 65 56 56 56 56 56  0  0  0 69  0
 0 63 63 77 77 79 79 35  0  0  0  0  0  0  0  0
80 80 80 77 80 79 79 74 79  0  0  0 80  0  0 80


70 70 80 80 80 80 80  0  0 47 47  0  0  0  0  0
69 69 80 80  0  0 80  0  0 47 47  0  0  0  0  0
69 69  0  0  0  0 80 80 23 47 47  0 63 63  0  0
80  0  0  0  0  0 80 80  0 47 47 13 63 63  0 80
80 35 35  0  0 70 80 80 80 47 47  0  0  0  0 80
18 35 35  0 35 70 74 23 47 47  0  0  0  0  0  0
35 35 35 35 35 70 79 80 80 47 47  0  0  0 80 80
80 80 35 35 76 79 79 80 23 23 47 47  0  0 80 80
80 80 75 71 75 75 80 80 80 23  0 47  0  0 80 80
80 80 75 71 75 75  0  0  0  0  0  0  0  0 80 80
80 68 75 75 75 75  0  0  0  0  0  0  0  0 80 80
80 68 75 75  0  0  0  0  0  0  0  0  0  0 79 79
77 78  0  0  0 80 80  0  0  0  0  0  0  0 80 80
80 50 74  0  0 80 80 80  0  0  0  0  0 80 80 80
74 74 74 80 80 80 80  0  0 00  0  0  0  0  0 80
74 74 80 80  0 80 80  0  0  0  0  0  0  0  0  0
```

FIGURE 5

```
69  0  0  0  0  0  0  0 75 75 75  5  5 19 69 69
 0 80 80  0  0  0  0  0 80 80  7  5 60 60  0  0
 0  0 80 80  0  0  0  0 80 80 77 60 60 60  0  0
 0  0 80 80 80  0 80 80 80 74 60 60 60 60  0  0
 0  0  0 80 80 80 80  0  0 75 60 64 64 60  0  0
 0  0  0 80 80 80 80  0  0  9  9  9  9  0  9  0
71  0 74 74 74 80 80  9  9  9  9  9  9  9  9 71
71 71 80 80 80 80 80  9  9  0 16 24  9  9 71 71
71 80 80 80 80 80  0  4  4 80 16 16 33 33 71 71
71 80 80 80  0  4  4  4 78 80 80 80 33 33 75 71
69 80 80  0  0  0  4  4 78 78 80 74 74 69 69 69
65 65 80 80  0  1  1  0 57 78 74 71 68 71 70 71
80 80  0  0 57 57 56 56 56 57 78 76 68 71 72 27
80 80  0 57 57 57 57 56 57 57  0 76 76 68 79 79
80 80  0  0  0 57 57 56 65 70 58 76 52 70 79 79
69  0  0  0  0  0  0  0 41 70 58 58  5 70 70 69
```

FIGURE 5

This figure shows 3 random networks with regular connections corresponding to 3 different matrices of boolean functions F.

For each network, the limit cycles corresponding to 80 different initial conditions have been calculated. For each element, we have printed the number of times (initial conditions) it was part of an oscillating subnet.

Some elements have been found to be always oscillating (80) and some always stable (0).

In a previous paper [8], we have proposed to use random boolean networks as models for the brain. We have already seen that resistance against amputation was one property shared by the brain and this model.

One can also see, in the evolution of the initially random network, a way by which random connections can get a structure, during the transition period and arrive at a configuration where some are degenerate (the connections between stable elements), and some are active or functional. These results could then give some support to a "theory of the epigenesis of neuronal networks by selective stabilization of synapses" (Changeux and Al [6]).

The initial redundancy of connections is altered through time until stabilization of those which participate in oscillating subnets and degeneracy of the others. Since it has been shown that some elements are always fixed (see figure 4), it should be the case that, in biological contexts, the degeneracy would always occur on the same connections.

We have seen that in the k=2 case, random boolean networks were generally remarkably stable. But, in the k=2 case, it is also possible to build "chaotic" networks. For this, it is sufficient to restrict the choice of boolean functions : let us assume that each element in the network can only perform a XOR or an "equivalence" function (n° 6 or 9 on table 1). Then the period of the network becomes very large, even non observable (it may approach 2^N). There exists no subnet any more (see Fogelman and Al ([7]).

These two functions have the property that they fully depend on their 2 inputs : the others 14 are "forcing" on one input (Kauffman [13]). There is one value of their input, which forces the value of the function, whatever the 2nd input. It has been shown that the proportion of "forcing" functions decreases rapidly towards o as k increases.

Hence networks with high values of k tend to have highly chaotic behavior. Since connectivity k in biological networks is generally high (thousands of synapses/neuron for example), the stability of such network cannot be obtained unless high specificity of the functions of elements (thus decreasing the proportion of non forcing elements).

VI - ASYNCHRONOUS NETWORKS

One of the main ingredients in the boolean networks studied so far is their parallelism : all automata are supposed to compute and change their state at the same time. It is quite obvious that natural systems do not work in this orderly fashion : the problem of synchronizing all the elements would require much too energy. One step towards biological relevance is then, to try to release this assumption.

R. Thomas [19] and P. Van Ham [22] have introduced a class of asynchronous boolean networks to describe complex systems in genetics. This model includes the possibility of differentiated delays for the elements of the network and results in a much wider range of behavior than the synchronous models. Some studies have been devoted also to the comparison of the boolean model to the more classical differential equations models. The two approaches appear complementary but yield behavior qualitatively similar-at least partially (see Thomas and Al [20]).

An asynchronous boolean network is a formal model involving a finite set of boolean variables linked together by boolean equations . The asynchronous feature is introduced in the following way. There are two classes of variables :

- flow variables χ_i represent the activity of a gene or a chimical reactant ...
- memory-variables x_i represent the result of the activity of variables χ_i. For example X_i would be a gene and x_i the concentration of one of the proteins synthesized by this gene activity.

The value of x_i is controlled by X_i through two delays ; δ_i and $\overline{\delta_i}$ (switch-on and switch-off delays).

Figure 6 represents such a relation for some couple (X_i, x_i).

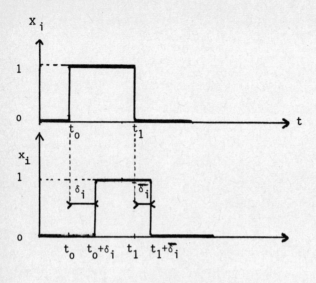

<u>FIGURE 6</u>

We can then represent an asynchronous boolean network by a set of boolean equations :

$$X_i = F_i (x_1, x_2, \ldots x_n) \qquad\qquad i=1\ldots n$$

and a set of delay-couples $(\delta_i, \overline{\delta_i}) \in R^2_+$

Let us consider now an example of asynchronous boolean network.

$$\begin{cases} X_1 = \overline{x_3} \\ X_2 = x_1 \\ X_3 = 1 \qquad \text{(so } X_3 \text{ is a tautology).} \end{cases}$$

The complete description of the system involves the delay vector $\delta = (\delta_1, \overline{\delta_1}, \delta_2, \overline{\delta_2}, \delta_3, \overline{\delta_3}) \in R^6_+$

Let us start with the truth-table which associates with each triple $(x_1, x_2, x_3) \in [0,1]^3$ a triple $(X_1, X_2, X_3) \in [0,1]^3$ given by the logical equations (see table 2).

x_1	x_2	x_3	X_1	X_2	X_3
$\bar{0}$	0	$\bar{0}$	1	0	1
0	0	1	(0	0	1)
0	$\bar{1}$	1	0	0	1
$\bar{0}$	$\bar{1}$	$\bar{0}$	1	0	1
1	1	$\bar{0}$	1	1	1
$\bar{1}$	1	1	0	1	1
$\bar{1}$	$\bar{0}$	1	0	1	1
1	$\bar{0}$	$\bar{0}$	1	1	1

TABLE 2

Numbers dotted by a dash mark an opposition between x_i and X_i. Circled states (001 in this example) are stable states (or limit cycle of period 1) : when the system has reached such a state, it will stay there forever.

It is possible to represent globally the evolution of the system by a transition graph (see figure 7) where nodes are the states of (x_1, x_2, x_3) and labeled arcs the different possible transitions between states (according to the different delays). For example, in the case shown in table 2, there are two arcs starting from state $\bar{0}0\bar{0}$:

$$\bar{0}\,0\,\bar{0} \xrightarrow{\delta_1} 1\,0\,\bar{0} \quad \text{or} \quad \bar{0}\,0\,\bar{0} \xrightarrow{\delta_3} \bar{0}\,0\,1$$

The selection between these different possible paths will be made according to the relative values of δ_1 and δ_3. (the first one if $\delta_1 < \delta_3$, the second if $\delta_3 < \delta_1$.)

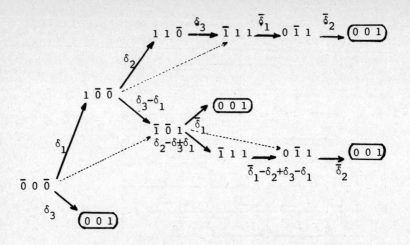

FIGURE 7

Generalizations of the model of asynchronous boolean network could
include stochastic delays or delays depending on the state of the system.
But even without such generalizations the behaviors exhibited by such networks
are extraordinarily diversified for the few states incorporated in the model.

Biological data in genetics have been analysed by these models and
the theoretical predictions checked by experimental programs ; for example,
immunity for phage λ or bacteriophage P 22 (see Thomas [21]).

VII – NETWORK MODELS OF DEVELOPMENT

Until now, we have presented models where the structure of the network
was fixed and determined before hand (even if this structure was supposed to
have been randomly assembled). In the case of the self-reproducing automata
of Von Neumann, the population of potential cells and connections is given
at the beginning, and, along the process, cells are activated along with
their pre-fixed connections. Cellular automata (as for example Conway's game Life,
Gardner [9]) are of this same type.

So none of these models is able to exhibit development capability ,i.e.
of creation of new cells and new connections.

One of the first who really presented a network model of development is Burks [5] in 1960. His main idea originated in the model of self reproduction by von Neumann [25]. But where von Neumann used 29-states automata, Burks needed about 30 000 !. To realize the reproduction, he uses a Turing machine which reads   the cellular map of the automaton and modifies it by addition deletion of cells. As in figure 8 below, cells constitute a set of circuits.

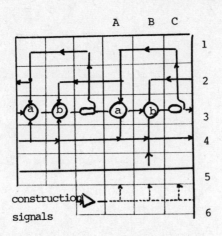

FIGURE 8

The purpose of this model was clearly technological and its adaptation to biological contexts seems questionnable. Moreover, the geometry of the cellular space (2-dimensional) is certainly very important in the properties of the model, which is thus hardly extendable.

Ten years ago, Apter [1] has developed a model of a self-constructing net : at the beginning there is a unique cell. This cell may duplicate and produce a daughter identical to itself. The "genetic program" of the cell is given by an oriented graph-drawn inside each cell (figure 9).

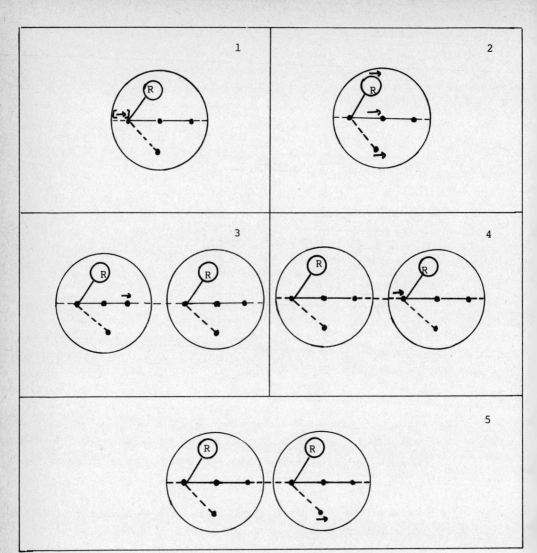

FIGURE 9

This graph includes different types of nodes and arrows. Pulses run along the arrows; when one pulse arrives at a particular node -Labelled R- then the whole cell duplicates, the daughter being connected to it by means of some arrows in their graphs : pulses keep running between cells.

The system is entirely deterministic, the final pattern depends only upon initial conditions.

Note that no distinction exists between internal pulses (cellular program) and external communications (cellular connections). This feature may be realistic but leads to very high difficulties in an inference process where the problem is to find initial conditions which would lead, after the development process of the network, to a "target" pattern.

Some developmental models are also used in botanics to model the development of plants. By means of parallel rewriting grammars, a process of morphogenesis is described which produces a plant in the form of a "word" in this grammar (see for example Lück [14]). These models are very difficult to handle and their asymptotic behavior quite impredictable before hand. Anyway their results seem to be very promising in a field where no qualitative models existed.

VIII - P ROBABILISTIC AUTOMATA NETWORK

Understanding the mechanisms by which networks of communicating cells are generated in embryogenesis and development is one of the challenges that the biologists are still facing today. The aim of the P robabilistic Automata Network model is to show that probabilistic programming may be more efficient than deterministic to account for the generations of such networks, as the number of cells and the diversity of their interactions become exceedingly large (see Milgram [16]).

The basic material of a P robabilistic Automata Network is a P robabilistic Network which is an Automaton (Q,Y,A) where Q is the set of states, Y set of inputs and $A(y_k)$ is a transition matrix for any $y_k \in Y$. The changes from one state to another are produced in a discrete manner : at every time unit, the automaton receives an input y_k and goes from state q_i for state q_j according to the probability $a_{i,j}(y_k)$ which is the generic element of matrix $A(y_k)$.

If, for every $y_k \in Y$, $A(y_k)$ has only 0 or 1 entries, we say that the automaton is deterministic.

To build an evolving network we have to give additional rules. These rules describe the behavior of the cells one versus the other and allows to generate the overall behavior of the network. As a consequence of there rules, there is an abstract causal loop (meta-loop) connecting the functioning of the automaton (local level) and the network (global level). (see Milgram-Atlan [17]).

Rule 1 : Every new cell is in its initial state "q_o" when it is created.

Rule 2 : Every cell reaching the state d (for "division") produces an additional cell which will appear at the next time unit.

Rule 3 : If a cell A_1 is in state "s" (for "source") and a cell A_2 is in state "g" (for "goal") a permanent connection is established from A_1 to A_2 and will appear at the next time unit.
(This rule can be applied simultaneously to a large number of cell pairs). For example if A_1, A_2, A_3 are in state s and A_4, A_5 in state g the following connections will be created :
$(A_1 A_4)$, $(A_1 A_5)$, $(A_2 A_4)$, $(A_2 A_5)$, $(A_3 A_4)$, $(A_3 A_5)$.

Rule 4 : The last rule relates the connection or lack of connection between the cells with the set of inputs in the automaton : the automaton of a cell is assigned the input $y = \alpha$ when it does not receive any connection and the input $y = \beta$ when it receives at least one connection.

At each step in the evolution of the network, several possibilities can occur and the whole evolution is equivalent to a set of choices among several directions. Since these choices have known probabilities, to each evolution of the network may be assigned (at least theoretically) a given probability. Let us present now an example ; consider the automaton with the transition matrices :

$Q = \{q_0, x, s, g, d\}$ $Y = \{\alpha, \beta\}$

	q_0	x	s	g	d
q_0	0	0	1	0	0
x	0	1	0	0	0
s	0	ε	0	$1-\varepsilon$	0
g	0	0	0	0	1
d	0	0	1	0	0

$y = \alpha$

	q_0	x	s	g	d
q_0	0	1	0	0	0
x	0	1	0	0	0
s	0	1	0	0	0
g	0	1	0	0	0
d	0	1	0	0	0

$y = \beta$

The produced network is as follows :

$$A_0 \leftarrow A_1 \leftarrow A_2 \leftarrow A_3 \leftarrow A_4 \cdots A_n$$

with : $\text{Prob } (n = k) = \varepsilon(1 - \varepsilon)^k$

$E[n] = \dfrac{1}{\varepsilon} - 1$ (E [n] stands for the mean value of n)

One can see that, for $\varepsilon \to 0$, $E[n] \to +\infty$
and that the deterministic case ($\varepsilon = 0$) leads to an infinite chain.

To generate more sophisticated networks (trees) on can combine several kinds of elementary automata. Let us generalize rules 2 and 3 as:

Rule 2' : Every cell reaching a state d $\in$ D produces an additional cell which will appear at the next time and be in state q_0.

Rule 3' : A connection may be established between cell A_i and cell A_j if A_i is in state s and A_j in a state g so that $(s,g) \in C$

Example : $Q = \{q_0, s, s', g, g', d, d', x\}$ $Y = \{\alpha, \beta\}$
$D = \{d, d'\}$
$C = \{(s,g), (s',g'), (g',g), (s,s')\}$

Transition matrices : $(\alpha + \beta = 1 ; 0 \leqslant \varepsilon \leqslant 1 ; \alpha, \beta \geqslant 0)$.

$= \alpha$

	q_0	s	g	d	g'	s'	d'	x
q_0	0	α	0	0	β	0	0	0
s	0	0	1	0	0	0	0	0
g	0	0	0	$1-\varepsilon$	0	0	0	ε
d	0	1	0	0	0	0	0	0
g'	0	0	0	0	0	1	0	0
s'	0	0	0	0	0	0	$1-\varepsilon$	ε
d'	0	0	0	0	1	0	0	0

For $y = \beta$, the transition matrix is a reset to state x as in the previous example.

This automaton generates a class of trees such as the following:

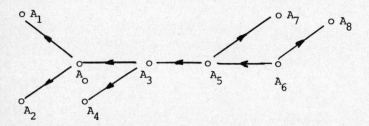

Some quantitative results about these structures can be derived from the study of the probabilities of the automata.

The use of probabilistic automata necessarily leads to some decreased accuracy in the resulting network as compared with what would be produced deterministically by using as large a number of states as necessary.

Nevertheless, some accuracy is still achieved and it is interesting to understand the mechanisms by which more or less of it is obtained.

IX CONCLUSION

Understanding the mechanisms by which networks of communicating cells are generated in embryogenesis and development is one of the challenges that the biologists are still facing today.

Because of the constitution of the biological systems in active elements well identified (such as neurons for exemple),it appears natural to use discrete models made of interacting elements.

The capability of the model to describe the morphogenesis process is then linked to the information amount ("genetic program") present in the compo-nents.In some cases,probabilistic programming may be more efficient than determi-nistic to account for the generation of biological nets,as the number of cells and diversity of their interactions become exceedingly large.

If we are searching for models with self-organization capabilities to account for phenomena of non directed learning at cellular and multicellular level,

we can choose either deterministic or probabilistic approach.Generally,determi-
nistic approach makes computations easier even when models are larger,complexity
being represented by a large number of elements rather than by a non-determinis-
tic feature.

Gregory Bateson said that "information is a difference that makes a
difference" and so,in our case,morphogenetic information is,at the beginning,a
selection among a large set of possibilities generated by a combinatoric scheme
which is arbitrary and meaningless,and that we call "randomized".

Now,most of the biologists admit that chance is not only a negative
term,a "noise".In an ecosysytem or a biological system,noise is always the intru-
sion of the environment,which has been found necessary in many cases to ensure
an accurate development (as,for exemple in retinotopy or somatotopy).

Probabilistic schemes are also often used to reduce an exceedingly
large number of elements of a deterministic model and in this case it is just a
trick to manage with too complex combinatoric problems.But we saw that they could
also be useful to allow for important simplifications in the models.

Scientific laws remain deterministic but the semantics of their statements can be probabilistic.

F. FOGELMAN-SOULIE
  U.E.R. de Mathématiques
  Université de Paris V
  12, rue Cujas
  75005 PARIS

M. MILGRAM
  Département M.A.I.
  Université de Technologie de Compiègne
  B.P. 233
  60206 COMPIEGNE CEDEX

G. WEISBUCH
  Département de Physique
  Case 901
  Faculté des Sciences de Luminy
  13288 MARSEILLE CEDEX

REFERENCES

[1] - M.J. APTER : The genesis of neural pattern - Advances in Cyber. and
        system Research.Gordon B. (1972)

[2] - W.R. ASHBY : Design for a brain - Chapman and Hall,London (1954)

[3] - H. ATLAN : L'organisation biologique et la théorie de l information
        Hermann (1972)

[4] - H.ATLAN - F. FOGELMAN-SOULIE - J. SALOMON - G. WEISBUCH :
        - Random boolean networks.Cybernetics and Systems.(1981).

[5] - A.W. BURKS : Computation, behavior and structure in fixed and growing
        automata in self-organizing systems - Yovitz et Cameron
        Ed. (1960)

[6] - J.P. CHANGEUX - P. COURREGE - A. DANCHIN : A theory of the epigenesis
        of neuronal networks by selective stabilization of Synapses.
        PNAS of USA Vol. 70, n° 10 (1973).

[7] - F. FOGELMAN-SOULIE - E. GOLES-CHACC et G. WEISBUCH :
        Specific roles of the different boolean mappings in
        random networks. Bull. math. Biol.to appear.

[8] - FOGELMAN-SOULIE : Les réseaux d'automates : une modélisation de systèmes
        biologiques ? Actes du 1er séminaire de Biologie
        théorique du CNRS - ENSTA.(1981).

[9] - M. GARDNER : Mathematical games. Scientific American Oct. 70 - Feb.71

[10] - E. GOLES-CHACC : Comportement oscillatoire d'une famille d'automates
        cellulaires non uniformes. Thèse Grenoble. (1980)

[11] - E. GOLES-CHACC : Comportement périodique des fonctions à seuil binaires
        et applications .Discrete Applied Math.3.(1981).

[12] - S. KAUFFMAN : Behavior of randomly constructed genetic nets. In towards
                    a theoretical biology. Vol. 3 - Ed. C.H. Waddington
                    Edinbrugh University Press (1970)

[13] - S. KAUFFMAN : Gene regulation networks : a theory for their global
                    structure and behaviors,in current topics in developmental
                    biology. Eds. Moscona AA and Monroy A. Vol. 6
                    Academic Press (1971).

[14] - H.B LÜCK   : Modèles discrets de la morphogénèse végétale:avec ou sans
                    interaction? in Elaboration et justification des modèles,
                    P. Delattre et M. Thellier,Editions Maloine,Paris.(1979).

[15] - W.S. MAC CULLOCH - W. PITTS : A logical calculus of the ideas
                    immanent in nervous activity.Bull;of Math·Biophysics.
                    5.(1943).

[16] - M. MILGRAM : Contribution aux réseaux d'automates - Thèse Compiègne (1982)

[17] - M. MILGRAM - ATLAN : Probabilistic automata as a model for epigenesis
                    of cellular networks.In preparation

[18] - H.A. SIMON : The Sciences of the artificial - Mit Press (1969).

[19] - R. THOMAS : Kinetic logic : a boolean approach to the analysis of
                    complex regulatory systems. Lecture Notes in Biomathematics
                    n° 29 - Springer Verlag - Berlin (1979)

[20] - R. THOMAS - G. NICOLIS et J. RICHELLE - P. VAN HAM :
                    General discussion on the simplifying assumptions. in methods
                    using logical, stochastic or differential equations. In
                    Thomas (1979).

[21] - R. THOMAS : Some biological examples in 'Thomas (1979).

[22] - P. VAN HAM : PhD thesis - Univ. libre de Bruxelles (1975)

[23] - H. VON FOERSTER : On self organizing systems and their environments. In
                    self organizing systems. Ed. Yovitz et Cameron
                    Pergamon Press (1960)

[24] - J. VON NEUMANN : Probabilistic logic and the synthesis of reliable
                       organisms from unreliable components.In automata
                       Studies. Ed. S.E. Shannon and J. Mac Carthy.
                       Princeton University Press - Princeton.(1956)

[25] - J. VON NEUMANN : Theory of self reproducing automata. Ed. A.W. Burks
                       University of Illinois Press.Urbana. (1966)

[26] - G. WEISBUCH - FOGELMAN-SOULIE F. : in preparation.

[27] - N. WIENER : Cybernetics or control and communication in the Animal
                  and the Machine. J. WILEY and Sons. (1948).

A CRITICAL DISCUSSION OF PLAUSIBLE MODELS FOR RELAY AND OSCILLATION OF CYCLIC AMP IN DICTYOSTELIUM CELLS

A. Goldbeter[1] and J.L. Martiel[2]

[1]Faculté des Sciences, Université Libre de Bruxelles,
C.P. 231, 1050 Brussels, Belgium, and [2]Chaire de Physique,
Institut National Agronomique, 75231 Paris, France

1. INTRODUCTION

Sustained oscillations arise in metabolic pathways as a result of enzyme regulation (1,2). A property shared by metabolic and other oscillatory systems, from the nerve membrane (3,4) to chemical clocks (5,6) such as the Belousov-Zhabotinsky reaction, is that they are excitable in a parameter domain close to that corresponding to sustained oscillations. Whereas autonomous oscillations occur around a nonequilibrium unstable steady state (7), excitability represents the property of a system, initially in a stable steady state, to amplify in a pulsatory manner suprathreshold perturbations in the concentration of some chemical intermediate. Oscillatory and excitable behavior thus originate from a common mechanism operating in different parameter domains; the requirements for both phenomena are therefore the same. In metabolic pathways, the prerequisites reduce to the existence of an appropriate nonlinear feedback process (2).

The purpose of this paper is twofold. First, we wish to explore several plausible sources of nonlinearity giving rise to oscillations and excitability in a biological system in which both types of phenomena are observed. The system to be considered is the mechanism which controls the periodic release and the relay of cyclic AMP (cAMP) signals during the aggregation phase that follows starvation in the cellular slime mold Dictyostelium discoideum. Several alternative mechanisms for relay and oscillation will be discussed, the set of which constitutes a partial catalogue of plausible nonlinearities causing excitable and oscillatory behavior in biochemical systems.

The second goal of the paper will be to contrast specific versus general properties of the various models, in order to pinpoint the theoretical results which may be relevant to experimental research even if the biochemistry of cAMP relay and oscillation is not yet known in full detail.

174

2. THE cAMP SIGNALLING SYSTEM OF D. DISCOIDEUM: A SUMMARY OF EXPERIMENTAL OBSERVATIONS

When D. discoideum amoebae come out of spores, they grow and divide as long as food is present. Upon starvation, they enter a developmental program which, after an interphase of some 8 h, leads to their aggregation and, finally, after migration of the aggregate which has by then formed a slug, to the formation of a fruiting body composed of a stalk surmounted by a mass of spores (8,9) (see Fig.1).

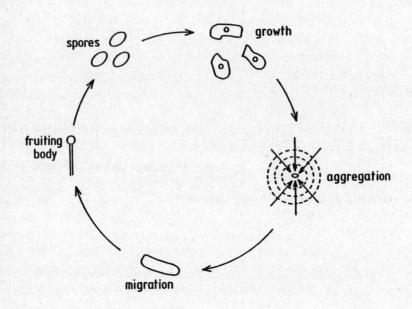

Fig.1. Life cycle of the slime mold Dictyostelium discoideum. The dashed, concentric lines denote the wavelike nature of the aggregation process.

One of the remarkable features of the aggregation process in D. discoideum and in some other slime mold species is that it is periodic (10,11). Time lapse movies have shown that amoebae aggregate around centers in concentric waves whose period is of the order of several minutes. To account for these observations, Shaffer (10) suggested that aggregation centers release periodically a chemical factor, the acrasin which, as shown by Bonner (8), controls the chemotactic response of the amoebae in the course of aggregation. In addition to postulating an autonomous production of periodic pulses of acrasin, Shaffer suggested that chemotactically responding cells are capable of relaying the chemical signal towards the periphery of the aggregation field, i.e. these cells synthetize a pulse of acrasin upon reception of an acrasin signal. As will be discussed below, the periodic synthesis and relay of acrasin can be identified, respectively, with the phenomena of oscillations and excitability (12). To date, they represent the best-known example of such behaviors in a biochemical system.

The two predictions made by Shaffer were later confirmed in a series of experiments on continuously stirred suspensions of D. discoideum cells (such a procedure permits a detailed kinetic study of the signalling mechanism since cells in suspensions are synchronized, which is not the case for cells aggregating on a solid support). Prior to these experiments, the acrasin of D. discoideum had been identified as being cyclic AMP (cAMP) (13), a chemical which plays a key role in hormonal control in higher organisms. Cell suspension studies showed that under slightly different conditions, D. discoideum amoebae are capable of generating autonomous cAMP pulses with a periodicity of several minutes (14), and of relaying sufficiently large pulses of cAMP (15).

The biochemical mechanism underlying cAMP relay and oscillation is still under investigation. A list of the components identified so far, and of the regulatory interactions which are agreed upon without being clarified yet at the molecular level, stands as follows (see ref. 16 for a review, and also Fig.2):

 (i) On the outer face of the plasma membrane — i.e. on the cell surface — amoebae possess receptors for cAMP.

 (ii) On the inner face of the membrane, an enzyme, adenylate cyclase, transforms ATP into cAMP.

(iii) Intracellular cAMP is transported into the extracellular medium where it is hydrolyzed by phosphodiesterase; the latter enzyme acts upon cAMP both in a membrane-bound form and in a form released by the cells into the extracellular medium.

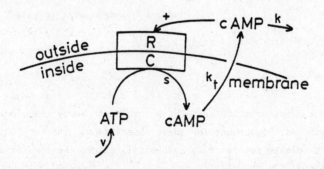

Fig.2. Regulation of the cAMP signalling system in D. discoideum. The sign + refers to the activation of adenylate cyclase (C) upon binding of cAMP to the cell surface receptor (R) (from ref.22)

(iv) Upon binding to the cell surface receptor, extracellular cAMP induces an increase in adenylate cyclase activity which results in the synthesis of intracellular cAMP, and in the subsequent increase in extracellular cAMP, owing to cAMP transport across the cell membrane.

The coupling mechanism by which adenylate cyclase is activated upon cAMP binding to the receptor is not yet known, but the existence of the positive feedback in cAMP synthesis is well established (16). Several alternative realisations of the positive feedback will be considered below, together with their implications for the dynamic behavior of the cAMP signalling system.

3. THE ROLE OF POSITIVE FEEDBACK IN THE MECHANISM OF OSCILLATION

The main ingredient in the theoretical modelling of the cAMP signalling system is the autocatalytic effect exerted by cAMP on its intracellular production. Such a role for positive feedback is not confined to Dictyostelium cells. Although much less frequent than negative feedback in biological regulations, positive feedback controls the operation of a variety of biological systems. When it occurs, it is frequently associated with self-organization phenomena such as excitability and oscillations. Thus the autocatalytic transport of Na^+ ions across the membrane plays a primary role in the excitable and rhythmic properties of many nerve cells and of pacemaker regions of the heart.

At the enzymatic level, other biochemical oscillations due to positive feedback are known. The best studied are glycolytic oscillations in yeast and muscle, which originate from the activation of phosphofructokinase by one of its reaction products (1,2). Finally, the autocatalytic production of an intermediate species in the Belousov-Zhabotinsky reaction is taken as responsible for both periodic and excitable behavior in this well-known oscillatory system (17). All these experimental results agree with predictions from nonequilibrium Thermodynamics (7) which point to autocatalysis as being one of the most efficient processes for inducing in open systems instabilities and the ensuing formation of dissipative structures in time and/or space.

Before turning to the modelling of the cAMP signalling system, it is useful to compare cAMP oscillations with glycolytic periodicities. The latter represent the prototype of metabolic oscillations. Whereas their function in yeast or muscle is less clear than the role of cAMP oscillations in the control of chemotaxis and differentiatic in D. discoideum amoebae, the molecular mechanism of instability in glycolysis is known in more detail. Phosphofructokinase is an allosteric enzyme, i.e. a protein composed of multiple subunits which may exist in at least two different conformational states. Co-operative interactions between the subunits lead to a nonlinear response to controlling ligands, resulting in sigmoid velocity curves for the enzyme reaction. In the concerted model for allosteric enzymes (18), all subunits undergo a concerted transition between the two conformational states R and T which may differ by their affinity for the ligand (the substrate, or an effector, either positive or negative) and/or by their catalytic activity. Positive feedback is achieved when a reaction product binds to a regulatory site on each of the enzyme subunits, with a higher affinity for the R state which, by convention, is taken as most reactive (see Fig.3). Activation thus occurs through pulling the R⇄T equilibrium towards the R state; as more product is being formed due to the subsequent enhancement in reaction rate, the conformational equilibrium is further shifted in favor of the R state: this is the basis for autocatalytic control through allosteric transition.

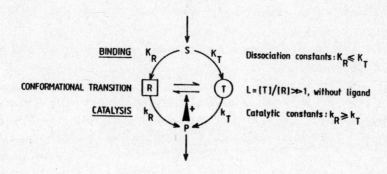

Fig.3. Positive feedback trough allosteric regulation (see text). This control mechanism is exemplified by the enzyme phospho-fructokinase, which is responsible for glycolytic oscillations.

Such a product-activated allosteric model has been analyzed for the phosphofructo-kinase reaction. The periodic behavior of this model, reviewed elsewhere (2,19-21), matches qualitatively most experiments on glycolytic oscillations in yeast extracts.

The mechanism by which extracellular cAMP controls adenylate cyclase in D. discoi-deum is not as clear as that which governs phosphofructokinase activity. A further difference stems from the compartmented nature of the cAMP signalling system in which the extracellular and intracellular volumes are separated by the cell membrane. Communication channels between the compartments include cAMP transport from inside to outside the cell, and activation of intracellular cAMP synthesis upon binding of extracellular cAMP to the receptor. Due to the coupling between receptor and enzyme, the number of possible activation mechanisms for adenylate cyclase is larger than for phosphofructokinase. The question arises as to whether the capability for excitable and oscillatory behavior in D. discoideum depends on the detailed mechanism of the activation process. To answer this question, we consider below three distinct mechanisms for enzyme activation:

1) Allosteric regulation;

2) Covalent modification;

3) Receptor-enzyme coupling.

Each of these mechanisms will be briefly discussed, and its predictions compared with observations on the experimental system.

There is a further motivation for studying several different mechanisms for adenylate cyclase control. Both in the excitable and oscillatory responses, a peak of cAMP consists of a rising and of a decreasing phase. If the rising phase results here from autocatalysis, reasons for the decrease can be manifold. Two such reasons will be discussed as different models based on the various activation mechanisms listed above are being considered. These are:
(a) Substrate limitation;
(b) Receptor desensitization.

The interest of these mechanisms goes beyond the particular case of D. discoideum amoebae. Finding the causes for the rising and decreasing phases is indeed one of the main problems which arise in the study of biological rhythms.

4. MODELS FOR THE cAMP SIGNALLING SYSTEM

4.1. Model based on allosteric regulation of adenylate cyclase
One of the simplest assumptions that can be made for the regulation of the compartmented system of Fig.2 is to treat the receptor and adenylate cyclase as the regulatory and catalytic sites of an allosteric protein (22). The receptor (regulatory) sites and the enzymatic (catalytic) sites face, respectively, the extracellular and intracellular volumes. When the protein complex is considered as a dimer, the time behavior of the cAMP signalling system is governed by a set of three ordinary differential equations (22):

$$d\alpha/dt = v - \sigma\Phi$$
$$d\beta/dt = q\sigma\Phi - k_t\beta$$
$$d\gamma/dt = (k_t\beta/h) - k_s\gamma \qquad \text{-1-}$$

with
$$\Phi = \alpha(1+\alpha)(1+\gamma)^2/(L+(1+\alpha)^2(1+\gamma)^2) \qquad \text{-2-}$$

Here, the three variables α, β, and γ denote the normalized concentrations of intracellular ATP, intracellular cAMP, and extracellular cAMP (see ref. 22 for further details on the equations and on the significance of the various parameters). For the following discussion, it is useful to specify that parameters v, σ, k_t, and k_s relate respectively to the constant input of substrate, maximum adenylate cyclase activity, transport of cAMP across the plasma membrane, and maximum phosphodiesterase activity.

Equations 1 admit a single steady-state solution. Linear stability analysis yields the conditions in which this steady state behaves as an unstable focus or node. Under these conditions the system undergoes sustained oscillations of the limit cycle type (20). The model is thus capable of accounting for the autonomous, periodic generation of cAMP pulses by the signalling system. The next property to be accounted for is relay. A most convenient way to demonstrate the link between relay and oscillation is to resort to the phase plane analysis of system 1. It is possible to carry out such an analysis in the (α, γ) phase plane after making a quasi-steady-state assumption for β, owing to the relatively large value of parameters q and k_t (12).

Most relevant to relay and oscillation is the fact that for suitable values of the parameters — e.g., for sufficiently large values of the allosteric constant L (see Fig.3) — the nullcline $d\gamma/dt=0$ in the (α, γ) plane is an S-shaped sigmoid (Fig.4). The steady state is located at the intersection of this sigmoid curve with the nullcline $d\alpha/dt=0$. Linear stability analysis shows (21) that the steady state is unstable whenever the slope $d\alpha/d\gamma$ in this point is less than $-(1/q)$. For $q \to \infty$, this condition shows that the steady state is unstable whenever it lies on the region of negative slope of the sigmoid nullcline; it is then enclosed by a limit cycle as shown in Fig. 4a.

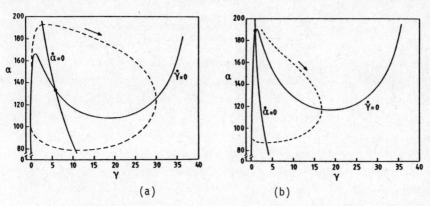

(a)   (b)

Fig.4. Limit cycle oscillations (a), and excitability upon suprathreshold perturbation (b), in a two-variable system derived from equations 1. The steady state is either stable or unstable depending on its position on the sigmoid nullcline $d\gamma/dt=0$ (see text).

The steady state is always stable when it lies on a region of positive slope of the sigmoid nuccline. To test the response of the system to the addition of an extra-cellular cAMP pulse — which corresponds to an instantaneous horizontal displacement to the right in the (α, γ) phase plane — one has to determine in this plane the trajectories followed by the system after such perturbation in γ. A most interesting situation arises when the steady state is located just to the left of the region of negative slope (Fig. 4b). Then, when subjected to small displacements away from the stable steady state — corresponding to the addition of tiny cAMP pulses — the system returns immediately to the steady state. When perturbed beyond a threshold, however, the system undergoes a large excursion in the phase plane before returning to the steady state. This phenomenon of excitability represents the pulsatory amplification of a suprathreshold perturbation. The phase plane analysis clearly shows how and why excitability is necessarily linked to the phenomenon of sustained oscillations. As previously shown by Fitzhugh for the nerve membrane (4), both phenomena require the existence of an S-shaped nullcline, and occur in contiguous regions of the parameter domain.

The model based on the allosteric regulation of adenylate cyclase thus accounts for the relay and oscillation of cAMP in D. discoideum cells (see Fig.5). From the theoretical point of view, aggregation centers are the cells which are the first to

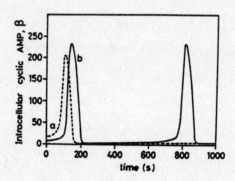

Fig.5. Relay (a) and oscillation (b) of cAMP in the model governed by equations 1 (redrawn from ref. 22).

enter the domain of self-sustained oscillations around an unstable steady state. The model also provides an explanation for the sequential transitions no relay-relay-oscillation observed during the interphase that follows starvation. In reason of its generality, which goes beyond the particular features of the models discussed here, the theoretical basis for the sequential transitions is discussed in section 5 below.

4.2. Model based on covalent modification

We consider here the situation — still hypothetical — in which adenylate cyclase is activated in an indirect manner, through a covalent modification catalyzed by a cAMP-dependent protein kinase. The simplest, non-compartmented, scheme of enzyme regulation (23) is then represented in Fig.6, where adenylate cyclase is phosphorylated by a protein kinase which is activated in a cooperative manner by cAMP (the latter process is observed in numerous phosphorylation systems (24)). Positive feedback occurs when the phosphorylated form of adenylate cyclase (E^*) has a larger affinity for the substrate ATP and/or a larger catalytic activity than the nonphosphorylated form (E). Here, the protein kinase is considered as being activated from K into K^* upon binding of two molecules of intracellular cAMP (23). The two variables of the model are then the intracellular concentrations of ATP and cAMP.

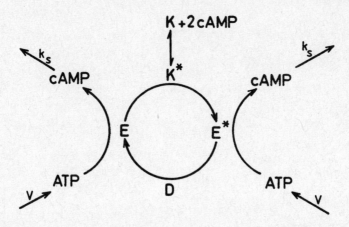

Fig.6. Autocatalytic regulation through covalent modification, illustrated by the putative activation of adenylate cyclase upon phosphorylation by a cAMP-dependent protein kinase (see text).

It is possible to construct models comprising three variables or more, which take into account explicitly the activation of adenylate cyclase upon binding of extracellular cAMP to the membrane receptor. At least two possibilities for activation of cAMP synthesis through protein modification then exist:

(i) It is observed that binding of extracellular cAMP to the receptor activates guanylate cyclase before adenylate cyclase; the intracellular cyclic GMP thus synthesized could activate an intracellular protein kinase (24) which would phosphorylate adenylate cyclase as shown in Fig.6.

(ii) Extracellular cAMP could activate a protein kinase which would phosphorylate the cAMP receptor, either intracellularly or extracellularly; the modified receptor would have an increased affinity for coupling with adenylate cyclase, with the result of an enhancement in cAMP synthesis.

Models based on either one of mechanisms (i) or (ii) constitute extensions of the basic mechanism of Fig.6, and exhibit the same modes of dynamic behavior. The kinetic equations which govern the time evolution of ATP and cAMP in the model of Fig.6 are (see ref. 23 for a detailed presentation):

$$d\alpha/dt = v - \sigma\Phi$$
$$d\gamma/dt = q\sigma\Phi - k_s\gamma \qquad\qquad -3-$$

These equations are similar in form to equations 1, but the rate function Φ for adenylate cyclase is now given by (see ref. 23):

$$\Phi = \alpha x(1+(\theta_1\lambda_1\lambda_2/Y_\gamma\lambda_3)) \qquad\qquad -4-$$

where the fraction of phosphorylated enzyme, x, is given by the relation:

$$x = (-A_2 + (A_2^2 + 4A_1A_3)^{1/2})/2A_1$$

with

$$A_1=\lambda_3(1+\alpha) + (\lambda_2(1+\alpha\theta_1)/Y_\gamma)$$
$$A_2=\lambda_3(\lambda_3(1+\alpha) +\theta_2 +\theta_3 - 1 + (\lambda_2/Y_\gamma)(1+\alpha\theta_1)) , \quad A_3=\lambda_3^2$$

(Parameters λ_1, λ_2, λ_3, θ_1, θ_2, θ_3 are defined in ref.23). Moreover, the saturation function for the binding of cAMP to protein kinase is defined by:

$$Y_\gamma = \gamma^2/(1+\gamma^2)$$

In the above equations, α and γ denote the normalized concentrations of ATP and cAMP.

Of special relevance to the present discussion is the fact that the nullcline $d\gamma/dt=0$ obtained from equation 3 in this model has also, for suitable parameter values, a sigmoid shape (see Fig. 7a), as in Fig.4 which was established for the case of allosteric regulation.

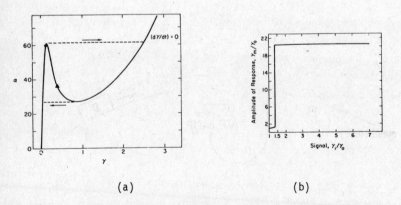

(a)   (b)

Fig.7. Limit cycle (a) obtained for equations 3 in the (α,γ)
plane when the unstable steady state ($\blacktriangle$) lies on the
region of negative slope of the $d\gamma/dt=0$ sigmoid null-

cline. (b): Dose-response curve showing a sharp threshold when the excitable steady state (●) is located to the left of the oscillatory domain on the nullcline of (a) (from ref.23).

The nonlinearity that gives the nullcline its sigmoid character originates here from the fact that the protein kinase is controlled by cAMP in a cooperative manner, as shown by the form of function Y_γ. Despite the radically different forms of the rate function Φ obtained for adenylate cyclase in the allosteric (equation 2) or covalent modification model (equation 4), we see that they give rise to similar portraits in the phase plane and, subsequently, to similar types of dynamic behavior, i.e. relay and oscillation.

4.3. Model based on receptor desensitization

The model we consider now departs from the preceding ones in two respects. First, adenylate cyclase is considered to be activated by cAMP neither through allosteric regulation, nor through covalent modification, but through formation of a complex with an active form of the cAMP receptor. Second, the substrate ATP is no more taken as the limiting factor responsible for the decreasing phase of the relay or oscillatory responses. Instead, this phenomenon originates here from the passage of the receptor into an inactive, desensitized state upon binding of cAMP.

Desensitization is a property exhibited by many receptors for a variety of hormones and neurotransmitters (25,26); it is reflected by the progressive decrease in the affinity for binding to the receptor when the latter is incubated during a sufficiently long time with its specific ligand. The phenomenon can actually occur through several mechanisms, but is reflected globally by an apparent decrease in the number of available receptor sites. Evidence for desensitization has been reported for the cAMP receptor in D. discoideum (27).

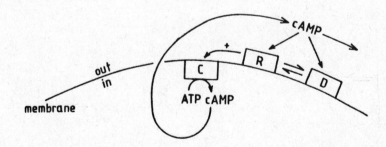

Fig.8. Modified model of Fig.2 showing the coupling of the cAMP receptor with adenylate cyclase; the active state of the receptor (R) is converted to a desensitized state (D) upon binding cAMP.

The model is based on the following assumptions (see Fig.8):

(a) The receptor exists under two conformations, active (R) and desensitized (D), which are interconverted in a reversible manner. In the absence of ligand, the ratio R/D=L is much larger than unity.

(b) Extracellular cAMP binds to the R and D states, but with a larger affinity for D ($c=K_R/K_D >1$).

(c) Only the R state forms a complex with adenylate cyclase and thereby activates the enzyme.

(d) The substrate ATP is taken as constant. As in the model of Fig.2, intracellular cAMP is transported across the plasma membrane into the extracellular medium where it is hydrolyzed by phophodiesterase.

The nonlinearity required for oscillatory behavior originates here from the cooperative binding of cAMP to the receptor. It could, alternatively, be due to a cooperative binding of the cAMP-receptor complex to the free form of adenylate cyclase. As in section 4.1, the system can be reduced to a system of two differential equations. The variables now are the normalized concentration of extracellular cAMP (γ) and the fraction ρ of free receptor in the active state R:

$$d\rho/dt = k_{-1}(-\rho + L\delta)$$
$$d\gamma/dt = \sigma\Phi - k_s\gamma \qquad\qquad -5-$$

with

$$\Phi = s(\epsilon\theta +\rho\gamma^2)/(\epsilon(1+\theta s) + \rho\gamma^2(1+s)).$$

The fraction δ of free receptor in the desensitized state is given by an expression of the form:

$$\delta = (1/(1+c^2\gamma^2)) (1-\rho(1+\gamma)^2-(\mu\rho\gamma^2(1+s)/(\epsilon(1+\theta s)+\rho\gamma^2(1+s)))$$

where s is the normalized, constant level of substrate ATP (k_{-1}, ϵ, θ , and μ are parameters related to kinetic properties and to total receptor and enzyme concentrations).

Here also, as in the preceding models, the nullcline $d\gamma/dt=0$ can have an S-shaped sigmoid form. Accordingly, excitable and oscillatory behavior are observed in the mode as shown in Fig.9 for the relay of a suprathreshold pulse of cAMP. Note here that the decrease in cAMP (γ) after a peak is brought about by a decrease in the amount of available receptor in active state (ρ), due to the desensitization process.

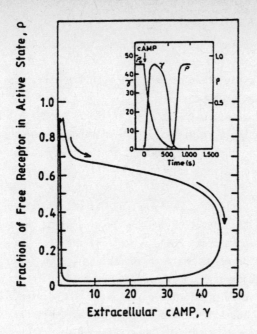

Fig.9. Phase plane trajectory for relay response in the model
based on receptor desensitization.

5. CONCLUSIONS

The analysis of several models based on the positive feedback exerted by cAMP
on its own production in D. discoideum shows that relay and oscillation of cAMP occur
in this system regardless of the molecular details of the feedback process. Once the
kinetic equations have a sufficient degree of nonlinearity, autocatalysis gives necessarily rise to excitable and oscillatory behavior. Phase plane analysis shows that
widely different phenomena such as allosteric regulation, covalent modification, and
receptor-enzyme coupling accompanied by receptor desensitization, are all capable,
when associated with positive feedback, to produce similar portraits based on the
existence of a S-shaped nullcline in the phase space. This occurs despite the fact
that the equations governing the evolution of the signalling system in the various
models have widely different forms.

It therefore appears that the existence of the positive feedback process ensures
the occurrence of excitability and oscillations, provided that interactions at the
receptor or enzyme levels are sufficiently nonlinear. When this condition is satisfied,
various molecular realisations of the feedback process can lead to similar types of
dynamic behavior. It should be noted that the actual feedback process in D. discoideum
could involve a combination of the above mechanisms 4.1-4.3, or other biochemical mechanisms not considered in the present paper, such as the regulation of adenylate

cyclase by an activator and an inhibitor which would be synthesized intracellularly, and sequentially, upon binding of cAMP to the receptor (28,29).

Although relay and oscillation of cAMP occur in the three models considered, these models differ by quantitative aspects and by specific predictions. Thus a phase shift between free and bound extracellular cAMP is obtained in model 4.3 but not in model 4.1. Only model 4.2 is associated with a periodic change in the phosphorylation level of some protein substrate. In the long term, such specific predictions should help in delineating which of the models gives best agreement with experimental data.

Experiments have recently been performed by Devreotes et al. (28,29) under condi-tions where the extracellular level of cAMP is held constant. No sharp threshold for stimulation by cAMP was found under these conditions for the relay response. We have studied the desensitization model analyzed in section 4.3 when the positive feedback loop exerted by cAMP is suppressed; this was done by holding the extracellular cAMP level at a fixed value. The results of simulations show that under these conditions, the dose response curve for relay loses the sharp threshold characteristic of excitable systems (see Fig.7b): autocatalysis by cAMP is a necessary prerequisite for a sharp excitation threshold. This view reconciles the data of Devreotes et al. with those obtained under natural conditions where the positive feedback is operating in Dictyostelium cells; the latter data support the existence of a threshold for relay.

Coming back to the sequence of developmental transitions no relay-relay-oscilla-tions observed during interphase, we can propose a mechanism for the transitions which is based on the fact that different behavioral domains, corresponding to different pa-rameter values in each of the above models for the cAMP signalling system. One can perform a linear stability analysis for the steady state in a space formed by two key parameters, namely, adenylate cyclase and phosphodiesterase (30). The results of such analysis are shown in Fig.10 for equations derived from those of model 4.1. In the dashed domain C, the system undergoes sustained oscillations in cAMP around an unstable steady state. In domain B, the steady state is stable but excitable, for a given initial perturbation in extracellular cAMP. Elsewhere in the plane there is a unique stable, non excitable steady state, except in region E where two stable steady states may coexist.

Starting from a low activity of adenylate cyclase and phosphodiesterase, one sees that a continuous increase in both activities will bring the signalling system succes-sively through the domains of no relay, relay, and autonomous oscillation (see arrow from A in Fig.10). Later, the system could quit the oscillatory domain upon further change in adenylate cyclase or phosphodiesterase activity (arrows toward B or D). Such an explanation for the sequence of developmental transitions is supported by the obser

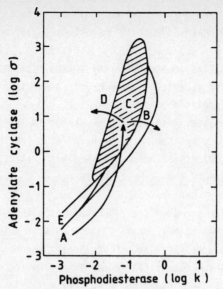

Fig.10. Developmental path for the transitions no relay-relay-oscillations in D. discoideum, based on a continuous variation in the activity of adenylate cyclase and phosphodiesterase (from ref.30).

vation that the activity of both adenylate cyclase and phosphodiesterase increases after starvation, prior to aggregation (30). The fact that a continuous variation in one or more key parameter(s) can lead to a succession of different behavioral modes is not restricted to any of the particular models 4.1-4.3, but is a property of any system capable of relay and oscillation. This view also extends to other behavioral modes corresponding, e.g., to spatiotemporal organization in morphogenesis.

Acknowledgments

The collaboration of T. Erneux and L.A. Segel in part of this work is gratefully acknowledged. J.L.M. was supported by a fellowship from D.G.R.S.T. (France).

REFERENCES

(1) Hess, B. & Boiteux, A. (1971) A. Rev. Biochem. 40, 237-58.

(2) Goldbeter, A. & Caplan, S.R. (1976) A. Rev. Biophys. Bioeng. 5, 449-76.

(3) Fessard, A. (1936) Les propriétés rythmiques de la matière vivante. Hermann, Paris.

(4) Fitzhugh, R. (1961) Biophys. J. 1, 445-66.

(5) Winfree, A.T. (1972) Science 175, 634-36.

(6) De Kepper, P. (1976) C.R. Acad. Sci., Paris, Ser.C 283, 25-28.

(7) Nicolis, G. & Prigogine, I. (1977) Self-Organization in Nonequilibrium Systems. Wiley-Interscience, New York.

(8) Bonner, J.T. (1967) The Cellular Slime Molds. Princeton Univ. Press.

(9) Loomis, W.F. (1975) Dictyostelium discoideum: A Developmental System. Academic

Press, New York.

(10) Shaffer, B. (1962) Adv. Morphogen. 2, 109-82.

(11) Gerisch, G. (1968) Curr. Top. Devel. Biol. 3, 157-97.

(12) Goldbeter, A., Erneux, T. & Segel, L.A. (1978) FEBS Lett. 89, 237-41.

(13) Konijn, T.M., van de Meene, J.G.C., Bonner, J.T. & Barkley, D.S. (1967) Proc. Nat. Acad. Sci. US 58, 1152-54.

(14) Gerisch, G. & Wick, U. (1975) Biochem. Biophys. Res. Comm. 65, 364-70.

(15) Roos, W., Nanjundiah, V., Malchow, D. & Gerisch, G. (1975) FEBS Lett. 53, 139-42.

(16) Gerisch, G. & Malchow, D. (1976) Adv. Cycl. Nucleot. Res. 7, 49-68.

(17) Tyson, J.J. (1976) The Belousov-Zhabotinsky Reaction. Lecture Notes in Biomathematics, Vol.10. Springer, Berlin.

(18) Monod, J., Wyman, J. & Changeux, J.P. (1965) J. Mol. Biol. 12, 88-118.

(19) Boiteux, A., Goldbeter, A. & Hess, B. (1975) Proc. Nat. Acad. Sci. US 72, 3829-33.

(20) Goldbeter, A. & Nicolis, G. (1976) Progr. Theoret. Biol. 4, 65-160.

(21) Goldbeter, A. (1980) In: Mathematical Models in Molecular and Cellular Biology (L.A. Segel, ed.) pp. 248-91. Cambridge Univ. Press.

(22) Goldbeter, A. & Segel, L.A. (1977) Proc. Nat. Acad. Sci. US 74, 1543-47.

(23) Martiel, J.L. & Goldbeter, A. (1981) Biochimie 63, 119-24.

(24) Krebs, E.G. & Beavo, J.A. (1979) A. Rev. Biochem. 48, 923-59.

(25) Katz, B. & Tehleff, S. (1957) J. Physiol. 138, 63-80.

(26) Heidmann, T. & Changeux, J.P. (1978) A. Rev. Biochem. 47, 317-57.

(27) Klein, C. (1979) J. Biol. Chem. 254, 12573-78.

(28) Devreotes, P.N. & Steck, T.L. (1979) J. Cell Biol. 80, 300-09.

(29) Dinauer, M.C., Steck, T.L. & Devreotes, P.N. (1980) J. Cell Biol. 86, 554-61.

(30) Goldbeter, A. & Segel, L.A. (1980) Differentiation 17, 127-35.

FULLY ASYNCHRONOUS LOGICAL DESCRIPTION OF NETWORKS COMPRISING FEEDBACK LOOPS

R. THOMAS

Laboratory of Genetics

University of Brussels (Belgium)

Summary

Much of the theoretical work on boolean networks and sequential automata deals with synchronous systems, partly because it is generally believed that the treatment of synchronous systems is desperately complicated. The purpose of this paper is to show (using methods developped before : Thomas, 1973 ; Thomas & Van Ham, 1974) that :
- a fully asynchronous logical description and treatment of this type of systems is feasible.
- that the description used here leads to a greatly enriched range of dynamical behaviours as compared with its synchronous homolog and even with other asynchronous logical descriptions.
- that, however rich, the range of dynamical behaviours is well-defined and perfectly analyzable (one does not find anything !).
- the formalism can be used to describe sequential automata (for a more formal analysis see Milgram (1982))
  synchronous if one uses equal delays.
  asynchronous if one ascribes a value to each of the time delays (two per variable).
  stochastic : if instead of ascribing to each delay a defined value one characterizes it by an average value and a distribution.
  "generalized" if one considers the value (or the average value) of each delay as a function of the state of the system.

Introduction

The systems we are dealing with consist of elements which influence the rate of production or of activity of each other. Our starting point was the study of sets of regulatory genes ; the function of each gene is to direct the synthesis of a specific product, and the various gene products influence the rate of synthesis of each other. Problems occuring in various other disciplines are in fact identical from the logical viewpoint, even though the nature of the elements and of the interactions between the elements are completely unrelated. Much of the content of this lecture can be found in scattered form elsewhere (notably in Thomas (1979) and Leclercq & Thomas (1981) from which the major example is taken). Parts of this text are common with a paper prepared at the same time (Thomas 1982), more developped but with a rather different objective.

The idea of treating complex systems of interacting elements in boolean
(logical) terms is far from new : see, for instance, in the particular
case of biological systems Rashevsky (1948), Sugita (1963), Kling & Székely (1968)
and especially Kauffman (1969, 1974) and Glass & Kauffman (1973).
Time has usually been introduced in logical formalisms by giving the logical values
of the variables "at time t + 1" as functions of their values "at time t". In practice, one tabulates the values at time t + 1 for each of the 2^n possible combinations
of values of the n variables at time t ; it is convenient to speak, for a network of
n variables, in terms of a n-vector whose value $\underline{x}_{t+1}$ at time t + 1 is given as a
function of its value $\underline{x}_t$ at time t. This version is a synchronous one ; where
$\underline{x}_{t+1}$ and $\underline{x}_t$ differ by the values of more than one variable, these values are
supposed to change   in a synchronous way at time t + 1 . The synchronous
treatment is very easy but extremely irrealistic. Among the efforts to render prac-
ticable a really* asynchronous treatment, I would like to mention especially the use
of differential equations comprising a boolean function (Glass,1975b;Tchuraev & Ratner,
1975), subsequently denoted as "PL" (piecewise linear ordinary differential) equations : Glass & Pasternak, 1978. The authors combine this quantitative description
with a logical analysis of the boolean moiety of their PL equations, using "state
transition diagrams" mapped on N-cubes (Glass 1975a), a development of the "toroid
maps" of Glass & Kauffman (1973).

The present paper deals with a purely logical, yet fully asynchronous method first
described in Thomas (1973) and Thomas & Van Ham (1974).

The logical variables and functions used.

Unlike other authors, we choose from the beginning to characterize each element i of
a system both by a logical variable α_i ("internal" variable) assciated with its
concentration (or, more generally,its level) and by a logical function a_i associated
with its rate of production (or, more generally, its flux). Variable α = 1 if the
concentration exceeds a functional threshold, α = 0 if not. Function a = 1 if the
rate of production (or activity) of the element is significant, a = 0 if not ; for
instance, in genetics a = 1 where a gene is "on", a = 0 where it is "off", and in
neurobiology a = 1 where a neurone is deshinibited, a = 0 where it is not.
There is a well-defined time relation between the values of a function a_i and its
assciated variable α_i. Let us examine this relation, taking as an example a gene

* using logical equations of the type :
$$x_i (t + \tau_i) = f_i [x_1, x_2, \ldots x_n (t)]$$
(Glass 1975a, after Kohavi 1970) is not a fully asynchronous treatment, if only because it does not allow for a distinct time delay depending on whether the variable
is on the point to switch on or off.

whose product is α . Clearly, in a steady state the logical values of a and α are the same : if a gene has been off (a = 0) for a long time, its product (which has a limited life span) will be "absent" (α = 0) ; if the gene has been on (a = 1) for a sufficient time, the product will be present (α = 1). If a change in the state of the variables results in a change of the value of a, α will adopt the new value of a, but only after a delay. In the meantime, the values of a and α will "disagree" until α has adopted the new value of a ; during this period, variable α is subject to an order to switch from its present value to the complementary value. For instance when a gene is switched on, the product will appear, but not until some minutes (necessary for the synthesis and accumulation of the product), and when the gene is switched off its product will disappear, but only after a delay which depends on its life span, diffusibility etc ...

Thus, we associate with each couple i (function a_i, variable α_i) two delays, one for the appearance, one for the disappearance of the product. Note that, formally, the relationship between a function a_i and its associated variable α_i is the same as the relation between a logical function Y_i and its memorization variables y_i, as used in sequential automata (Huffman,1954 ; Florine,1964);one difference is that a function Y_i and its memorization variable y_i are one and the same thing "seen" at different times while our function a_i and the corresponding variable α_i represent qualitatively distinct things (a rate of production and a concentration, respectively).

An important feature of our method is the simplifying assumption that when, starting from a situation in which $a_i = \alpha_i$, one changes the value of a_i, the value of α_i will change after a characteristic delay unless a counter order (an additional change of the value of a_i) is given before the delay has elapsed ; and if such a counter order has taken place before the order has been executed, we reason as if the order had been merely cancelled (see Thomas & Van Ham, 1974 and Van Ham, 1975). As all simplifying assumptions, this rule may introduce distorsions in particular cases ; however, the gain in simplificity by far compensates these occasional distorsions.

Logical equations.

Our logical equations usually describe systems by relating the logical values of the functions a_i (rates of production) with the values of the internal variables α_i (concentrations) and of input variables such as temperature (T) :

$$a_i = \phi_i (\alpha_1, \alpha_2, ... \alpha_i, ..., \alpha_n ; T, ...)$$

in which ϕ_i is a boolean function. In a vectorial notation :

$$\underline{a} = \phi (\underline{\alpha} ; T).$$

If one compares these equations to the logical equations frequently used which relate the situation at time t + 1 to the situation at time t, one may ask where time is hidden in our equations. In fact, it is present in an <u>implicit</u> way (just as in the differential equations used in chemical kinetics) because one relates <u>rates</u> of production to concentrations. Time is, on the other hand, present in an <u>explicit</u> way as time delays which relate changes in the logical value of each concentration α_i with previous changes in the value of the corresponding rate of synthesis a_i .

Here is an example, taken from Leclercq and Thomas (1981), of a logical scheme and the corresponding logical equations. The logical scheme (left) represents a system comprising two conjugated feedback loops, a negative one and a positive one. For instance $\beta \longrightarrow \alpha$ means that the condition for the synthesis of α is the absence of β , and

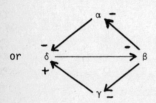

$$\begin{array}{c} \alpha \\ \text{or} \xrightarrow{\quad} \delta \\ \gamma \end{array}$$ means that δ is synthesized iff α is absent or (inclusive) γ is present.

The corresponding set of logical equations is :

$$a = \bar{\beta}$$
$$b = \bar{\delta}$$
$$c = \bar{\beta}$$
$$d = \bar{\alpha} + \gamma$$

in which $\bar{\beta}$ means (not β) and + is the logical sum (inclusive or).

<u>State tables.</u>

From the logical equations which describe a system, we derive a state table which gives the values of the functions a_i for each of the 2^n combinations of values of the n variables α_i (Thomas, 1973) . In spite of a superficial similitude, these tables deeply differ from the classical ones because instead of tabulating $\underline{x}_{t+1}$ as a function of $\underline{x}_t$ we tabulate the logical values of the rates of production (fluxes) for each combination of values of the concentrations ; thus, the boolean "vector" in the right column is usually <u>not</u> the next state for the boolean vector at the same line in the left column.Table 1 is the state table corresponding to the logical scheme and equations given above.

Table 1.

α β γ δ	a b c d
$\bar{0}\ \bar{0}\ \bar{0}\ \bar{0}$	1 1 1 1
$\bar{0}\ 0\ \bar{0}\ 1$	1 0 1 1
$\bar{0}\ 0\ 1\ 1$	1 0 1 1
$\bar{0}\ \bar{0}\ 1\ \bar{0}$	1 1 1 1
0 1 1 $\bar{0}$	0 1 0 1
0 $\bar{1}\ \bar{1}$ 1	0 0 0 1
0 $\bar{1}$ 0 1	0 0 0 1
0 1 0 $\bar{0}$	0 1 0 1
$\bar{1}$ 1 0 0	0 1 0 0
$\bar{1}$ 1 0 $\bar{1}$	0 0 0 0
$\bar{1}\ \bar{1}\ \bar{1}$ 1	0 0 0 1
$\bar{1}$ 1 $\bar{1}\ \bar{0}$	0 1 0 1
1 $\bar{0}$ 1 $\bar{0}$	1 1 1 1
1 0 1 1	1 0 1 1
1 0 0 $\bar{1}$	1 0 1 0
1 $\bar{0}\ \bar{0}$ 0	1 1 1 0

Table 1. State table
For each of the 2^4 combinations of values of the 4 variables, this state table gives the values of the associated functions, as provided by the logical equations :

$$a = \bar{\beta}$$
$$b = \bar{\delta}$$
$$c = \bar{\beta}$$
$$d = \bar{\alpha} + \gamma$$

Where vectors $\underset{\sim}{\alpha}$ and $\underline{a}$ are the same, in other words where the value of each function "agrees" with the value of the corresponding variable, one deals with a stable state since no variable is requested to change its value. For instance, in Table 1, for α β γ δ = 1 0 1 1 one has also a b c d = 1 0 1 1 ; this is a stable state and we write ⟨1 0 1 1⟩. For the other states, one or more function "disagrees" with the corresponding variable, whose value in thus requested to change. We draw the attention on this situation by writing a dash over the values of the variables which disagree with the corresponding functions. For instance, where αβγδ|abcd=1110/0101 we write $\bar{1}$ 1 $\bar{1}\ \bar{0}$. This compact notation depicts the fact that variables α and γ are requested to switch from 1 to 0 and variable δ from 0 to 1.

Graph of the sequences of states.

In a synchronous system, the state following $\bar{1}$ 1 $\bar{1}\ \bar{0}$ would be 0 1 0 1 , with a synchronous change of the values of three variables. We reason rather (Thomas,1973) that either of the orders will be executed, thus leading in the present case to either of three possible next states :

$$\bar{1}\ 1\ \bar{1}\ \bar{0} \quad \xrightarrow{\bar{\alpha}} \quad 0\ 1\ \bar{1}\ \bar{0}$$
$$\xrightarrow{\bar{\gamma}} \quad \bar{1}\ 1\ 0\ \bar{0}$$
$$\xrightarrow{\delta} \quad \bar{1}\ \bar{1}\ \bar{1}\ 1$$

where the dashes in the right members are taken from the state table.

(Usually, we do not consider explicity the possibility that two or more commutations take place in exact simultaneity Should this happen, the situation would be taken into account automatically in the simulations, however).

Consider, for instance, transition $\bar{1}\,1\,\bar{1}\,\bar{0} \xrightarrow{\;\;\overline{\gamma}\;\;} \bar{1}\,1\,0\,0$, in which variable γ switches from 1 to 0 . In the resultant state $\bar{1}\,1\,0\,0$, the order $\bar{\alpha}$ is still present but the order δ has disappeared ; and in accordance with the rule mentioned p. 3 we reason as if this order to synthesize δ had been merely cancelled, because a counter-order (involved in the transition $\bar{1}\,1\,\bar{1}\,\bar{0}\xrightarrow{\;\;\overline{\gamma}\;\;}\bar{1}\,1\,0\,0$) has taken place before the order has been executed.

In this way, one can derive graphs of the sequences of states. When pro-ceeding to this construction, it is essential to realize that <u>different occurences of a same boolean state may correspond to non-identical situations</u>. For instance, in the sequence :

$$\bar{0}\bar{0}\bar{0}\bar{0}\xrightarrow{\;\alpha\;}1\underset{11}{\bar{0}}\bar{0}0\xrightarrow{\;\beta\;}\bar{1}100\xrightarrow{\;\bar{\alpha}\;}0100\xrightarrow{\;\delta\;}0\bar{1}01\xrightarrow{\;\bar{\beta}\;}\bar{0}0\underset{1}{\bar{0}}1\xrightarrow{\;\alpha\;}1\bar{0}\bar{1}\xrightarrow{\;\bar{\delta}\;}1\underset{2}{\bar{0}}\bar{0}0\xrightarrow{\;\beta\;}\bar{1}100\longrightarrow\ldots$$

the binary state $1\,\bar{0}\,\bar{0}\,0$ occurs twice.

However, these states are <u>not</u> equivalent since in the first case both orders β and γ were already present in the former state ($\bar{0}\,\bar{0}\,\bar{0}\,\bar{0}$) while in the second case order β was not yet present in the former state ($1\,0\,\bar{0}\,\bar{1}$) but the order γ was already present two steps ahead (state $\bar{0}\,0\,\bar{0}\,1$). This can be expressed by subscripts (Leclercq & Thomas, 1981) which indicate whether (and for how many steps) an order was already present in former states ; thus in the first case we write $1\,\underset{1\,1}{\bar{0}}\,\bar{0}\,0$ and in the second case $1\,\underset{2}{\bar{0}}\,\bar{0}\,0$. Two states with different subscripts <u>are</u> different ; two states with the same index <u>may</u> be identical (as, for instance, in the two occurences of the boo-lean state $\bar{1}\,1\,0\,0$, which has <u>no</u> subscript in either case ; in both cases, the delay $t_{\bar{\alpha}}$ begins to run exactly at the onset of state $\bar{1}\,1\,0\,0$).

<u>Conditions of the various sequences of states ; logical stability analysis.</u>

Which pathway will be effectively followed, depends on the relative values of the time delays. Simple cases have been treated in Thomas (1973) and Thomas & Van Ham (1974). Let us come back to our example. In a situation like

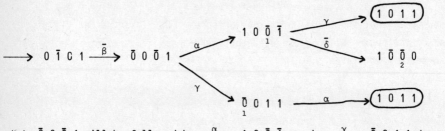

state $\bar{0}\,0\,\bar{0}\,1$ will be followed by $\xrightarrow{\;\alpha\;} 1\,0\,\underset{1}{\bar{0}}\,\bar{1}$ or by $\xrightarrow{\;\gamma\;} \underset{1}{\bar{0}}\,0\,1\,1$ depending simply on whether the time delay t_α is shorter or longer than t_γ. From $1\,0\,\bar{0}\,\bar{1}$, the system may proceed to $\xrightarrow{\gamma}$ ($1\,0\,1\,1$) or to $\xrightarrow{\bar{\delta}}$ $1\,\bar{0}\,\bar{0}\,0$. In this case, the situation is slightly more complicated because the order to synthesize γ was already present during the preceeding period whereas the order $\bar{\delta}$ has been given only at the onset of state $1\,0\,\bar{0}\,\bar{1}$; thus, the decision depends on whether $t_\gamma < t_\alpha + t_{\bar{\delta}}$ or vice versa (here, the signe + is the arithmetic, not the logical, sum!). With each fork in the graph of the sequences of states, one can associate inequalities (one for a <u>bifurca-</u><u>tion</u>, three for a <u>trifurcation</u>, etc...) between the time delays or their entire linear combinations. Thus, with any sequence of states one can associate a set of inequalities which give the conditions necessary and sufficient for this sequence to be followed.

In particular, when one finds a state which has already been found upsteam (with the same subscript   if any), one may determine in which conditions this trajectory can be followed as a cycle.

Without entering into details, let us mention that one finds stable and unstable cycles. <u>Stable cycles</u> are so named because in the 2n dimensional space of the delays their domain of stability occupies a 2n dimensional variety ; one can thus modify the value of one or more delay(within certain limits) without leaving the domain of stability of the cycle.

<u>Unstable</u> cycles are characterized by the fact that among the relations between the delays there is one (or more) equality ; it ensues that the domain of stability is a 2n-1 dimensional variety in the 2n dimensional space of the delays, and any modification of one of the delays involved in an equality leads the system to leave the cycle.

We do <u>not</u> consider as cycles situations like the following :

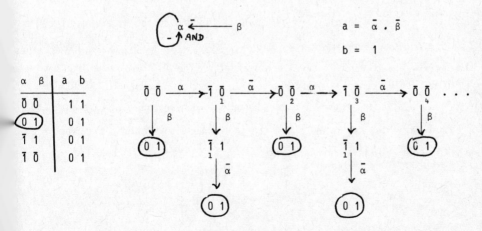

in which the successive occurences of $\bar{0}\,\bar{0}$ (or of $\bar{1}\,\bar{0}$) are different, as shown by the increasing value of their subscript. One easily sees that there can be for some time an oscillation $\bar{0}\,\bar{0} \underset{\bar{\alpha}}{\overset{\alpha}{\rightleftharpoons}} \bar{1}\,\bar{0}$ if the time delay t_β is long enough, but sooner or later one will fall into the stable state $(0\ 1)$. This is apparently the logical equivalent of a <u>damped oscillation</u>.

As an example of our stability analysis, let us examine the simplest cyclic trajectory in the double-loop system already considered above :

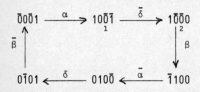

At the level of state $\bar{0}0\bar{0}1$, there is a fork :

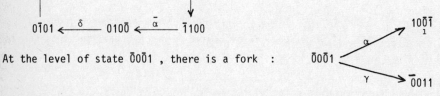

Whether the first or the second choice is adopted depends on whether or not $t_\alpha < t_\gamma$. We pose $m \equiv t_\alpha < t_\gamma$; $m = 1$ if the statement "$t_\alpha < t_\gamma$" is true, $m = 0$ if not. At the level of state $10\bar{0}\bar{1}$ there is a second fork :

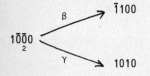

Whether the first or the second choice is adopted depends on whether or not $t_\gamma < t_\alpha + t_{\bar{\delta}}$. We pose $n \equiv t_\gamma < t_\alpha + t_{\bar{\delta}}$. At the level of state $1\bar{0}\bar{0}0_2$ there is a third and last fork :

$$1\bar{0}\bar{0}0_2 \begin{cases} \xrightarrow{\beta} \bar{1}100 \\ \xrightarrow{\gamma} 1010 \end{cases}$$

Whether the first or the second choice is adopted depends on whether or not $t_\alpha + t_{\bar{\delta}} + t_\beta < t_\gamma$. We pose $p \equiv t_\alpha + t_{\bar{\delta}} + t_\beta < t_\gamma$. Thus, the conditions to remain in this cyclic trajectory are : $m\,\bar{n}\,p$. However, one can take advantage of the fact that variables m, n and p are not independent to simplify the expression of the conditions of stability of the cycle :

$$
\begin{aligned}
m &\equiv t_\alpha < t_\gamma \\
n &\equiv t_\gamma < t_\alpha + t_{\bar{\delta}} \\
p &\equiv t_\alpha + t_{\bar{\delta}} + t_\beta < t_\gamma
\end{aligned}
\left.\begin{aligned} &\text{Thus, } \bar{n} \to m \\ &\text{Thus, } p \to \bar{n} \end{aligned}\right.
$$

Clearly, if $p \rightarrow \bar{n}$ and $\bar{n} \rightarrow m$, the conditions $m \bar{n} p$ reduce to p . Thus the only condition to remain in this trajectory is : $t_\alpha + t_{\bar\delta} + t_\beta < t_\gamma$.

For more information about this logical stability analysis see Thomas (1979 , Chapt.6 ; 1982) and Leclercq & Thomas (1981). Most of the procedure has been automatized (Van Ham & De Hoeck, 1979 ; Van Ham, in preparation).

The final states.

The graph of the sequences of states may lead to one or more final states or attractors,which may be <u>stable states</u> , already detected at the level of the state tables or <u>stable cycles</u> (presumably also "strange" attractors, i.e. chaotic situations).

As far as we can tell, a necessary (but not sufficient) condition for multiple attractors is that the logical structure comprise at least one positive loop, and a necessary (but not sufficient) condition for a stable periodic behaviour is the presence of at least one negative loop in the logical structure.For instance, a simple positive loop can provide for two attractors (in this case, two stable states). In order to have <u>both</u> multiple attractors and sustained oscillations, one needs at least two loops, a positive and a negative ones;the system taken as an example in this paper provides for two attractors, a stable state and a stable cycle. Note that except for very simple systems a stable cycle may display various sequences of boolean states depending on the values of the time delays (just in the same way as, in the continuous description, a limit cycle has various shapes depending on the values of the parameters) ; among these variants one may find cycles with multiple periodicities : see Leclercq & Thomas 1981 and Thomas 1982.
For instance the family of trajectories :

$$
\left[10\bar{1}0 \xrightarrow{\beta} \bar{1}1\bar{1}0 \xrightarrow{\delta} \bar{1}\bar{1}\bar{1}1 \xrightarrow{\bar\gamma} \bar{1}\bar{1}0\bar{1} \xrightarrow{\bar\beta} 10\bar{1} \xrightarrow{\bar\delta} 1\bar{0}0\bar{0} \right]_m
$$

$$
\downarrow \gamma \qquad\qquad\qquad\qquad\qquad\qquad \downarrow \beta
$$

$$
1\bar{0}0\bar{0} \xleftarrow{\bar\delta} 10\bar{0}\bar{1} \xleftarrow{\alpha} \bar{0}00\bar{1} \xleftarrow{\bar\beta} 0\bar{1}01 \xleftarrow{\delta} 010\bar{0} \xleftarrow{\bar\alpha} \bar{1}100
$$

in which m can take any integer value including 0. When m = 0 , one rejoins the simple case chosen above for the logical stability analysis ; as for the sequence between brackets, it is the unstable cycle of the system.

On the relation between this discrete description and the continuous description using differential equations.

The differential equations used for the description of regulatory systems are most frequently of the type :

$$\dot{x}_i = f_i \ (x_1, x_2, \ldots x_n) - k_{-i} \ x_i$$, in which f_i is a sigmoid function and $- k_{-i} \ x_i$ is a term of decay, assumed to be proportional to the concentration of the substance (Goodwin, 1965 , Griffith 1968 and others). As pointed out e.g. by Walter (1967) and by Glass & Kauffman (1972, 1973) these functions tend to step functions as the sigmoid becomes steeper and steeper.

In order to make a parallel between this type of differential equations and our logical equations, it is convenient to re-write the differential equation :

$$\dot{x}_i + k_{-i} \ x_i = f_i \ (x_1, x_2, \ldots x_n)$$

and remark that the two members are homologous respectively, to the two members of our logical equations.

$$a_i = \phi_i \ (\alpha_1, \alpha_2, \ldots \alpha_n)$$

Our functions a_i are the logical equivalents, not of the time derivatives $\dot{x}_i$, but of $\dot{x}_1 + k_{-i} \ x_i$, which represents the gross rate of synthesis of x_i (not corrected for the decay term $- k_{-i} \ x_i$).

In the continuous formalism, the determination of the trajectories involves an integration, which can be made analytically only in very simple cases, but has to be made numerically in most practical situations ; when this is the case, it may be difficult to have a general idea of the dynamical possibilities of the system.

Our logical treatment can also proceed without ascribing any numerical value to the time delays (this is the "analytical" approach) ; or, one can ascribe values to the delays (this is the "numerical" approach, for which one can use the logical simulator "Delphine" : Van Ham, 1979 or computer programs : Van Ham & Dehoeck, 1979).

A key of the efficiency of the method (and the reason why it can deal with complex systems) is that the set of trajectories consistent with a logical structure can always be obtained in the analytical mode :

a) for each state, one knows from the state table which next states are conceivable in the system.
b) any sequence can be analyzed in order to see in which conditions (if any) it will be followed.

As regards the correspondance between the previsions of our boolean description and of the continuous description, one does not expect them to fit entirely, in view of the different simplifying assumptions. An important paper by Glass and Kauffman (1972) shows, however, that in the cases chosen the transition from a sigmoid interaction to a Heaviside (that is all - or - none) interaction does not alter the qualitative dynamics of the system.   There are some problems ; for instance, what is described in boolean descriptions as a stable cycle may be in the continuous description a limit cycle or a stable steady state depending on the values of the parameters or delays.   This problem was analyzed with a deep insight by Richelle (1977, 1979, 1980) ;see also Thomas, Nicolis, Richelle and Van Ham, 1979. Let us simply recall here that in living processes the occurrence of macro-molecular syntheses practically forces one to take incompressible time lags into account, and once this is done the constraints for obtaining permanent oscillations are largely relaxed ; another simple consideration is that where the logical analysis predicts a permanent oscillation and the continuous analysis a stable steady state, the former may be right at the level of the individual cells and the latter at the level of the population.

In the example used throughout this paper, the logical analysis predicts a choice between two attractors (a stable state and a stable cycle), depending on the initial   state and values of the time delays (with the theoretical possibility of an unstable cycle between the two attractors).   The translation into the continuous language is   : for proper values of the parameters there is a choice (depending on the initial state and values of the parameters) between two attractors. One of them is a stable state and the second is a limit cycle or a stable steady state depending on the values of the parameters ; and between these two attractors there is an unstable steady state.   The continuous system is already too complex to be treated analytically .   However, starting from the logical analysis, it has been possible to find values of the parameters   such that the continuous system has indeed the choice between a stable steady state and a limit cycle, depending on the initial state ; we found also values of the parameters such that the cycle has a multiple periodicity, a possibility suggested by our boolean analysis (Leclercq & Thomas, 1981).

The reverse operation : given a set of interacting elements, find the types of connections which will permit a given behaviour.

In this case there is, needless to say , a multiplicity of solutions. This inductive (or synthetic) pathway is usually lead in an essentially intuitive way;see however Huffman (1954) and Florine (1964)for the "synthesis" of logical machines.This type of problems has been treated in the case of neuronal networks:given a set of neurones and their phase diagram, find interactions, as simple as possible, which will permit (or impose) this phase diagram (Thomas, 1979). Another simple problem (interactions providing for three stable states) has been treated for a three - variable system (Thomas, 1981) and since for a two - variable system (unpublished).   A more sophisticated case (a four - dimensional system with two cyclic attractors operating in opposite directions) will be described in Thomas (1982). In each of these cases, it has been checked that in the continuous system derived from the logical equations there are values of the parameters which lead to the wanted dynamics.

References

Florine, J. (1964). La synthèse des machines logiques. (Presses académiques Europé--ennes, Bruxelles), 345 pp.
Glass, L. (1975a) J. theor. Biol. 54, 85-107.
Glass, L. (1975b) J. Chem. Phys. 63, 1325-1335.
Glass, L. & Kauffman, S.A. (1972) J. theor. Biol. 34, 219-237.
Glass, L. & Kauffman, S.A. (1973) J. theor. Biol. 39, 103-129.
Glass, L. & Pasternak, J.S. (1978) Bull. Math. Biol. 40, 27-44.
Goodwin, B.C. (1965) Adv. Enzyme Regulation, 3, 425.
Griffith, J.S. (1968) J. theor. Biol. 20, 202-216.
Huffman, D.A. (1954) J. Franklin Inst. 257, 161-189.
Kauffman, S.A. (1969) J. theor. Biol. 22, 437-467.
Kauffman, S.A. (1974) J. theor. Biol. 44, 167-190.
Kling, U. & Székely, G. (1968) Kybernetik 5, 89-103.
Kohavi (1970) Switching and Finite Automata, Chap.II. New York : Mc Graw-Hill.
Leclercq, J. & Thomas, R. (1981) Bull. Cl. Sci. Acad. Roy. Belg. 67, 190-225.
Leussler, A. & Van Ham, P. (1979) Lecture Notes in Biomathematics 29, 62-106.
Rashevsky, N. (1948) Mathematical Biophysics, The University of Chicago Press.
Richelle, J. (1977) Bull. Classe Sci. Acad. Roy. Belg. 63, 534-546.
Richelle, J. (1979) Lecture Notes in Biomathematics 29, 281-325.
Richelle, J. (1981) Mémoires Acad. Roy. Belg. 67, 890-912.
Sugita, M. (1963) J. theor. Biol. 4, 179-192.
Tchuraev, R.N. & Ratner, V.A. (1975) in "Studies on Mathematical Genetics (V.A. Ratner, ed.) p.5. Inst. Cytol. Genet. Press, Novosibirsk (in Russian).
Thomas, R. (1973) J. theor. Biol. 42, 563-585.
Thomas, R. (1978) J. theor. Biol. 73, 631-656.
Thomas, R. (1979) Lecture Notes in Biomathematics 29, 107, 142 & 354-401.
Thomas, R. (1981) Springer Series in Synergetics 9, 180-193.
Thomas, R. (1982) Adv. Phys. Chem. (in press)
Thomas, R., Nicolis, G., Richelle, J. & Van Ham, P. (1979) Lecture Notes in Biomathe--mathics 29, 345-352.
Thomas, R. & Van Ham, P. (1974) Biochimie 56, 1529-1547.
Van Ham, P. (1975) Thesis, University of Brussels.
Van Ham, P. (1979) Lecture Notes in Biomathematics 29, 143-148.
Van Ham, P. & Dehoeck, J.L. (1979) Lecture Note in Biomathematics 29, 149-163.
Walter, C. (1967) in Quantitative Biology of Metabolism (A. Locker, ed ; Springer) pp.38-44.
Milgram, M. (1982) Thesis Université de Compiègne France

Acknowledgements

This work was carried out under contract Euratom-ULB, with an agreement between the Belgian Government and the Université libre de Bruxelles concerning priority action for collective basic research and with the help of the "Fonds de la Recherche Fonda-mentale Collective".

THE ROTOR IN REACTION-DIFFUSION PROBLEMS
AND IN SUDDEN CARDIAC DEATH

Arthur T. Winfree
Department of Biological Sciences
Purdue University
West Lafayette, Indiana 47907

1. Abstract.

For many years it has been speculated that some forms of heart failure derive ultimately from the instigation of rotating waves in the excitable neuro-electric tissue of the ventricle. I show here that exactly such a peculiar event can easily arise by the action of a spatially graded perturbation on a nerve-like medium which has recently conducted a periodically recurrent wave. The arguments are only geometrical, computational, and heuristic, and they only establish appropriate initial conditions, without specifying conditions to guarantee persistence of the wave so initiated. However, a diversity of experimental examples encourage the belief that mathematical labors in this direction might be rewarded with a stability proof.

2. Excitable Media.

My purpose here is to exhibit a parallelism between certain aspects of heart physiology and corresponding aspects of physical chemistry in the Belousov-Zhabotinsky reagent. Its basic features have been noted before, but we can now additionally connect the earlier story to topological aspects of phase shifting in limit-cycle oscillators (1).

Krinskii (2), Troy (3), and Winfree (4,5) have drawn attention to the mathematical correspondence between Belousov-Zhabotinsky solution and other excitable media, e.g., neural membranes. In a nutshell, all exhibit a globally attracting steady-state not far from a saddle-like region of flow beyond which trajectories execute a large excursion before inevitably returning to the steady state. In spontaneously oscillating excitable media, matters stand much the same except that trajectories only GRAZE the steady state and pass on to another excursion without assistance from any external stimulus (or, if you like, a chronic stimulus is built into the spontaneous dynamics).

3. Excitability Spatially Coupled by Diffusion.

We now redirect our interest from the ordinary differential equations of spatially homogeneous kinetics in a stirred tank reactor to the partial differential equations of a spatially extended medium. The striking similarity between chemical excitability and neuroelectric excitability remains and is even enhanced. In the chemical case, a Laplacian operator is added to the local kinetics to represent molecular diffusion. In the neuroelectric case, the same operator is added to represent electric current flow along potential gradients.

4. Phase Resetting Limit-Cycle Oscillators.

Consider first a spatially homogeneous bioelectric membrane, spontaneously oscillating as in a pacemaker neuron. A discrete perturbation kicks its state point off the attracting limit cycle, to which it presently returns with some discrepancy of timing relative to an unperturbed control. This offset of timing depends on both the timing and the magnitude of the stimulus. This dependence is best described by a 3-dimensional plot that resembles a screw surface (6,7). Figure 1 shows the contour map of one such surface. This one was calculated from the Hodgkin-Huxley equations of rhythmically firing squid axon subjected to a current pulse (8,9).

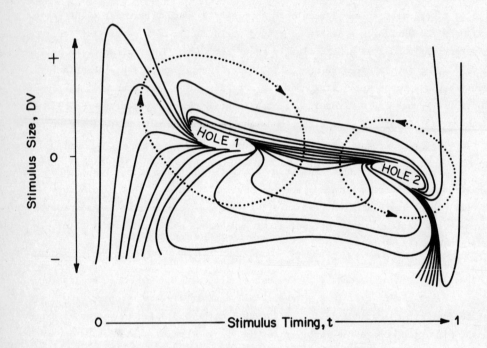

Figure 1.   This contour map shows loci on the plane of stimulus size (zero in the middle, positive above, negative below) and stimulus timing (spanning one full cycle left to right) which result in resetting a Hodgkin-Huxley pacemaker to the same phase. Phase values on these contours vary through one full cycle clockwise around HOLE 1 and counterclockwise around HOLE 2. For detail see (9,16,17).

5. Black Holes.

The essential qualitative feature of this contour map for present purposes is the CONVERGENCE of contour lines to a BLACK HOLE in the half-plane of positive stimuli and to another in the complementary half-plane of negative stimuli. Each contour line joins the two BLACK HOLES. The BLACK HOLE may be arbitrarily small, even as

small as an isolated point singularity bringing together all the contour lines. This
curiosity is well understood theoretically — indeed, it was predicted from theory
(10) — and seems now to find experimental confirmation as well (11,12).

The topological analysis of attracting limit cycle kinetics leads to the inference (13) that the same qualitative pattern will be found when the corresponding
measurements are carried out on the FKN model (14) or an actual Belousov-Zhabotinsky
solution in a CSTR (e.g., using ultraviolet irradiation or bromide injections). This
remains to be verified.

6. Phase Resetting in a Spatial Gradient.

Now consider the implications for a spatially extended thin layer of excitable
medium, subjected to a spatially graded stimulus. Imagine a train of parallel plane
waves (ideally "pseudo-waves," i.e., phase gradients little affected by diffusion of
molecules or electric potential; see (13) page 305). Let each wavefront extend north-
south, the wave proceeding from east to west. A perturbation falling on the medium
(e.g., ultraviolet light or acetylcholine from a widely branching vagus nerve) finds
volume elements at various phases in the cycle according to distance behind the
nearest wavefront to the left — exactly as described by the horizontal axis in Figure
1. The vertical axis in Figure 1 represents stimulus magnitude, from zero to infinity
in the upper half-plane. In the chemical analogue, we might achieve that arrangement
by grading the UV irradiance from zero upward to some extreme.

According to the scheme of Figure 1, this should result in resetting the phase
of parochial oscillation in each volume element, according to its initial phase and
the local exposure. The contour lines of Figure 1 then represent loci of uniform
phase, i.e., of identical time-until-turning-from-red-to-blue or time-until-bioelec-
tric-discharge. They therefore represent the successive positions of a wavefront
(specifically, of a "pseudo-wave"). This locus apparently rotates about an ambigu-
ously-phased pivot point once in every period of the spontaneous oscillation.

7. Does Spatial Coupling Allow or Preclude Stable Wave Circulation?

This hand-waving argument ignores the spatial coupling of adjacent volume elements, blithely pretending that the autonomous ordinary differential equation is unaffected by molecular diffusion (in the case of the Belousov-Zhabotinsky reaction)
or by electric currents (in the case of neural membranes). This might be an excellent
approximation were the experiment conducted on a gargantuan scale with correspondingly
shallow gradients of timing and of perturbation magnitude.

But even in this situation, contour lines AFTER perturbation converge to the
boundary of a BLACK HOLE. Whether the latter be a finite disk or a mere point, contour lines approach infinite density there (15), so the gradients of phase AFTER perturbation exceed any pre-established limit. Consequently, the Laplacian term MUST
be reckoned with. Can it alter the TOPOLOGICAL configuration of the wave grandly
rotating along the horizon? If not, then we have created a "reverberator," a "rotor."

I know no mathematical proof but believe this to be the case.

8. Rotating Waves in Excitable Cardiac Tissue.

In the case of neural media, graded stimuli do commonly fall upon sheets of periodically firing cells, spatially graded in their timing. The heart is such an organ. Electric currents and vagal arborizations (in the atria) provide such stimuli. Perniciously stable rotating waves have been initiated in heart muscle by procedures similar to that idealized above (see 16,17 for citations). There is some speculation that this constitutes one mode of SUDDEN CARDIAC DEATH, a mysteriously abrupt and lethally catastrophic onset of arrhythmia in the normal healthy heart (16,17).

9. Experimentally Stable Rotors.

In emphasizing continuity and homogeneity, the arguments presented here differ from the pioneering insights of Moe et al. (18,19,20) and of Krinskii (2,21,22) which emphasized heterogeneity and discontinuities. I believe that turbulence is implicit even in the equations of voltage and permeability for membranes of smoothly-graded properties. Moe et al. (op. cit.) implicitly argued along these lines by comparing fibrillation to hydrodynamic turbulence, even writing a mathematical expression analogous to the Reynolds' number.

Rozenstraukh et al. (23) make an argument of this sort using vagal stimulation of the atrium to introduce a TEMPORARY inhomogeneity, much as we here use a graded stimulus. Gulko and Petrov (24) also computed a stable rotor in a homogeneous Hodgkin-Huxley-like medium. The rotor computed by Shcherbunov et al. (25) was among the first using continuous media described by continuous partial differential equation (the Noble equation), but the computation included a parameter gradient, and the rotor proved quickly unstable. Others, without parameter gradients, prove stable (26,27). Analogous vorticity in an electrochemical excitable medium (28,29) was observed in Lillie's iron wire preparation of a half century ago, extended to two dimensions by replacing the single wire with a mesh. A spatially graded stimulus was applied in the wake of a wave to initiate a rotor.

Are vorticity and turbulence latent even in simple homogeneous excitable media? An answer was attempted (30) by lowering a large iron SPHERE into a vat of nitric acid — such an unlikely scene in a medical school that the experimenters took the trouble to film it. The spherical surface eliminated the edge effects inevitable to Nagumo's independent experiment with a flat iron gridwork and admitted the possibility of "circus waves" along closed great-circle paths. The movies, kindly loaned to me by Professor Guyton, show much disorganized wave motion, but I believe it consists mostly of simple waves from a point origin, complicated by convection and bubbling of the nitric acid. The experiment would have to be tried again under gravity-free conditions to serve its intended purpose.

A more convenient chemical analog of excitable media was invented in the U.S.S.R. (31). The remarkable similarity of its kinetics to the Hodgkin-Huxley kinetics has become the subject of many technical papers by mathematicians and physical chemists (3,5,13,32-34).

Krinskii (21,22) came very close to anticipating these rotating excitations on purely theoretical grounds. It is perhaps hair-splitting for me to refer to them as "rotors" rather than by his much earlier term "reverberators." I do so only to emphasize that rotors can be understood in the continuous terms of kinetics and diffusion, whereas the original reverberator was specifically a consequence of discontinuity and inhomogeneity either in the physical medium or in the time course of its excitation at any point. The lifetime of a reverberator and its prospects of multiplying were determined by those factors. Discontinuity and inhomogeneity are real properties of myocardium and undoubtedly do much to condition the detailed development of vorticity; but the point I wish to emphasize here is that they are not the essential causes of vorticity. The rotor can be induced and is stable even in perfectly homogeneous media with smooth kinetics.

Now going back to the individual rotor, it is of interest to enquire about the state of the membrane near its center, about which the wave pivots. In the earliest experiments with circulating waves (35-38), there was no center; circulation on a ring was ensured by punching a hole in the medium. The pulmonary vasculature plays the role of a hole in arguments about atrial flutter as a "circus wave" (39). In experiments (40-42) a wave of spreading depression rotates persistently in a sheet of neurons, but the center of the rotation is an inexcitable lesion — functionally a hole. The first mathematical analysis (43) required a hole of a certain minimum circumference around which a normal action potential might circulate indefinitely. The hole can be replaced by a discontinuity of much smaller dimensions in the case of a more heart-like medium with a prolonged excited state (22,44). By all these subterfuges, the question was evaded, "What is going on at the center of a rotating wave? Is the medium there always refractory? If so, why doesn't it recover to excitability? If not, why doesn't the wave short-circuit through the excitable center?"

Allessie et al. (45-47) were the first to deliberately create and document a rotor in real myocardium (the left atrium of a rabbit) and to focus attention on its center. They observed irregular incursions of wavelets from the excitation circulating around the center, passing through the center while attenuating, and finally dying out in the still-refractory tissue on the far side. This irregularity might not be due to structural and functional inhomogeneity in the preparation. Even in ideally homogeneous and isotropic excitable media the center can behave irregularly (24,48-52). The causes of this irregularity are not yet understood, but the consequence is that the inner endpoint of the wave lashes about unpredictably and the rotor wanders around. This behavior seems to contribute to the mutual extinction of clockwise and counterclockwise rotors packed too close together. It may therefore be important to study in connection with recovery from fibrillation.

ACKNOWLEDGMENTS

This work was supported by the United States National Science Foundation under grant CHE-77-24649 and by the Institute for Natural Philosophy.

REFERENCES

1. A. T. Winfree, Arch. Biochem. Biophys. 149:388 (1972).
2. V. I. Krinskii, Pharmac. Ther. B. 3:539 (1978).
3. W. C. Troy, Theor. Chem. 4:133 (1978).
4. A. T. Winfree, Adv. Biol. Med. Phys. 16:115 (1977).
5. A. T. Winfree, Lecture Notes in Biomathematics 2:243 (1974).
6. A. T. Winfree, Lectures on Mathematics in the Life Sciences 2:109 (1970).
7. A. T. Winfree, J. Theor. Biol. 28:327 (1970).
8. E. Best, Biophys. J. 27:87 (1979).
9. A. T. Winfree, Lectures in Applied Mathematics 19:265 (1981).
10. A. T. Winfree, Science 197:761 (1977).
11. R. Guttman, S. Lewis, and J. Rinzel, J. Physiol. (London) 305:377 (1980).
12. J. Jalife, and C. Antzelevitch, Science 206:695 (1979).
13. A. T. Winfree, The Geometry of Biological Time, Springer, New York (1980).
14. R. J. Field, E. Koros, and R. M. Noyes, J. Amer. Chem. Soc. 94:8649 (1972).
15. J. Guckenheimer, J. Math. Biol. 1:259 (1976).
16. A. T. Winfree, in Cardiac Rate and Rhythm, H. Jongsma and L. Bouman, eds., in press.
17. A. T. Winfree, Scientific American, in press.
18. G. K. Moe, and J. A. Abildskov, Amer. Heart J. 58:59 (1959).
19. G. K. Moe, Arch. Int. Pharmacodyn. 140:183 (1962).
20. G. K. Moe, W. C. Rheinboldt, and J. A. Abildskov, Amer. Heart J. 67:200 (1964).
21. V. I. Krinskii, Biofizika 11:676 (1966).
22. V. I. Krinskii, Prob. Kibernetiki 20:59 (1968).
23. L. V. Rozenshtraukh, A. V. Kholopov, and A. V. Yushmanova, Biofizika 15:690 (1970).
24. F. B. Gulko, and A. A. Petrov, Biofizika 17:261 (1972).
25. A. I. Shcherbunov, N. I. Kukushkin, and M. E. Saxon, Biofizika 18:519 (1973).
26. L. V. Reshodko, and J. Bures, Biol. Cyb. 18:181 (1975).
27. H. R. Karfunkel, Dissertation, Universitaet zu Tubingen (1975).
28. J. Nagumo, R. Suzuki, and S. Sato, Notes of Professional Group on Nonlinear Theory of IECE (Japan), February 26, 1963.
29. R. Suzuki, Adv. Biophys. 9:115 (1976).
30. E. E. Smith, and A. C. Guyton, Physiologist 4:112 (1961).
31. A. N. Zaikin, and A. M. Zhabotinsky, Nature 225:535 (1970).
32. A. T. Winfree, in Theoretical Chemistry, 4, H. Eyring and D. Henderson, eds., Academic Press, New York (1978).
33. J. J. Tyson, Lecture Notes in Biomathematics, Vol. 10, S. Levin, ed., Springer-Verlag, Berlin (1976).
34. R. J. Field, and W. C. Troy, SIAM J. Appl. Math. 37:561 (1979).
35. A. G. Mayer, Papers of the Tortugas Lab. of the Carnegie Inst. of Wash. 1:115 (1908).
36. A. G. Mayer, Papers of the Tortugas Lab. of the Carnegie Inst. of Wash. 6:25 (1914).
37. W. E. Garrey, Amer. J. Physiol. 33:397 (1914).
38. G. R. Mines, Trans. R. Soc. Can. 4:43 (1914).
39. G. R. Stibitz, and D. A. Rytand, Circulation 37:75 (1968).
40. M. Shibata, and J. Bures, J. Neurophys. 35:381 (1973).
41. M. Shibata, and J. Bures, J. Neurobiol. 5:107 (1974).
42. H. Martins-Ferreira, G. de Oliveiro Castro, C. J. Struchinea, and P. S. Rodriques, J. Neurophys. 37:773 (1974).
43. N. Wiener, and A. Rosenblueth, Arch. Inst. Cardiologia de Mexico 16:205 (1946).
44. I. S. Balakhovskii, Biophysics 10:1175 (1965).
45. M. A. Allessie, F. I. M. Bonke, and F. J. G. Schopman, Circ. Res. 33:54 (1973).
46. M. A. Allessie, F. I. M. Bonke, and F. J. G. Schopman, Circ. Res. 39:168 (1976).

47. M. A. Allessie, F. I. M. Bonke, and F. J. G. Schopman, Circ. Res. 41:9 (1977).
48. A. T. Winfree, Science 175:634 (1972).
49. O. E. Rössler, Zeit. Naturforsch. 31a:1168 (1976).
50. O. E. Rössler, in Synergetics, H. Haken, ed., Lecture Notes in Physics, Springer-Verlag, Berlin (1978).
51. O. E. Rössler, and C. Kahlert, Z. Naturforsch. 34a:565 (1979).
52. Y. Kuramoto, Prog. Theor. Phys. 64 (supplement):346 (1978).

CHAPTER 3

DETERMINISTIC MODELLING OF RHYTHMS

SPATIO TEMPORAL OSCILLATIONS OF A CELLULAR
AUTOMATON IN EXCITABLE MEDIA

J.P. ALLOUCHE et C. REDER
U.E.R. de Mathématiques et d'Informatique
Université de Bordeaux I
33405 TALENCE CEDEX

§ 0 - Introduction.

Cellular automata usually consist of an infinite planar grid of square cells ; every cell can take numerical values and "transition rules" permit to construct at each (discrete) time step the new generation of cells, knowing the previous ones (see for instance [2] or [7]).

The terminology : "cellular", "dead or living configuration", "generation" or "game of life", "garden of Eden" ... is the traditional one. But of course we do not pretend that our cells have any biological reality.

The particular automaton we study here is a deterministic one which was proposed in [4] (see also [1], [3], [5], [6]). Its interest lies in giving a simple model generating a spatio temporal structure which looks like the one we can observe in the "BZZ reaction" (see figure 7 below and p. 313 in [8]).

In part one of this article, we give the definition of the studied automaton. We shall see in the second part that every configuration generated by this automaton has temporal periodicity with only one possible period.

In the last part, we define a notion of "wave-front" and use it to describe the spatio temporal structure of the plan : there is essentially only one type of pattern. (*)

§ 1 - "Rule of the game".

Given two integers N and e, with $1 \leqslant e \leqslant N-2$, take an infinite planar grid, each cell of which can be in the states $0, 1, 2, \ldots, N-1$. Call $1, 2, \ldots, e$ the "excited" states and define the following transition rules :

(A) If a cell is in state i $(1 \leqslant i \leqslant N-2)$, its state at the next generation is $i+1$; if a cell is in state $N-1$, its next state is 0.

_____

(*) In this paper, we give no proofs of the announced results. We refer the reader to [1].

(B)   If a cell is in the 0-state, there are two cases :

        - if one of the four neighbouring cells is excited, the next
          state is 1 ;

        - if none of the neighbouring cells is excited, the next state
          is 0 .

Figure 1 : the four neighbouring cells of the cell   c

Remarks :   (A) is a reaction rule: starting from an homogeneous initial condition,
the evolution of every cell is just governed by this rule and if no external perturbation occurs, every cell of the grid will reach the 0-state after a short time and remains in this steady state.

    (B) is clearly a diffusion rule.

    Notice the difference with a reaction diffusion system : here the reaction
and diffusion rules do not act simultaneously ; so it is easier to study the behaviour
of the system.

    Define "dead" and "living" configurations as follows : a configuration is
dead if, given one cell (or equivalently any finite number of cells), it reaches in
finite time the 0-state and remains in this steady state ; otherwise, the configuration
is said to be a living one.

§ 2 - Temporal structure of a living configuration.

    In what follows, we shall suppose that N is greater than or equal to 5 ,
e is greater than or equal to 2 , and that the configurations we study are living
ones.

    It was proved in [6] that, starting from an initial condition involving only
a finite number of non-zero cells, there exists a "period" T   such that the process
is ultimately T-periodic in any bounded region of the plan.

The rather surprising result we prove in [1] is that this period T is equal to N , the number of states . (But this result is false if e is equal to 1).

§ 3 - <u>Spatial structure of a living configuration</u>.

Starting as previously from an initial condition involving only a finite number of non-zero cells, we want to study the spatial structure of the plane outside some bounded region including the initially non-zero cells and for a fixed generation. (We suppose of course that the configuration is a living one and that the transient regime is ended).

Let R be a rectangle including the initially non-zero cells and their neighbours.

Using the results of [1], we can easily deduce what happens on the "normal cones" of the rectangle R (see figures 2 and 3) :

- on a horizontal or vertical half straight line originating from a cell of an edge of R and normal to this edge :

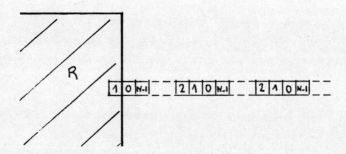

Figure 2

- on the angular sector defined by the two horizontal and vertical half
straight lines originating from a cell of a wedge of R :

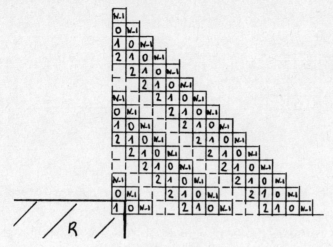

Figure 3

(In the figures 2 and 3 the states of the cells of the normal cones of R are given
up to a constant modulo N).

Thus we can observe a spatial periodicity of the cells in the plan.

How to describe the global structure ?

Let us define a "wave front" as a chain of cells $c_o, c_1, \ldots, c_n$ such that
every cell is in the 1-state, and for every i , c_i and c_{i+1} are "almost neighbouring" cells.

Figure 4 : the eight almost neighbouring cells of the cell c

This wave front can be represented as the broken line obtained by drawing straight segments from the center of c_i to the center of c_{i+1}

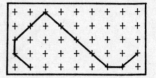

Figure 5

We shall say that a wave-front is "circular" if this broken line is a closed simple curve, whose interior contains R and is "almost convex" (i.e. its intersection with any straight line of slope 1 or -1 is convex).

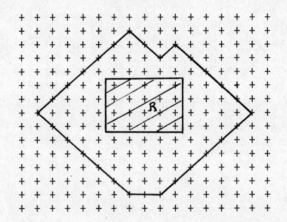

Figure 6 : example of circular wave front

We summarize the spatial behaviour of the automaton (in case $N \geq 5$, $e \geq 2$) as follows :

   Outside a bounded region including those cells whose distance to the rectangle R is less than the perimeter of R , there are only circular "parallel" wave fronts, the distance between two consecutives waves is exactly N (the number of states) and these wave fronts are expanding with speed 1 .

In particular, no wave front is a spiral pattern.

215

DATE=56

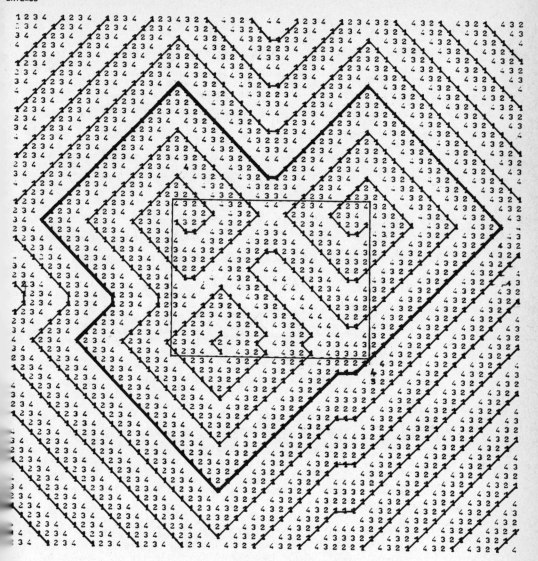

Figure 7 : Example of wave fronts

The designed rectangle satisfy the condition of this paragraph.

The first circular wave front is drawn thicker.

Conclusion :

Why did we only study what happens outside a bounded region of the plan ? Let us explain our point of view. Imagine that the automaton represents the evolution of a chemical "excitable" reaction in a Petri dish ; at the beginning of the experiment, the medium is homogeneous and in the steady state. Put a dust in the dish. Suppose we observe the mixture far enough from the initially disturbed area. According to our model, we will observe after some length of time either the steady state again or a both in time and space periodic phenomenon provoked by circular wave fronts. And in the later case, the period does not depend on the initial disturbance.

Opposed to this situation, we could imagine that there are many disturbances distributed in the dish. In that case, we could not look far from "the" disturbance and thus our results say nothing about the spatial patterns but still claim the existence of exactly one possible temporal period.

REFERENCES

[1] J.P. ALLOUCHE, C. REDER : "Période des oscillations d'un automate cellulaire". (C.R.A.S., t.294,1982) and an article in preparation.

[2] A.W. BURKS : "Essays on cellular automata". (Univ. of Illinois Press).

[3] P. CIPIERE, C. LOBRY, C. REDER : "A propos de réactions chimiques oscillantes". (Publi. A.A.I. Bordeaux, oct.1979, n° 7914).

[4] J.M. GREENBERG, S.P. HASTINGS : "Spatial patterns for discrete models of diffusion in excitable media". (SIAM J. of Appl. Math., vol.34, n°3, May 1978).

[5] J.M. GREENBERG, B.D. HASSARD, S.P. HASTINGS : "Pattern formation and periodic structures in systems modeled by reaction-diffusion equations". (Bull. of the Am. Math. Soc., vol.84, n°6, Nov.1978).

[6] J.M. GREENBERG, C. GREENE, S.P. HASTINGS : "A combinatorial problem arising in the study of reaction-diffusion equations". (SIAM J. Alg. Discr. Meth., vol.1, n°1, March 1980).

[7] F. ROBERT : "Itérations discrètes : une étude métrique". (I.M.P. Grenoble)

[8] A. WINFREE : "The geometry of biological time". (Biomathematics, vol.8, Springer-Verlag).

———

On the use of renormalization technics in the study of discrete population models in one dimension

M. COSNARD and A. EBERHARD

There exists an extensive litterature concerning first order difference equations as models of the simplest systems used in biology, ecology, economics,... In this context the relation of the magnitude of the population (il we use biological terminology) in generation t+1 with this in generation t is given by :

$$x_{t+1} = f(x_t)$$

where f is density dependent, i.e. a nonlinear application. We refer the reader to the survey paper of R.May [14] as an introduction to the subject and to the books of I. Gumowski and C. Mira [12][13] for a mathematical study.

Another domain of application of these models is in mathematical physics in order to study the transition to turbulence. Original works have been done in this way and recently M. Feigenbaum [7], [8], [9] proposed an explanation based on cascades of bifurcations of cycles of order 2^i in cycles of order 2^{i+1} and related universal constants. He introduced a very powerful operator from the renormalization theory and proposed fine conjectures on the role of this operator. We do not want to present a survey of Feigenbaum's theory which can be found in his papers and in a more global form in P. Collet and J.P. Eckmann [2]. However we shall study some iterative properties of the renormalization operator in order to obtain new results on the iterative behavior of different classes of models.

1 - BASIC DEFINITIONS AND RESULTS

In the sequel we shall work with continuous models and normalized populations. Hence f will be a continuous application from I into itself.

First of all we introduce the renormalization operator. Let τ be an affine transformation from I into itself. We say that f is renormalizable if f^2 leaves invariant the interval $\tau(I)$, i.e. $f^2(\tau(I)) \subseteq \tau(I)$. If f is renormalizable we define the renormalized

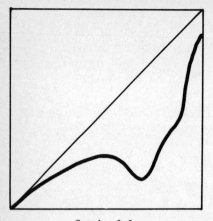

Graph of f

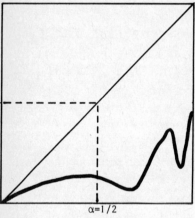

$\alpha = 1/2$

Graph of f^2

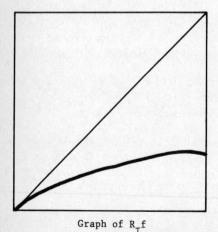

Graph of $R_\tau f$

FIGURE 1

application as the image of f through the renormalization operator R_τ , defined as follows :

$$R_\tau f = \tau^{-1} \circ f^2 \circ \tau$$

An important property of R_τ is that the renormalized application is topologically conjugated to f^2 . Therefore the two applications possess the same iterative behavior. A geometric explanation of this fact is the following : the graph of $R_\tau f$ in $I \times I$ is homothetic to the graph of f^2 in $\tau(I) \times \tau(I)$ through the similarity induced by τ .

Our aim in this paper is to study iterative properties of R_τ and, more precisely, to show explicit fixed-points. We shall distinguish two cases according as f and τ have the same fixed point or not.

2. f AND τ HAVE THE SAME FIXED POINT

Without loss of generality we assume that 0 is the common fixed point

$$\tau(x) = \alpha x \quad , \quad f(0) = 0$$

Hence the renormalization operator is given by : $R_\tau f(x) = \frac{1}{\alpha} f^2(\alpha x)$. The problem is of interest only if we add two assumptions : $0 < \alpha < 1$ and $f'(0) = 1$, (if $0 \leq f'(0) < 1$, $R^n f$ converges uniformly to 0 and if $f'(0)$ does not exist we cannot conclude).
We shall consider $I = [0,1]$. So we deduce that f^2 is renormalizable if and only if $f([0,\alpha]) \subseteq [0,\alpha]$ (see figure 1).

DEFINITION : <u>Let</u> β <u>be a positive real. We say that</u> f <u>admits at</u> 0 <u>an asymptotic development of order</u> $1+\beta$ <u>if there exists a continuous application</u> t <u>such that</u>

$$\forall \, x \in [0,1] \quad f(x) = x-ax^{1+\beta} + x^{1+\beta}t(x)$$

<u>with</u> $a > 0$ <u>and</u> $t(0) = 0$.

The set of such applications will be called P_a^β. The first result is consequence of a direct calculation.

PROPOSITION : <u>If</u> f <u>is a renormalizable element of</u> P_a^β <u>for</u> a,β <u>two positive reals, then</u> $R_\tau f$ <u>belongs to</u> $P_{a'}^\beta$, <u>with</u> $a' = 2\alpha^\beta a$.

A direct corollary is that, if α equals $\alpha^* = (\frac{1}{2})^{1/\beta}$, then a' equals a and $R_\tau f$ is also an element of P_a^β. Another obvious property is that R_τ admits two trivial fixed points : the null function and the identity (recall that f is a fixed point of R_τ if $R_\tau f = f$). But if α equals α^* it can possess more.

PROPOSITION : <u>Let</u> a,β <u>be two positive reals and</u> $\alpha = \alpha^* = (\frac{1}{2})^{1/\beta}$.

<u>Then</u> $\quad f_{a,\beta}(x) = x(1+a\beta x^\beta)^{-1/\beta}$

<u>is a fixed point of</u> R_τ <u>in</u> P_a^β.

An important particular case of the preceding result is obtained for $\beta = 1$ (i.e. $\alpha^* = \frac{1}{2}$). $f_{a,1}(x) = x(1+ax)^{-1}$ is fixed point of R_τ in P_a^1 (applications with a negative second derivative in 0). The other fixed points are related to $f_{a,1}$ in the following way : if we set $S_\beta(x) = x^\beta$ then $f_{a,\beta}$ and $f_{a\beta,1}$ are conjugated by δ_β, i.e. $f_{a,\beta} = S_\beta^{-1} \circ f_{a\beta,1} \circ S_\beta$.

Let us study the iterative behavior of the renormalization operator. If f is an element of P_a^β for some positive a and β, we are concerned in the behavior of the sequence $R_\tau^n f$, $n \in \mathbb{N}$.

THEOREM 1 : <u>Let</u> a,β <u>be two positive reals. If</u> f <u>is an element of</u> P_a^β <u>then</u> :

i) <u>if</u> $\alpha < \alpha^*$ $R_\tau^n f$ <u>converges uniformly to the identity</u>

ii) <u>if</u> $\alpha = \alpha^*$ $R_\tau^n f$ <u>converges uniformly to</u> $f_{a,\beta}$

iii) <u>if</u> $\alpha > \alpha^*$ $R_\tau^n f$ <u>converges uniformly to the null function.</u>

The proof can be found in Cosnard [5]. Theorem 1 can be interpreted in terms of bifurcations. To simplify we assume that $\beta = 1$: we consider the set of applications with a negative second derivative at 0. If $\alpha < \frac{1}{2}$ the renormalization operator R_τ possesses a globally attracting fixed point (the identity) and a repulsive fixed point (the null function). $\alpha = \frac{1}{2}$ is a bifurcation value : the identity losses its attractivity and an infinite number of attractive fixed points $(f_{a,1})$ appears ; the domain of attraction of $f_{a,1}$ is P_a^1. When $\alpha > \frac{1}{2}$, the preceding fixed points disappear, the null function becomes globally attractive and the identity remains repulsive.

In terms of population models, theorem 1 gives us a normalized law in case of extinction of the population.

COROLLARY : Let f belongs to P_a^β for positive β and a . When n goes to infinity $f^{2^n}(x)$ behaves like

$$2^{-n/\beta} f_{a,\beta}(2^{n/\beta}x) = \frac{x}{(1+a\beta 2^n x^\beta)^{1/\beta}}$$

i.e., $\lim\limits_{n \to +\infty} \sup\limits_{x \in [0,1]} |f^{2^n}(x) - 2^{-n/\beta} f_{a,\beta}(2^{n/\beta}x)| = 0$

3. f AND τ HAVE DIFFERENT FIXED POINTS

In this part we shall assume that f is an even application from $[-1,+1]$ into itself, strictly decreasing on $[0,1]$ with $f(0) = 1$. Moreover we shall choose $\tau(x) = -\alpha X$, where α is taken in $]0,1[$.

The most famous logistic model of this kind is $f_\mu(x) = 1 - \mu x^2$ where $\mu \in [0,2]$. The iterative behavior of such a function can be very complicated. We refer the reader to R. May [14] and P. Collet and J.P. Eckmann [2] to obtain more informations about the interesting theory developped on the subject.

Hence the renormalization is given by : $R_\tau f(x) = -\frac{1}{\alpha} f^2(-\alpha x)$. We shall first be concerned in the construction of fixed points of R_τ. In contrast with the preceding case we shall not give the analytic expression of the fixed points, but only an algorithm to obtain them. The results we present are related with those obtained by P. Collet, J.P. Eckmann and O.E. Lanford [3], M. Feigenbaum [7], [8], [9] and M. Campanino and H. Epstein [1].

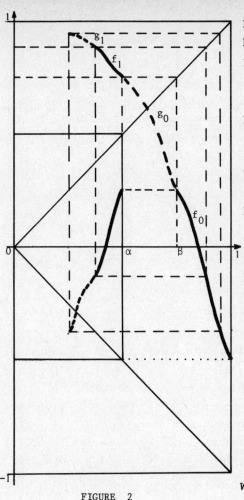

FIGURE 2

Let β belong to $]\alpha,1[$ and f_o be a strictly decreasing homeomorphism from $[\beta,1]$ in $[-\alpha,\alpha^2]$.

For $i=1,2,\ldots$,we define f_i by $\forall x \in [\alpha^i\beta,\alpha^i]$

$$f_i(x) = f_o^{-1}[-\alpha f_{i-1}(\tfrac{x}{\alpha})]$$

Without difficulty we can see that f_i is a strictly decreasing homeomorphism.

Let g_o be a continuous decreasing application (the assumption that g be decreasing is only used for simplicity, the necessary conditions on g are in reality less stringent) on $[\alpha,\beta]$ such that

$$g_o(\beta) = f_o(\beta) \ , \ g_o(\alpha) = f_1(\alpha)$$

For $i=1,2,\ldots$ we define g_i by

$$\forall x \in [\alpha^{i+1},\alpha^i\beta] \ ,$$

$$g_i(x) = f_o^{-1}[-\alpha g_{i-1}(\tfrac{x}{\alpha})]$$

We set :

$$\forall x \in [-1,+1] \ , \ F(x) = \begin{cases} f_i(|x|) & \text{if } \exists i \ |x| \in [\alpha^i\beta,\alpha^i] \\ g_i(|x|) & \text{if } \exists i \ |x| \in [\alpha^{i+1},\alpha^i\beta] \\ 1 & \text{if } x = 0 \end{cases}$$

Figure 2 gives an illustration of the construction of f .

THEOREM 2 : The constructed application F is a fixed point of the renormalization operator :

$$R_\tau F = F \iff F(x) = -\frac{1}{\alpha} F^2(-\alpha x)$$

See figure 3 for examples of solutions.

If we add some assumptions about f_o and g_o we get k-times continuously differentiable solutions ; see M. Cosnard [6]. But we

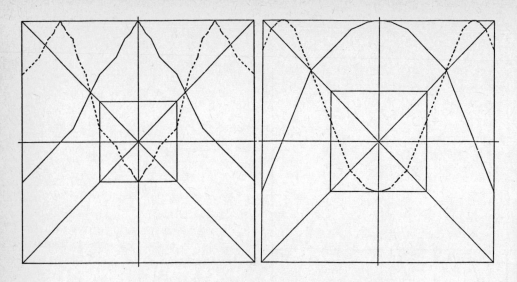

Two piecewise linear solutions
FIGURE 3

could not succeed in obtaining analytic solutions (Feigenbaum's conjecture is based on such a solution). The existence of an analytic fixed point has been proved by M. Campanino and H. Epstein [1] using a different technic (figure 4 shows an example of a C^1 solution).

It is not very difficult to obtain a kind of reciprocal of the theorem 2 : let f be an even continuous fixed point of R_τ , strictly decreasing on [0,1] and such that f(0) = 1 ; if we define $\alpha = -f(1)$, $\beta = f^{-1}(\alpha^2)$, f_0 and g_0 as the restrictions of f to $[\alpha,1]$ and $[\beta,\alpha]$ respectively, then the constructed application F is equal to f on [-1,+1] .

We shall now study some properties of the fixed points of R_τ in order to describe their iterative behavior. Let f be as in the reciprocal of theorem 2. We can remark that if x belongs to $[-1,-\alpha[$, then $f(x) \in [-\alpha,1]$ and so $f^n(x)$ leaves $[-1,-\alpha[$ and never returns in it. So we restrict the study of f on $[-\alpha,1]$ and divide it in three parts : $L = [-\alpha,1] = J_1 \cup K_0 \cup J_0$ with

$J_1 = [-\alpha,\alpha^2]$, $K_0 =]\alpha^2,\beta[$ and $J_0 = [\beta,1]$. From the choice of f we know that :

$$\forall \ x \in L \ , \quad f(x) = \tau^{-1} \circ f^2 \circ \tau(x)$$

which is equivalent to the following :

$$\forall \ x \in \tau(L) = J_1 \ , \quad f^2(x) = \tau \circ f \circ \tau^{-1}(x) \tag{1}$$

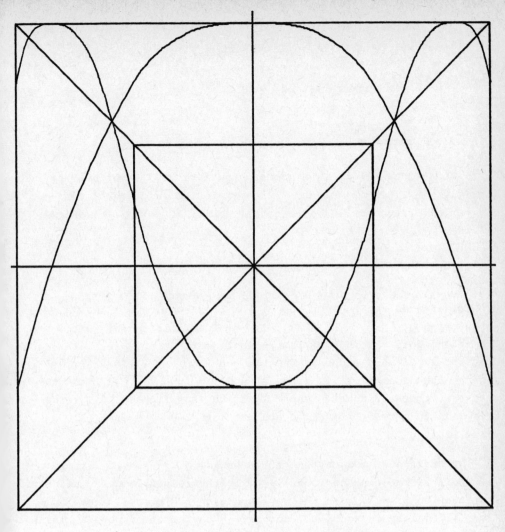

A   C^1 solution of the renormalization equation

It is constructed using the algorithm introduced
in the preceding pages : f_o and g_o are pieces
of hyperbolas. Note that the derivative at 0 is
equal to 0.
In the upper right and left corners, we can remark
that the graph of f^2 is not exactly the same as
the graph of f . In fact relation (3) is verified
but θ is a nonlinear application.

FIGURE 4

So f^2 and f are topologically conjugated and the dynamic of f^2 on J_1 is identical to that of f on L which is given by the following scheme :

$$(2)$$

Let us now define an homeomorphism θ from J_o into L by : $\theta = \tau^{-1} \circ f_o$. Then we get on J_o an analogous relation of conjugation which will be called θ -renormalization or nonlinear renormalization :

PROPOSITION : $\forall \; x \in J_o$, $f^2(x) = \theta^{-1} \circ f \circ \theta(x)$ $\qquad(3)$

The proof is a direct consequence of the construction of f . In general the graph of f in $J_o \times J_o$ is not identical to this of f in $L \times L$ (see figure 4). In fact θ is nonlinear. In the particular case where f_o is linear, and only in this case, θ is a linear transformation and the graphs of f upon L and f^2 upon J_o are the same : we say that there is double renormalization (see figure 3). This case corresponds to a renormalization operator studied by Tresser and Coullet [21].

From this we deduce that the dynamic of f^2 on J_o is identical to (2). Composing θ and τ^{-1} by themselves we get cascades of conjugation relations on the corresponding subintervals (see [6]).
It is easy to know the iterative behavior of f on K_o since f is a continuous decreasing application from K_o into $K_o \cup J_o$. This dynamic is transported by the preceding relations to subintervals of J_o and J_1 . Using these facts we can prove the following result.

THEOREM 3 : 1. For all $i \in \mathbb{N}$, f possesses at least one cycle of order 2^i ;
2. f admits no cycle of order different of a power of 2 ;
3. There exists a Cantor set J which is invariant and minimal by f ;
4. J is an attractor for a set of non zero measure of points in L ;
5. The sequences $f^n(x)$ which do not converge to J , converge to the cycles of order 2^i .

The proof is long and can be found in [6]. In the examples we have studied, the Lebesgue measure of J is always equal to 0 , but we do not know if it is true in the general case. However it can be seen that the theorem is valid without any assumption on f such as negative Schwarzian derivative [18], [10], [17], [3].

If we restrict us to the population models problem, theorem 3 gives us an easy way to construct a model such that for almost every initial data, the population sequence is aperiodic and converges to a Cantor set.

REFERENCES

[1]   M. CAMPANINO and H. EPSTEIN, "On the existence of Feigenbaum's fixed point", I.H.E.S. preprint P/80/35 (1980).

[2]   P. COLLET and J.P. ECKMANN, Iterated maps on the interval as dynamical systems , Birkhäuser, Boston-Basel-Stuttgart (1980).

[3]   P. COLLET, J.P. ECKMANN and O.E. LANFORD, "Universal properties of maps on an interval", Commun. Math. Phys. 76 (1980), 211-254.

[4]   G.R. CONWAY, "Mathematical models in applied ecology", Nature 269 (1977), 291-297.

[5]   M. COSNARD, "Comportement d'itérations d'un opérateur de renormalisation", (1981) to appear in RAIRO Anal. Num.

[6]   M. COSNARD, "Etude des solutions de l'équation fonctionnelle de Feigenbaum" (1981) to appear.

[7]   M. FEIGENBAUM, "Quantitative universality for a class of non linear transformations", J. Stat. Phys. 19 (1978) 25-52.

[8]   M. FEIGENBAUM, "The universal metric properties of non-linear transformations", J. Stat. Phys. 21 (1979), 669-706.

[9]   M. FEIGENBAUM, "The transition to aperiodic behavior in turbulent systems", Commun. Math. Phys. 77 (1980), 65-86.

[10] J. GUCKENHEIMER, "Sensitive dependence to initial conditions for one dimensional maps", Commun. Math. Phys. 70 (1979), 133-160.

[11] J. GUCKENHEIMER, G. OSTER and A. IPAKTCHI, "The dynamics of density dependent population models", J. Math. Biology 4 (1977), 101-147.

[12] I. GUMOWSKI and C. MIRA, Recurrences and discrete dynamic systems, Lectures Notes in Math. 809 (1980).

[13] I. GUMOWSKI and C. MIRA, Dynamique chaotique, CEPADUES Edition, Toulouse (1980).

[14] R.M. MAY, "Simple mathematical models with very complicated dynamics", Nature 261 (1976), 459-467.

[15] J.A. MEYER, "Sur la structuration des systèmes écologiques", in La Morphogenèse, de la biologie aux mathématiques, Maloine Editeur Paris (1980), 173-178.

[16] M. MISIUREWICZ, "Absolutely continuous measures for certain maps of an interval", IHES Preprint M/79/293 (1979).

[17] M. MISIUREWICZ, "Invariant measures for continuous transformation of [0,1] with zero topological entropy", Lecture Notes in Math. 729, (1980), 144-152.

[18] D. SINGER, "Stable orbits and bifurcation of maps of the interval", SIAM J. Appl. Math. 35 (1978) 260-267.

[19] S. SMALE and R.F. WILLIAMS, "The qualitative analysis of a difference equation of population growth", J. Math. Biology 3 (1976), 1-4.

[20] C. TRESSER and P. COULLET, "Itérations d'endomorphismes et groupe de renormalisation", C.R. Acad. Sc. Paris 287 (1978), 577-580.

[21] S. USHIKI, M. YAMAGUTI and H. MATANO, "Discrete population models and chaos", Lecture Notes in Num. Appl. Anal. 2 (1980) 1-25.

M. COSNARD et A. EBERHARD
Laboratoire IMAG
Université de Grenoble 1
B.P. 53 X
38041 GRENOBLE cédex
France.

HYDRODYNAMICS AND CELL DIVISION

G.H.COTTET Labo.Ana.Numer.PARIS VI
4place Jussieu 75230

Y.MADAY Labo.Math. PARIS XII
Av.G.deGAULLE Creteil

1. ABSTRACT.

We present here prerequisites for cell division with hydro-
dynamical arguments. The model we study concerns a spherical cell filled
with a homogeneous viscous, incompressible, Newtonien fluid whose boundary
is covered whith a surfactant directly responsible of surface tension.
We analyse the behaviour óf the cell during it's growth. We prove the
existence of a critical size after which non uniform flows áppear in the
cytoplasm and surfactant accumulate along an equatorial line which can be
seen as a mitotic ring.

2.THE EQUATIONS GOVERNING THE MODEL.

Let us define $\vec{\hat{u}}$ (resp. $\hat{p}$) as the velocity (resp. the pressure)
in the sphere Ω_R of radius R, $\hat{c}$ the concentration of surfactant on the
boundary Γ_R $\hat{\sigma}$ the surface tension, $\hat{D}$ the surface diffusivity of the surfactant and $\hat{\nu}$ the viscosity of the fluid.

It is convenient to introduce dimensionless variable in order to
work on Ω_1 , hence the variable will be defined by:

$$\vec{\hat{u}} = \frac{\overline{\hat{c}}}{\hat{\nu}}\, \vec{u}$$

$$\hat{p} = \frac{2\overline{\hat{\sigma}}}{R} + \frac{\overline{\hat{c}}}{R}\, p$$

$$\hat{c} = \overline{\hat{c}}\, c ,$$

$$\hat{\sigma} = \overline{\hat{\sigma}} + \overline{\hat{c}}\, \sigma , \quad \hat{D} = \frac{\overline{\hat{c}} R D}{\nu}$$

where for a function q we denote by $\overline{q}$ the mean-value $\displaystyle\int_{\Gamma_1} q$

The equations governing the problem are then:

the Navier-Stokes equations in Ω_1 for $\vec{u}$ and $p(\vec{u}=(u_i)_{i=1,\dots 3})$

$$\frac{\partial \vec{u}}{\partial t} - 2\frac{\partial}{\partial x_j}D_{ij}\vec{u} + \left(\frac{\nu}{c}\right)^2 \vec{R}(\vec{u}.\vec{\nabla})u_i + \frac{\partial p}{\partial x_i} = 0 \quad i = 1,2,3. \tag{2.1}$$

$$\vec{\nabla}.\vec{u} = 0 \tag{2.2}$$

where $D_{ij}\vec{u}$ denotes the tensor $(\frac{\partial u_i}{\partial x_j} + \frac{\partial u_j}{\partial x_i})$ and $\vec{\nabla}$ the vector $(\frac{\partial}{\partial x_i})_{i=1,2,3}$.

On the boundary, the condition of zero flux and equilibrium of tangential stresses impose that :

$$\Sigma u_i . n_i = 0 \tag{2.3}$$

$$2\Sigma D_{ij}\vec{u}\, n_i \tau_j^k = \frac{\partial \sigma}{\partial \tau k}, \quad k = 1,2 \tag{2.4}$$

where n_i (resp. τ_i^k) denote the components of the vector normal to the boundary (resp. the two tangential vectors) and $\frac{\partial}{\partial \tau k}$ are the tangential derivative operators.

Moreover the concentration is coupled with the velocity by the following equations :

$$\frac{\partial c}{\partial t} + \frac{\partial(\vec{u}.n)}{\partial n}c + (\vec{u}.\tau^k)\frac{\partial c}{\partial \tau k} - D\frac{\partial^2 c}{\partial \tau^2} = 0 \tag{2.5}$$

The effect of the surfactant on σ is given by the following law $\sigma = f(c)$, where f is a positive, growing fonction.

We first get the following result:

THEOREM 2.1. For law values of R (say $R < R_o$, $R > 0$)[*]the equilibrium solutions of (2.1),...,(2.5) are the couples $(\vec{u}(M) = \vec{b} \wedge \vec{OM}$, $c = c_0$) where $\vec{b}$ is a given vector of $\mathbb{R}^3$, c_0 a given positive number and O is the center of Ω_1.

These solutions can be seen as rigid motions of the cytoplasm inducting an uniform distribution of surfactant along the surface.

[*] Remember the relation between D (the parameter in (2.5), and R.

Our purpose is now to study the loss of stability of these solutions (which we shall call trivial) when R increases . There are two non linearities that can be responsible of such instabilities; usually in hydrodynamic the non linearity occuring in (2.1) from the convective term $(\vec{u}.\vec{\nabla})\vec{u}$ is the only agent responsible, nethertheless our hypotheses will be to assume that the main effect in surface are due to the non linearity present in the equation (2.5) assuring the conservation of mass in surface. Hence, at first, we shall neglect the effect of the convective terms .

3.ANALYSE OF THE INSTABILITIES.

Let us suppose that an instability occurs when the cell has the axial symmetry of vector $\vec{b}$ (i.e. $\vec{u} = \vec{b} \wedge \vec{OM}$). We shall restrict the problem of stability to this one : look for instability responding to pertubation having the axial symmetry of $\vec{b}$. The justification of this point will be discussed in the last paragraph.

Now if we write $\vec{u}$ in the spherical coordonates of axes $\vec{b}$ (see.fig 1) denoting by u,v,w the component of $\vec{u}$ in this system , we verify that these new unknows are independant of ϕ, hence the problem can be simplified to a two dimensional one.

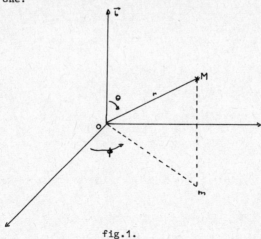

fig.1.

The linearised problem deducted from (2.1),....,(2.5)can be stated in the simple following form:

Over $(0,1)X(0,\pi)$:

$$- \frac{\partial \bar{p}}{\partial r} + \frac{1}{r^2} [\frac{\partial^2}{\partial r^2}(r^2 u) + \frac{\partial}{\partial \eta}((1-\eta^2) \frac{\partial u}{\partial \eta})] = 0 \qquad (3.1)$$

$$\frac{\partial}{\partial \eta} [(1-\eta^2) \frac{\partial p}{\partial \eta}] + \frac{\partial}{\partial r} \frac{\partial p}{\partial r} = 0 \qquad (3.2)$$

$$\frac{\partial^2}{\partial r^2} (rw) + \frac{1}{r} \frac{\partial}{\partial \eta} [(1-\eta^2) \frac{\partial w}{\partial \eta}] = 0 \qquad (3.3)$$

$$\frac{1}{r^2} \frac{\partial}{\partial r}(r^2 u) + \frac{1}{r\sin \theta} \frac{\partial}{\partial \theta}(v\sin \theta) = 0 \qquad (3.4)$$

Where we have set $\eta = \cos \theta$ .The conditions over Γ_1 are then :

$$u = 0 \qquad (3.5)$$

$$- \frac{\partial}{\partial r} [\frac{1}{r^2} \frac{\partial}{\partial r} (r^2 u)] + \frac{\partial}{\partial \eta} [(1-\eta^2) \frac{\partial c}{\partial \eta}] = \frac{\partial}{\partial \eta} [(1-\eta^2) \frac{\partial c}{\partial \eta}] f'(c_0) \qquad (3.6)$$

$$(3.7)$$

$$\frac{\partial}{\partial r} (\frac{w}{r}) = 0$$

$$c_0 [- \frac{\partial}{\partial r}(r^2 u) + 2u] - D \frac{\partial}{\partial \eta} [(1-\eta^2) \frac{\partial c}{\partial \eta}] = 0 \qquad (3.8)$$

By developping along the suitable basis of Legendre polynomials P_N we can explicit the non trivial solutions of the system (3.1),....,(3.8) and thus determine the stability of the equilibrium.

THEOREM 3.1.

The first instability occurs for $D=D_c=1/3$. Indeed the mode

$$
\begin{cases}
u_1 = (1-r^2) \cos \theta \\[2mm]
p_1 = 10r \cos \theta \\[2mm]
c_1 = (3/f'(c_0)) \cos \theta
\end{cases}
$$

is unstable for this value of D.

Moreover it emerges from D two branches of solutions: the trivial branch will become unstable and a branch of stable equilibrium which can be locally written in the form:

$u = \lambda(D-D_c)u_1 + \varepsilon (D-D_c)$; $p = \lambda(D-D_c)p_1 + \varepsilon (D-D_c)$; $c = \lambda(D-D_c)c_1 + \varepsilon (D-D_c)$: Where $\varepsilon (x)$ tends to 0 as x tends to 0, and λ is a real constant.

REMARK :

1) It is important to note that D is independent of $\vec{b}$

2) Using the terminology of the bifurcation theory (see e.g.(1)) we can say that, from the point of view of the plane symmetry the cell was presenting before D_c , the bifurcation that appears at D_c is a symmetry breaking one, while, of course, it preserves the $\vec{b}$-axial symmetry (see fig.2).

It is easy to see that the main consequence of this bifurcation will be an accumulation of surfactant at one of the poles and a new balance of pressures between the two poles.

Although these observations are of interest in studying the cell life (it makes think to ameboid movement and migration) it seems to be no relevant with the cell division. Hence we must add an assumption which takes into account the intern structure of the cell.

Whe shall suppose that there exists a surface inside the cell which is globally submitted to no constraint from the fluid ; the interpretation of this assumption will be given in the last paragraph. The new condition imposed to the fluid can be written:

$$\int_s (p-2\frac{\partial u}{\partial r})\cos\theta \ ds = 0 \qquad\qquad (3.9)$$

Taking for S a surface which has both $\vec{b}$ axis symmetry and symmetry with regard to the equatorial plane, it is easy to observe that the mode P_1 cannot verify the condition (3.9).So we obtain the following result:

THEOREM 3.2

Under the condition (3.9), the first instability occurs for $D=D_c \approx\frac{1}{3}$. It emerges from D_c a non trivial branch of bifurcation, stable, along which the equilibrium can be locally written:

$$u=\lambda(D-D_c)u_2+\epsilon(D-D_c); \quad p=\lambda(D-D_c)p_2+\epsilon(D-D_c); \quad c=\lambda(D-D_c)c_2+\epsilon(D-D_c).$$

$$\begin{cases} u_2=(r-r\ )P_2(\cos\ ) \\ p_2=\alpha r^2 P_2(\cos\ \theta) \\ c_2=\beta P_2(\cos\ \theta) \end{cases}$$

$$P_2(\eta)=\frac{3\eta^2-1}{2}\ ,\ \alpha\ \text{and}\ \beta\ \text{two constants}\ (\beta>0).$$

At the opposite of what happened in the previous situation, the present bifurcation is symmetry preserving relati vely both to the equatorial plane $(\theta=\frac{\pi}{2})$ and $\vec{b}$ axis.

The stable configurations of flow and concentration are now, for $D>D_c$: an accumulation of surfactant in the equatorial plane, a symmetric increase of dynamic pressure near the poles and decrease of this pressure in the equatorial plane.(see fig.3).

All these facts are what we shall call the hydrodinamical prerequisites for cell division.

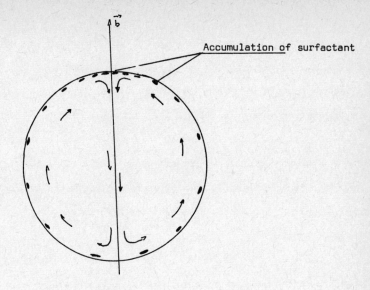

Fig.2

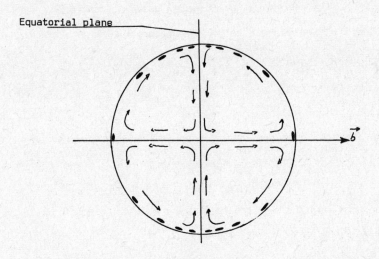

Fig.3

5.DISCUSSION.

It is now time to consider our model from a " physiologist's" point of view. The rigid motion can be seen as a sleeping state of the cell (obtained for exemple in a poor environment) which is not the state generally observed in a cell culture ;nethertheless we can con ider that just before D_c it has actually reached this symmetric state (this is the meaning of the mathematical concept of asymptotic state) that one, beeing backed up by the existence of the mitotic apparatus. Hence the pertubations guiding the cell to the stable branch of the bifurcation will be created by the above orientations.

The surface S introduced in the condition (3.9) can be seen as the boundary of the mitotic apparatus which behaves as the squeleton of the cell, jointly with the membrane of the cell. Intuitively, the bifurcation described in theorem 3.1. and fig.2. will push this apparatus towards one ofthe poles of the cell and hence has to be rejected, just as any bifurcation following the instability of a mode P_{2N+1}.

We must add that the values of D_c we find have physiological sense (D_c corresponds to an R_c of about 10^{-4} cm ; for a viscosity of about 10 cm^2/s. , and a surface diffusivity of about $10^{-7} cm^2$/s)

An improvement of interest of this model would be to restore the convection terms in the definition of the equilibrium. In fact, although accor- ding to our hypothesis,the main non linear effects do not come from the convective non linearity, it seems very drastic to neglect the convectivity, whose effects will be, without any doubt, to introduce coupling between modes P_2, P_4,...

To finish with, we may hope to follow the actual bifurcation of the cell (i.e.: observe the real cleavage of the cell) if we are able to derive a mathematical formalization of the problem relaxing the sphericity constraint, together with the condition of flux nul(condition which expresses that the cell is isolated from its environment).

235

REFERENCES

(1)H.FUJII & M.YAMAGUTI: Strutures of singularities and its numerical realization in nonlinear elasticity;Jour.Math. KYOTO Univ. 20.3 1980

(2)H.P.GREENSPAN: On the dynamic of the cell cleavage; J.Theor.Biol. 65,1977

(3) H.P.GREENSPAN :On the deformation of a viscous droplet caused by variable
surface tension; Stud. App. Math. 57,45 58 , 1977

ON THE SOLUTIONS
of
Some DIFFERENTIAL EQUATION in $\mathbf{R}^3$
with
SMALL PARAMETER

C. LOBRY   F. MAZAT

A first version of this note was written in November 1981.
Later we met E. BENOIT and we discovered that he had done independently similar work, but motivated by a different problem. Thus we suppressed most of
the first mathematical developments which will appear elsewhere under the
signature of BENOIT and decided to concentrate ourselves on motivations and
to provide illustrations from computer.

The well known system of equations called "Oregonator" and
the question of existence of chotic behaviour for such systems is at the
origin of our interest in "singularly pertubed differential equations".
The main point of this paper was discovered when we tried to make more
rigorous some speculations stated in a paper with LOZI (8) - see also (7).
We acknoledge E. BENOIT, R. LOZI, and C. REDER for discussions on this, and
related, subjects.

I INTRODUCTION : Differential equations of the form:

$$
\begin{cases}
\dfrac{dx}{dt} = f(x,y) & x \in R^n \\[2ex]
\dfrac{dy}{dt} = \dfrac{1}{\epsilon}g(x,y) & y \in R^m
\end{cases}
$$

have always interested mathematicians. In recent years the case n = 2 m = 1 (or more)
has been proposed by various authors as being likely to furnish exemples of differential equations whose behaviour is complex (chaotic) . Without claiming to be
exaustive and apologizing to those not cited, we quote: ARGEMI (1) , LOZI (7)
RÖSSLER (12) (13) , TAKENS (14) (15), TYSON (17).

Implicitely all these authors use the supposed smallness of ϵ in passing from the differential equation above to the constrained equation:

$$\begin{cases} \dfrac{dx}{dt} & = & f(x,y) \\[2ex] 0 & = & g(x,y) \end{cases}$$

where they claim to observe the behaviour at the limit of the initial differential equation.

The remark made in this note, although extremely elementary, does not seem to have been made by the authors cited . It questions the fact that constrained equations (in the sense of TAKENS) are always a faithful approximation of differential equations with small parameters. Of course this does not remove any of the interest from constrained differential equations as such.

We shall try to clarify the situation by refering to ROBISON's Nonstandard Analysis (11), by using the notion of reals which are infinitely small. In doing so we are only taking up an idea of REEB who has shown its richness. (See lecture 580 of P. CARTIER at the Bourbaki seminar).

II THE EQUATION (E_ϵ)

Let (E_ϵ) be the following differential system:

$$(E_\epsilon) \qquad \begin{cases} \dfrac{dx}{dt} & = & 1 \\[2ex] \dfrac{dy}{dt} & = & 2x \\[2ex] \dfrac{dz}{dt} & = & \dfrac{1}{\epsilon}\,(y - z^2) \end{cases}$$

Theorem : The mapping $t \longrightarrow (x(t)=t, y(t)=t^2-\epsilon , z(t)=-t)$ is a solution of (E_ϵ) .

Proof: It is a verification.

The rest of this note is devoted to show that this proposition should be taken seriously.

III <u>CONSTRAINED DIFFERENTIAL EQUATIONS.</u>

In this paragraph we quickly recall what a constrained differential equations is in the sense of TAKENS (14). We just adapt to the special case of $\mathbb{R}^3$ the general definitions of (14).

Let us consider the differential system in $\mathbb{R}^3$:

$$(F_\varepsilon) \quad \begin{cases} \dfrac{dx}{dt} &= \quad f(x,y,z) \\[2ex] \dfrac{dy}{dt} &= \quad g(x,y,z) \\[2ex] \dfrac{dz}{dt} &= \quad \dfrac{1}{\varepsilon}h(x,y,z) \end{cases}$$

We shall denote by S the set of zeros of the function h which we suppose to be a submanifold of $\mathbb{R}^3$ without singularity. The manifold S is called the "slow manifold" of the system (F_ε) . The stable (respectively unstable) part of the slow manifold, which we denote by S_{min} (see (14) for the motivation), is the set of points (x,y,z) of S where the tangent plane to S is not vertical and the gradient of h is directed downward (thus h is negative above the surface and positive below) - (respectively upward for the unstable part S_{max})- The points of S where the tangent plane is vertical form the apparent contour of S (in the direction Oz).

It is well known that points of the apparent contour are either "fold" or "cusp" points (for generic surfaces). We are only concerned here with folds. If x and y are just parameters, not dynamically coupled with z, one recognizes the basic elements of THOM's catastrophe theory (16). The remarks which follow are therefore pertinent every time that a system evolves rapidly towards a minimum of a potential and that this potential depends itself slowly on the state of the system.

DEFINITION (from TAKENS): A solution of the constrained differential equation:

$$(F_c) \quad \begin{cases} \dfrac{dx}{dt} & = \quad f(x,y,z) \\[2em] \dfrac{dy}{dt} & = \quad g(x,y,z) \\[2em] 0 & = \quad h(x,y,z) \end{cases}$$

is a curve $t \longrightarrow (x(t),y(t),z(t))$ such that for every t_0 in the interval of definition the limits :

$$\text{Lim } (x(t),y(t),z(t)) \quad = \quad (x(t_0^-),y(t_0^-),z(t_0^-))$$
$$t \longrightarrow t_0 \text{ , } t < t_0$$

$$\text{Lim } (x(t),y(t),z(t)) \quad = \quad (x(t_0^+),y(t_0^+),z(t_0^+))$$
$$t \longrightarrow t_0 \text{ , } t > t_0$$

exist and satisfy the following conditions :

i) If the two limits are equal, then their commun value is $(x(t_0),y(t_0),z(t_0))$, belongs to S_{min} , the derivative exists and we have:

$$\frac{dx}{dt}(t_0) \quad = \quad f(x(t_0),y(t_0),z(t_0))$$

$$\frac{dy}{dt}(t_0) \quad = \quad g(x(t_0),y(t_0),z(t_0))$$

ii) If the two limits are different then they only differ by their last component:

$$(x(t_0^-),y(t_0^-)) \quad = \quad (x(t_0^+),y(t_0^+)) \quad ; \quad z(t_0^-) \neq z(t_0^+)$$

and in the interior of the segment :

$$\left[(x(t_0^-),y(t_0^-),z(t_0^-)) \quad ; \quad (x(t_0^+),y(t_0^+),z(t_0^+)) \right]$$

the function h does not vanish and has the sign of $z(t_0^+) - z(t_0^-)$

We obtain a continuous path if we add to the mapping $t \longrightarrow (x(t),y(t),z(t))$ the vertical segments which join the two points of dicontinuity, and , if necessary, we can add to the ends of the path so formed, unlimited vertical semi-segments if S_{min} is no longer met.

We show on the next picture typical trajectories of the constrained differential equation (E_c) corresponding to (E_ε). (Notice that in order to make the picture readable the choice of axes is special)

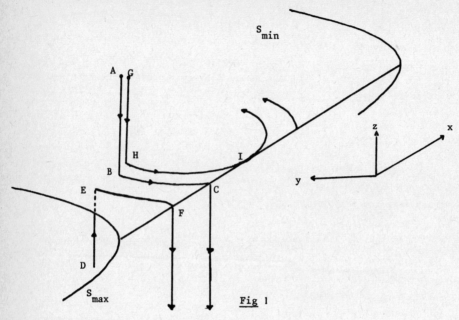

Fig 1

A trajectory starts from A, falls on S_{min} at B follows S_{min} up to the fold line where it falls down to infinity.

A trajectory from D jump to S_{min} at point E, follows the surface and falls down at F.

The trajectory from G is very special: it is just tangent to the fold line at I . Notice that there is no continuous dependance with respect to initial conditions : Very close to G we have trajectories which fall down and trajectories which remain on S_{min}.

There is no problem to draw the trajectories in this example. In general (i.e. for generic f,g,h) it is possible to draw the trajectories without any ambiguity; one has to consider all the possible singularities. This has been done in (14) . In the present note the only singularities we are going to consider are those of type n° 5 or n° 9 of (14). We emphasize that the phenomenum described here has nothing to do with the so called "funnels" which are related to some other kind of singularities.

Local models for the two types of singularities we consider are:

$$\begin{cases} \dfrac{dx}{dt} &= 0 \\[2em] \dfrac{dy}{dt} &= -1 \\[2em] 0 &= (y - z^2) \end{cases}$$

for the first one, and precisely the equation (E_c) which corresponds to (E_ε) by setting $\dfrac{dz}{dt} = 0$, in the same way (F_c) corresponds to (F_ε).

It is apparent from the picture (fig 1) that no solution of (E_c) is close to the surface S_{max}, and it is clear why: From the definition of the solution of a constrained differential equation no solution can stay near S_{max} . This is perfectly reasonnable : If h = -grad V such points wi ll physically correspond to unstable extremums of the potential. But nevertheless , the solution of the "theorem" in & 1 is a solution of (E_ε) which, even if ε is very small, is not close to any solution of (E_c) . See picture below :

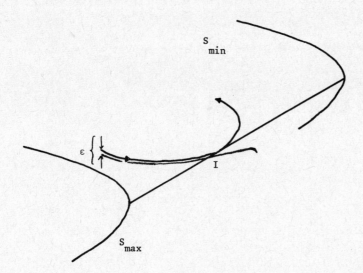

fig 2

242

At this point one can argue that we are not interested in convergence of any individual trajectory of (E_ε) to some trajectory of (E_c) but rather by the convergence of phase portaits. If a trajectory like :

$$t \longrightarrow (x(t) = t,\ y(t) = t^2 - \varepsilon\ ,\ z(t) = -t)$$

is more and more unstable, no matter if it disappears in the limit !!! This seems reasonable, but is not, because the trajectory may be very attracting on a first part and very unstable later. Consider the following exemple, which we recognize as being non generic with respect to the second equation, but which has explicit solutions .

$$\begin{cases} \dfrac{dx}{dt} = 1 \\[2mm] \dfrac{dy}{dt} = +\dfrac{1}{\varepsilon}\ xy \end{cases}$$

The trajectory $t \longrightarrow (x(t) = t\ ,\ y(t) = 0)$ is very unstable for positive t. But , if we choose $\varepsilon = 0.01$, every trajectory which starts at a point x_0, y_0 with $x_0 < -1$ will satisfy $y(t) < 0.4\ 10^{-4}$ for every t such that: $-0.9 < t < 0.9$. Below we show the phase portrait of this equation. Notice that every trajectory which is close to y = 0 at some negative x_0 will remains close to y = 0 in the future up to $-x_0$.

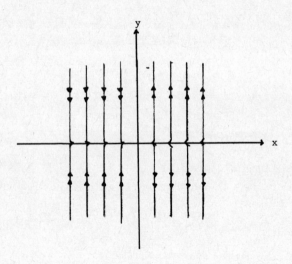

fig 3

At this point we shall not go further. Our opinion is that Non Standard Analysis is more suitable to describe the phase portrait of (F_ε) when ε is small.

IV THE EQUATION (F_ε) WITH ε INFINETESIMAL.

We consider the equation (F_ε) with ε ifinitely small real number different from zero. The mathematician who is interested in mathematical foundations and practice of Nonstandard Analysis is refered to (9) (10) (11). To the non mathematician reader we claim that his intuition about infinitesimals is perfectly sufficient.

Theorem: (By Non Standard techniques) Every standard result about (F_ε) , and especially continuous dependence with respect to initial conditions, is true even if ε is infinitely small - but non zero .

The space $\mathbb{R}^3$ contains standard and non standard points. Every point in $\mathbb{R}^3$ is infinitely close to a standard point which is unique (this is only true for points which are at a limited distance from the origin), this point is called the "shadow". The shadow of x is denoted by $^\circ x$. It is reasonnable to think to the "shadows" as points which are visible with naked eyes, and to think to the points which are infinitely close to some point as points belonging to the microscopic structure, and accessible only to microscopes.

With the same notation as in & III we define the slow manifold S as the set of zeros of h(x,y,z), define S_{max} and S_{min} in the same way and assume that h is generic.

Definition: Constrained arcs of (F_ε) .
A constrained arc of (F_ε) is either the image of a maximal solution of

$$
\begin{cases}
\dfrac{dx}{dt} & = \quad 0 \\[2em]
\dfrac{dy}{dt} & = \quad 0 \\[2em]
\dfrac{dz}{dt} & = \quad \text{sign } h(x,y,z)
\end{cases}
$$

on the open set R^3 S, either the image of a maximal solution on S_{max} or S_{min} of the projection of the vector field (f,g,h) on S_{max} (or S_{min}). Constrained arcs are oriented by the underlying flows.

<u>Definition</u>: A constrained solution is a continuous path composed of a succession of constrained arcs with compatible orientation.

On the picture below we show some constrained solutions of (E_ε). Contrary to solutions of the "constrained equation" (E_c) we have not uniqueness of solutions.

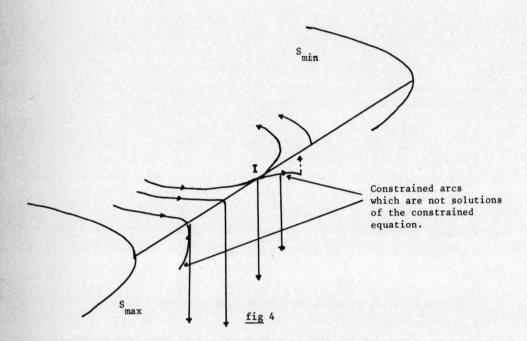

S_{min}

Constrained arcs
which are not solutions
of the constrained
equation.

S_{max}

<u>fig</u> 4

The general theory of relationship between the "shadows" of solutions of (F_ε) and "constrained solutions" of the same equations is rather complete in the case of two dimention systems: See paper by BENOIT, CALLOT, M. and F. DIENER (3) and the bibliography of (6). In R^3 the situation is more complex and no general theory is yet available. There are some partial results (see (4)(5)). In the last paragraphs we explain some of them on a specific example.

V AN EXAMPLE

We consider a system of the form (F_ε), with f,g,h defined as follows:

$$f(x,y,z) = a(z)f_1(x,y) + (1-a(z))f_2(x,y)$$
$$g(x,y,z) = a(z)g_1(x,y) + (1-a(z))g_2(x,y)$$

with:

$$f_1(x,y) = \alpha(x-x_0) - (y-y_0)$$
$$g_1(x,y) = (x-x_0) + \alpha(y-y_0) \qquad \alpha > 0$$

$f_2(x,y)$ not specified but of the order of 1
$g_2(x,y)$ $= +1$

and a function a(z) having a graph of the following form:

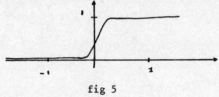

fig 5

The last function is defined by :

$$h(x,y,z) = (y - \frac{z^3}{3} + z)$$

On the next figure we show the constrained solutions of this equation. One sees that we have exactly two types of singular points corresponding to the models we described in &III. The picture emphasizes the lack of uniqueness from the point denoted by C.

We shall use the constrained arcs to describe the solutions of (F_ε).

i) Let (x_1,y_1,z_1) be an initial condition not infinitely close to the slow manifold S. Then the shadow of the corresponding solution is exactly the constrained arc through (x_1,y_1,z_1) until the solution is infinitely close to S or, if not, until the solution is infinitely large. Then there are two possibilities:

246

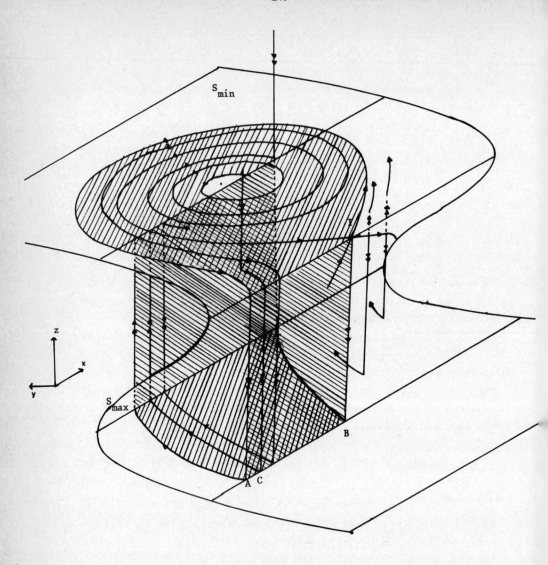

Fig 6

ii-a) The trajectory tends to a point infinitely close to the apparent contour, then go to point iii)

ii-b) The trajectory tends to a point of S_{min} not in the apparent contour, then the shadow is contained in the constrained arc through this point. There are two possibilities: the constrained arc tends to a point on the apparent contour or not; we do not dicuss the second case (which is impossible on our exemple with α positive) then:

iii-a) The point in question has a local model of the form, after a change of coordinates :

$$\frac{dx}{dt} = 0$$

$$\frac{dy}{dt} = -1$$

$$\frac{dz}{dt} = \frac{1}{\varepsilon} (y - z^2)$$

which means that trajectory on S_{min} is transverse to the fold, then the shadow of the trajectory after this point is contrained through the <u>unique</u> constrained arc with the same orientation from this point.

iii-b) The point in question has a local model given by (E_ε) then there are two constrained arcs from this point with the correct orientation and moreover from the one which is drown on S_{min} at any point starts a new constrained arc correctly oriented. By a suitable choice of the initial condition (up to some infinitesimal) there is a trajectory whose shadow is any of the possible choices.

<u>Few words about the proof</u>: Point i) to iii-a) are proved by straightforeward adaptations of the methods of (3). Point iii-b) is somewhat different. The existence of a trajectory with a precribed shadow is given by a continuity argument.

A more precise analysis of iii-b) is possible using the local model (E_ε) - actually it is better to consider a more general model which is essentially the same but is "generic" which is not the case for (E_ε) see (5)- and its explicit solution. This solution is called "Canard" (See (3) to find an explanation of this terminology) ; it plays a central role in a finer analysis. It is proved (see (4)) that this "Canard" is very unstable, in the sense that a solution which remains close to it for an appreciable time must be close to the order of $\exp(- \frac{k}{\varepsilon})$ - Recall the exemple in &III.

One sees on fig 6 that the behaviour of solutions is rather complicate. A solution goes alternatively upward and downward in an apparently unpredictable way. As noticed by ROSSLER and TAKENS we see that this type of differential equations are good candidates for modelling of "chaotic" behaviour. A rigorous mathematical description of the asymptotic behaviour of this equation is delicate. It relies very much on properties of iterations of dicontinuous mappings of the interval (see KEENER (18)) and properties of the "Canard". For instance it is possible to prove that every standard interval contained in the segment [A,B) in fig 6 contains initials conditions for solutions which run along the "Canard" for an appreciable duration. This is the case for initial conditions infinitely close to point C for instance.

VI COMPUTER EXPERIMENTS

We propose (fig 7-11) five computer experiments on the preceding example for various values of the parameters. The parameter ε is fixed at 0.1 . It is very sriking to observe the power of prediction of the theory with ε infinitesimal even in this case.

Fig 7   The heavy line from A to B is a "Canard". One can appreciate the extreme instability with respect to initial conditions. In order to follow the "Canard" from A to B the initial condition must be specified up to 10^{-12}. Notice that the computer certainly dont say : 0.3646045871060 is an initial condition for a "Canard", it just says that, not to far from this point, may be 10^{-4}, 10^{-6}, with the same extreme sensibility to initial condition, there is an initial condition for a "Canard". Nevertheless we are sure of the existence of the "Canard" from A_1 to A_{15} by continuity.

Fig 8   In this experiment we look for a long range behavior. At point A we have two initial conditions A_1 and A_2 which are very close together. We follow them. They are indistinguisable, they turn around the unstable focus, fall down at point B, come back at C, fall down a new time at D, come back at E, turn around up to F and then separate. Notice that they do not separate just at F which should be the case for the constrained equation, but somewhat further.

Fig 9   It the same than the preceding one with some extra initial conditions in the neighbourhood of A.

Fig 10 - Fig 11   The two systems are the same except a slight change in the dynamics for the part which is on the low part of the slow manifold. In one case the trajectory will come back to the focus, in the other one it will drift slowly away from it.

CONCLUSION. In some sense nothing is very new in this paper.

Existence of strange behaviours of differential equations caused by:

- Small parameter
- Re-injection of the solution in the neighbourhood of an unstable focus

was known for a long time, at least by Levinson (in the late forties) by Sil'nikov (in the sixties) and more systematically reintroduced later by Rössler, Takens and other.

But, nevertheless our feeling is that, thanks to the methods of Non Standard Analysis introduced by Benoit, M. and F. Diener, Callot and other people from the "Reeb school" in Strasbourg, and thanks also to modern computer facilities,we have now powerfull tools to get better insight into the behaviour of, to paraphrase the title of a celebrated paper of May, "simple differential equations in R^3 with complicated dynamics".

C. Lobry

1 rue Jacques Bounin
06 100 Nice (France)

F. Mazat

25 rue G. Bizet

33 400 Talence (France)

Fig 7

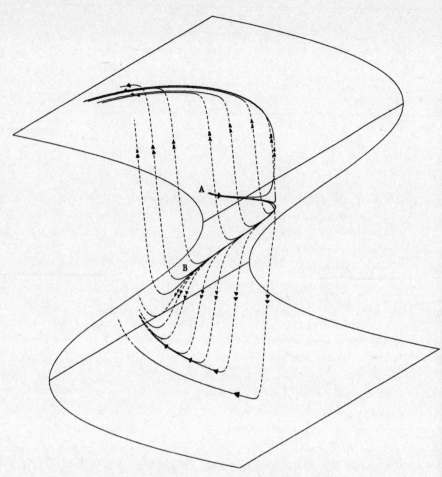

* 0 < T < 3.2

* CONDITIONS INITIALES :

      Y0=0.95 , Z0=1.3

Λ1 : X0=0.35   * Λ2 : X0=0.364   * Λ3 : X0=0.3646

Λ4 : X0=0.3646045   * Λ5 : X0=0.364604585   * Λ6 : X0=0.3646045871

Λ7 : X0=0.3646045871055   * Λ8 : X0=0.3646045871060   * Λ9 : X0=0.3646045871064

Λ10: X0=0.364604587107   * Λ11: X0=0.36460458711   * Λ12: X0=0.3646045872

Λ13: X0=0.364604589   * Λ14: X0=0.3646047   * Λ15: X0=0.366

Fig 8

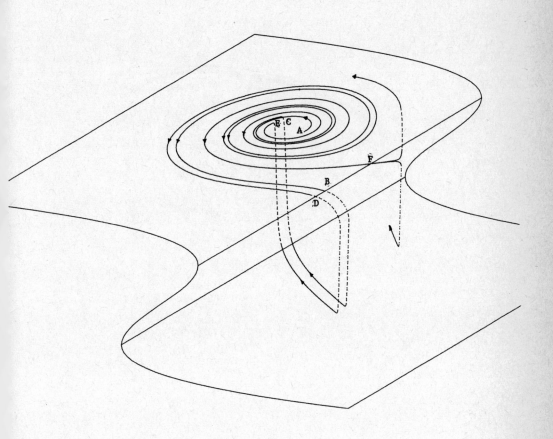

* 0 < T < 58

* CONDITIONS INITIALES :

   A1 : X0=0.0070 * Y0=-0.579 * Z0=1.9

   A2 : X0=0.0071 * Y0=-0.579 * Z0=1.9

Fig 9

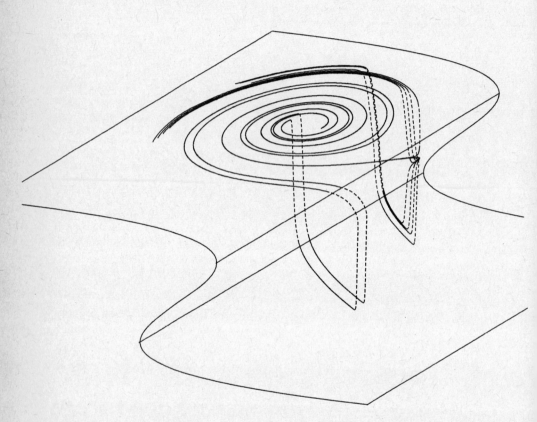

* O < T < 60

* CONDITIONS INITIALES :

       Y0=-0.579 , Z0=1.9

A1 : X0=0.0070   * A2 : X0=0.007067

A3 : X0=0.0070674   * A4 : X0=0.007067447

A5 : X0=0.00706745   * A6 : X0=0.0070675

A7 : X0=0.007068   * A8 : X0=0.0071

Fig 10

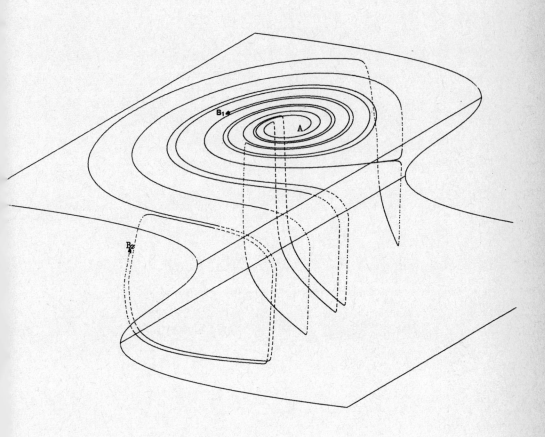

* 0 < T < 70

* CONDITIONS INITIALES :

A $\begin{cases} \text{A1 : XO=0.0070 * YO=-0.579 * ZO=1.9} \\ \text{A2 : XO=0.0071 * YO=-0.579 * ZO=1.9} \end{cases}$

Fig 11

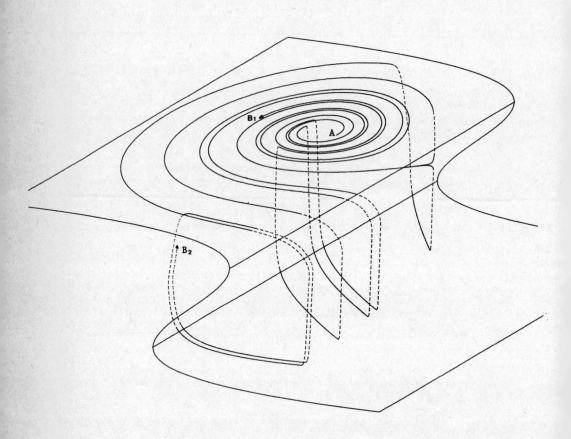

* 0 < T < 70

* CONDITIONS INITIALES :

A { A1 : X0=0.0070 * Y0=-0.579 * Z0=1.9

A2 : X0=0.0071 * Y0=-0.579 * Z0=1.9

REFERENCES

(1) ARGEMI, J. : Approche qualitative d'un problème de perturbations singulières dans R^4. Dans Equadiff 1978, R.CONTI, G.SESTIN, G.VILLARI ed. pp 333 340.

(2) ARGEMI J. et B. ROSSETTO : Solutions périodiques discontinues pour l'approximations singulière d'un modèle neurophysiologique dans R^4. Prépublication.

(3) BENOIT E., J.L. CALLOT, M.et F. DIENER:Chasse au Canard, Collectanea Mathematica vol 31, 1980.

(4) BENOIT E. Travail sur l'équation de Van der Pol en cours de rédaction...

(5) BENOIT E. et C. LOBRY : Canards de R^3, soumis aux C.R.A.S.

(6) CARTIER P. : Perturbations singulières des équations différentielles ordinaires et Analyse Non Standard, Séminaire Bourbaki, exposé n° 580.

(7) LOZI R.:Sur un modèle mathématique de la suite de bifurcation de motifs dans la réaction de BELOUSOV ZHABOTINSKI. C.R.A.S. à paraitre.

(8) LOZI R. et C. LOBRY : Bifurcation of "motifs" in falillies of "Mixed Two-vectors fields". Synergetics

(9) LUTZ R. et M. GOZE : Nonstandard Analysis , Lecture Notes in Mathematics n° 881

(10) NELSON E. : Internal Set Theory , Bul A.M.S. vol 83, 1977, pp 1165-1198.

(11) ROBINSON A : Non Standard Analysis, North Holland, Amsterdam 1966.

(12) ROSSLER O. : Chaos in abstract kinetics: Two prototypes, Bull of Math. Biology, 39, 1977, pp 237-253.

(13) ROSSLER O. : Continuous chaos, four prototype equations. N.Y.A.S. 1979, pp 376-392.

(14) TAKENS F. : Constrained equations; a study of implicit differential equations and their discontinuous solutions. Lecture Notes in Math. n° 525, pp 141-234.

(15) TAKENS F. : Iplicit differential equations; some opens problems? Lecture Notes in Math. n° 535, pp 237-253.

(16) THOM R. : Stabilité structurelle et morphogénèse. Benjamin 1972.

(17) TYSON J. : On the appearance of chaos in a model of the Belousov reaction. J.of Math. Biology, 5, 1978 pp 551-562.

(18) KEENER J.P. : Chaotic behaviour in piecewise continuous difference equations. Trans. Amer. Math. Soc. Vol 261, 1980 pp 589-604.

SELF-PULSING IN RING-LASERS

H. Ohno and H. Haken

Institut für theoretische Physik
Universität Stuttgart
Pfaffenwaldring 57/IV
7000 Stuttgart 80

As this conference deals with nonlinear systems that show periodic behaviour we want to consider the seemingly simple physical model of a ring-laser. The active material is assumed to consist of homogeneously broadened two-level atoms in a ring cavity, one mode of which beeing in perfect resonance with the transition frequency ω_0 of the atoms. Confining ourselves to only one direction of propagation for the electric field, the basic equations of motion take the following form [1,2,5]

$$\partial_t P + \gamma_\perp P = (-iM/(3\hbar))ED + \Gamma_P,$$

$$1 \qquad \partial_t D + \gamma_\parallel D = \gamma_\parallel d_0 + (2i/\hbar)[EP^* - E^*P] + \Gamma_D,$$

$$[\partial_t + c\partial_x + \kappa]E = (i\omega_0/2)P + \Gamma_E.$$

The atoms are described by their polarization density $P(x,t)$ and inversion density $D(x,t)$, their equations of motion are derived from the quantum mechanical treatment of a two level atom in an external field $E(x,t)$. The electric field, on the other hand, is governed by Maxwells equations for an electric field driven by (given) atomic dipoles. The damping constants $\gamma_\parallel$ and $\gamma_\perp$ are introduced heuristically to simulate the finite lifetime of the excited state of the atoms and their natural linewidth, i.e. the spontaneous emission. κ is the damping of the electric field in the cavity. M is the absolute square of the dipol matrix element corresponding to the atomic transition. d_0 describes the pumping process, i.e. the flow of energy into the atomic system, such as to produce, in the absence of the electric field, a fixed inversion in the atoms. This unsaturated inversion will be the control parameter for our system. ∂_t and ∂_x denote the derivatives with respect to time and the one relevant spatial coordinate x. As we treat a ring-cavity, all quantities have to be periodic in the cavity length L

2           $E(x+L,t) = E(x,t), \quad P(x+L,t) = P(x,t), \quad D(x+L,t) = D(x,t)$

Note that in deriving eqs. (1) the rapidly oscillating parts of the electric field and the polarization density have already been eliminated [5], leaving us with a set of first order differential equations for the slowly varying amplitudes E and P. Γ_P, Γ_D and Γ_E are fluctuating forces introduced to ascertain quantum mechanical consistency in the equations (1). As usual, we assume these fluctuations gaussian and delta-correlated in space and time [5,10]. Equations (1) are the starting point of semiclassical laser laser theory, and although their solutions are well known it will be useful to discuss these solutions in some details [1-5].

First we neglect the fluctuations in (1) and look for the stationary solutions. If the pump is lower than a certain critical value given below, the only possible stationary solutions of (1) read

3           $E_{cw} = P_{cw} = 0, \quad D_{cw} = d_o.$

The atoms take the inversion as given by the external pumping process, but there is no radiation field in the cavity. If, on the other hand, the pump is larger than the critical value, a nonzero solution is possible

$$E_{cw}{}^2 = (c\hbar\omega_o/(8\kappa))[d_o - d_{thr}], \quad P_{cw} = (2i\kappa/(c\omega_o))E_{cw},$$

4           $$D_{cw} = d_{thr} = 6\hbar\kappa\gamma_\perp/(c\omega_o M).$$

d_{thr} denotes the threshold value of the pump. The suffixes cw are to indicate the continous-wave solutions, i.e. the usual laser action. Without fluctuations, our laser would emit a single, infinitely long wave of frequency ω_o. This result is, of course, quite unphysical, below threshold the laser should emit thermal light, and above threshold, the emitted radiation should have a nonzero, although very narrow, linewidth. As is well known [5], this is achieved by keeping the fluctuations in equations (1). Thus, at the first laser threshold, fluctuations are necessary to obtain physically reasonable results.

In order to simplify the notation, we now normalize the atomic variables and the electric field to their cw-values. In addition, we scale time and spatial coordinate to units of $\gamma_\perp^{-1}$ and $c\gamma_\perp^{-1}$, respectively. Then the equations (1) take the form

$$[\partial_t + \partial_x + \kappa]E = \kappa P + F_E,$$

5
$$[\partial_t + \gamma]D = \gamma(1+\lambda) - \gamma\lambda EP + F_D,$$

$$[\partial_t + 1]P = ED + F_P.$$

As was shown in the literature [1,2,14], it is sufficient to consider only real amplitudes E and P, if fluctuations are neglected. Keeping the noise terms, this assumption is justified for times small compared to the phase-diffusion time, as will transpire below. λ is a normalized pump parameter given by $(d-d_{thr})/d_{thr}$; κ and γ are dimensionless damping constants (units $\gamma_\perp$). The cw solutions are now given by E=P=D=1.

To investigate the stability of the cw solutions, we now perform a usual linear stability analysis by explicitely introducing the deviations of E, D and P from their cw values

6
$$(E, D, P) = 1 + (e, d, p)$$

and decomposing equations (5) into their linear and nonlinear parts

7
$$[\partial_t + K(\partial_x)]q = (0, -\gamma\lambda ep, ed) + f, \qquad q = (e, d, p),$$

where the linear matrix K is given by

8
$$K(\partial_x) = \begin{pmatrix} \partial_x+\kappa & 0 & -\kappa \\ \gamma\lambda & \gamma & \gamma\lambda \\ -1 & -1 & 1 \end{pmatrix}.$$

Neglecting the nonlinearities and fluctuations, we try a solution of (7) in the form

9
$$(e, d, p) \equiv q = q_o \exp(\beta t + ikx).$$

The corresponding eigenvalue problem has been discussed in the literature [1,3] and we merely summarize its results. If the pump parameter λ is small, all eigenvalues β have negative real parts, i.e. the cw solutions are stable. For large values of λ, two different situations may occur, depending on the magnitude of the cavity loss κ. For large κ and properly chosen cavity length (which means properly chosen possible wavenumbers k) two modes with k=0 may become unstable; the electric field undergoes spatially homogeneous oscillations which may show chaotic temporal behaviour. This case is precisely equivalent to the Lorenz model of turbulence [11-14]. We confine ourselves to the case of small cavity losses κ. Then the instability occurs provided

10
$$\lambda > \lambda_c = 4 + 3\gamma + 2[2(1+\gamma)(2+\gamma)]^{1/2}.$$

If the cavity length (or, equivalently, the possible wavenumbers k) is chosen properly, and if the pump is not too high above the critical value (10), then there occurs one critical mode (real part = 0) with a frequency (imaginary part) given by

11
$$\beta_c^2 = \gamma(\gamma - 3\lambda_c)/2$$

at a critical wavenumber k_c

12
$$ik_c = -\beta_c - \kappa\gamma(\lambda_c+\gamma)/[2\beta_c(1+\gamma)].$$

In the following we assume the cavity length chosen such that the wavelength corresponding to k_c fits one time into the cavity, i.e. we have one pulse running inside the cavity.
To investigate the solutions of (7) above this second threshold, we now have to include the nonlinear terms (and, eventually, the fluctuations). To this end we make the following hypothesis [6-10]

13
$$q = \sum \xi_{k,j}(t)0^j(k)\exp(ikx)\exp(i\omega_k t), \qquad \omega_k = Im(\beta_c)k/k_c .$$

The sum runs over all possible wavenumbers k and all eigenvalues j. The oscillation with ω_k was introduced to make the expansion coefficient $\xi_{k,j}$ a slowly varying amplitude. The constant vectors $0^j(k)$ are the right-hand-side eigenvectors of the linear matrix K as given by (8)

14    $K(ik)0^j(k) = -\beta_j(k)0^j(k)$, $\bar{0}^j(k)K(ik) = -\beta_j(k)\bar{0}^j(k)$.

The left-hand-side eigenvectors $\bar{0}$ are needed in the following and are also defined above. It is then a straightforward procedure [6-10,15-17] to transform the equations (5) into equations for the modes $\xi_{k,j}(t)$

15    $\partial_t \xi_{k,j}(t) = -\gamma_{kj}\xi_{k,j} + \sum_{q,l,m} \Omega^{jlm}_{q,k-q} \xi_{q,l}\xi_{k-q,m} + \eta$

where the coefficients are given by

16    $\gamma_{kj} = \omega_k - \beta_j(k)$, $\Omega^{jlm}_{q,k-q} = \bar{0}^j(k):g:0^l(q):0^m(k-q)$.

The colons indicate the tensorial product of the eigenvectors 0, $\bar{0}$ with the nonlinear coupling tensor in (7). Note that the linear parts in (15) contain essentially the real parts of the eigenvalues β. The basic assumptions for treating the system of equations (14) are now as follows [6,7,10]. First we seperate the equations into into those for the stable modes ξ_s

16    $\partial_t \xi_s = \gamma_s \xi_s + \Omega\xi\xi + \Omega\xi\xi_s + \dots + \eta_s$

and the single unstable mode ξ

17    $\partial_t \xi = b\xi + \Omega\xi\xi_s + \Omega\xi_s\xi_s + \eta$, $\beta = Re(\beta_c)$.

For sake of simplicity, we dropped all unnecessary indices in (16), (17). Due to the nonlinearities, the unstable mode is coupled to the stable modes as indicated in (17), the stable modes couple among themselves and are (for k=0, k=2k_c) driven by the first nonlinear term in (16). Again the fluctuations η would have to be included. In the vicinity of the second threshold, the real part b of the critical eigenvalue β_c becomes very small, whereas the real parts of the stable eigenvalues do not change appreciably. But this means that the motion of the unstable mode becomes very much slower than the motion of the stable modes, which are in turn <u>driven</u> by the unstable mode. This allows us to apply the adiabatic elimination principle [10]: In (16), we may treat the unstable mode ξ as temporally constant and apply the following iteration scheme. As a 0-th order approximation we keep only the terms directly driven by the unstable mode

18
$$\partial_t \xi_s^0 = \gamma_s \xi_s^0 + \Omega \xi \xi, \text{ for } k=0, \ k=2k_c$$

and in the next step we take the modes driven by the modes (18)

19
$$\partial_t \xi_s^1 = \gamma_s \xi_s^1 + \Omega \xi \xi_s^0, \text{ for } k=k_c, \ k=3k_c.$$

As has been shown in the literature [5-10], the adiabatic approximation is equivalent to neglecting the derivatives in (18),(19), which allows to solve these equations immediately

20
$$\xi_s^0 = (-1/\gamma_s)\Omega\xi\xi, \qquad \xi_s^1 = (-1/\gamma_s)\Omega\xi(-1/\gamma_s)\Omega\xi\xi$$

where again we suppressed all indices. Note that there are modes which are of second order in ξ ($k=0$, $k=2k_c$) and of third order ($k=k_c$, $k=3k_c$). These expressions now have to be inserted into the equation for the unstable mode (17), giving rise to higher nonlinearities which eventually will have to stabilize the whole system.

Two remarks have to be made about the solutions (20). First, the fluctuations occuring in (16) have been neglected for the stable modes. This can be justified by treating the problem in terms of a Fokker-Planck equation for the modes and performing an approximation which is equivalent to the steps outlined above [6,7,10]. It can be shown that the corresponding iteration scheme for the stationary solution of this Fokker-Planck equation yields precisely the results (20). Another, although much weaker, argument is that the stable modes have to stabilize the system by the nonlinearities mentioned above, and this is achieved by the solutions (20). If, on the other hand, noise would be included in (20), this would yield multiplicative stochastic forces in the equation for the unstable mode, which eventually would lead to a negligible shift in the critical pump λ_c. In addition, we cancelled the homogeneous solutions of (16) in deriving (20), this gives correct results for times which are large compared to γ_s^{-1}, i.e. the lifetime of the stable modes.

In principle, our iteration scheme can be performed for arbitrary high orders of accuracy, which eventually would give expressions for all modes ξ_s and the corresponding nonlinearities in the equation for the unstable mode, which dominates the behaviour of the whole system and is therefor called the order-parameter of the system. If we confine ourselves to (20), we end up with the following equation

21
$$\partial_t \xi = \beta\xi + \Phi|\xi|^2\xi - \Psi|\xi|^4\xi + \eta$$

which is called the generalized Ginzburg-Landau-equation of our system. Φ and Ψ are rather lengthy expressions in the eigenvectors 0, $\bar{0}$ and the coupling tensor g. Their explicit form is unimportant for our purposes and is therefor not given here.

The discussion of the solutions of (21) is now straightforward. First we split the coefficients Φ and Ψ into real and imaginary parts and decompose ξ into modulus and phase

22
$$\Phi = \phi + i\Phi_i, \qquad \Psi = \psi + i\Psi_i, \qquad \xi = R(t)\exp(i\rho(t))$$

which immediately gives

23
$$\partial_t R = bR + \phi R^3 - \psi R^5 + \eta_R, \qquad \partial_t \rho = \Phi_i R^2 - \Psi_i R^4 + \eta_\rho/R,$$

where η_R and η_ρ are the radial and tangential parts of the fluctuations η in (21). The minus sign in (23) is shown explicitly to indicate the sign of the real part of Ψ, which therefor stabilizes the system. The sign of ϕ, however, depends on the length of the cavity [17]. Changing this length from values lower than the critical length (as defined by k_c, eq. (12)) to larger values one gets a transition from negative ϕ to positive ϕ. But this means, if the r.h.s of (23) is interpreted as the derivative of a potential $V(R)$

$$24 \qquad \partial_t R = - \partial_R V(R)$$

that we may switch from a second order nonequilibrium phasetransition ($\phi < 0$) to a first order transition ($\phi > 0$) [3-5,10]. In the second order case, the cw solution is stable up to $\lambda = \lambda_c$ and then becomes unstable. In the first order case, for $\lambda < \lambda_c$ the cw solutions are stable. For $\lambda < \lambda_c$, due to the positiv cubic term in (23), a metastable state with $R \neq 0$ occurs which eventually, for $\lambda > \lambda_c$, will be the only stable state. This state can be readily determined by the zeros of (24), all stable modes are given by the iteration (20), and thus the fields E, D and P may be calculated using (13). The corresponding results (without noise) are in very good agreement with numerical calculations on this model [1,15]. The fluctuating terms in (23) have now three main effects on the solutions to (23). First, they kick the system out of an unstable state and thus yield the buildup of the pulses above threshold $\lambda = \lambda_c$. Second, they produce a finite lifetime for the metastable state mentioned above, this lifetime can be estimated by using a simple model for the decay of this metastable state [18]

$$25 \qquad \text{decay rate} = \exp[-(V_M - V_o)/Q] + \exp[-(V_M - V_1)/Q]],$$

where V_o and V_1 are the values of the potential at R=0 and the metastable state, respectively; V_M is the height of the potential barrier inbetween. Q is the correlation coefficient of n_R. Numerical calculations for the case $V_o = V_1$ show that the lifetime of the metastable state is by orders of magnitude bigger than the round-trip time of the pulses, i.e. if the system is in the metastable state, it will remain there for rather long times, in this sense, the amplitude fluctuations are negligible.

The last effect produced by the fluctuations is a phase diffusion for ξ as there is no restoring force for the phase in (23). This diffusion leads to a variance of the phases which grows proportional to time

26
$$\langle \rho^2 \rangle - \langle \rho \rangle^2 \simeq Qt/R_0^2$$

where Q is again the correlation coefficient of the fluctuations and R_0 is the state under consideration, for the metastable state this phasediffusion is rather slow as compared to the roundtrip time of the pulses and thus may again be neglected.

As we mentioned in the beginning, fluctuations play a decisive role at the first laser threshold, neglecting them would cause unphysical results. But these fluctuations are determined by quantum properties of light and matter, i.e. they have to simulate spontaneous emission. The second threshold in the laser is determined by the nonlinear dynamics in the system, and as the noise terms have, at least in a good approximation, the same strength as at the first threshold, their influence becomes less and less important, if the pumping power is increased. Thus, at least for times small to those given by (25), (26), at the second threshold noise terms may be safely neglected.

references

[1]   H. Risken and K. Nummedal; J.Appl.Phys. 39(1968)4662
[2]   H. Risken and K. Nummedal; Phys.Lett. 26A(1968)275
[3]   R.Graham and H. Haken; Z.Phys. 213(1968)420
[4]   R.Graham and H. Haken; Z.Phys. 237(1970)31
[5]   H. Haken: "Laser Theory", Encyclopedia of Physics XXV/2c
      Springer, Berlin 1970
[6]   H. Haken; Z.Phys. B21(1975)105
[7]   H. Haken; Z.Phys. B22(1975)69
[8]   H. Haken; Z.Phys. B30(1978)423
[9]   H. Haken; Z.Phys. B29(1978)61
[10] H. Haken: "Synergetics. An Introduction"
      2nd ed., Springer, Berlin 1978
[11] E.N. Lorenz; J.Atmos.Sci. 20(1963)130
[12] H. Haken; Phys.Lett. 53A(1975)77
[13] H. Haken and A. Wunderlin; Phys.Lett. 62A(1977)133
[14] R. Graham; Phys.Lett. 58A(1976)440
[15] H. Haken and H. Ohno; Opt.Comm. 16(1976)205
[16] H. Ohno and H. Haken; Phys.Lett. 59A(1976)261
[17] H. Haken and H. Ohno; Opt.Comm. 26(1978)117
[18] R. Landauer and J.W.F. Woo in "Synergetics", ed. H. Haken,
      Teubner, Stuttgart 1973

NUMERICAL ANALYSIS OF THE BEHAVIOUR OF AN ALMOST PERIODIC SOLUTION TO A PERIODIC DIFFERENTIAL EQUATION, AN EXAMPLE OF SUCCESSIVE BIFURCATIONS OF INVARIANT TORI.

Elaine THOULOUZE-PRATT
Université de Provence
3, place Victor-Hugo
1331 Marseille cédex 3-France

I- INTRODUCTION.

Most problems related to nonlinear forced oscillations that engineers
are faced with can generally be reduced to the study of smooth differential systems such as

$$\dot{X} = F(X,t,\lambda) \qquad (1)$$

periodic with respect to time and dependant on a parameter λ. Among
steady state responses of these systems, time periodic solutions have
been extensively dealt with from a theoretical point of view as well as
a numerical and experimental one, whereas bounded but non-periodic solutions are still being investigated. A theoretical aspect may be found
in the work of Moser [1],[2], Cartwright [3], Bogolyubov and Mitropolskii
[4] whereas numerical or quantitative results are rare. These bounded
oscillations may however lead to defective behaviour of a physical system if they reach large amplitudes and therefore it is of some interest
to be able to study them *a priori*. A method of investigation of such oscillations is given in § II, the results rendered by this method applied to
an example are found in § III. These results turn out to be richer than
expected : they give evidence of successive bifurcations of the initial
torus of solutions into double, quadruple, etc... tori ; § IV contains
the numerical evidence above mentionned.

II- A METHOD OF ANALYSIS.

Our purpose was not at the beginning to study all steady state responses to equation (1) but only almost periodic solutions. It is known
that if there exists an invariant torus of solutions to (1) then there
exists an almost periodic solution.

The problem was then how to analyse the possibility of the existence
of such an invariant torus. An approach was given in THOULOUZE-PRATT [5]

266

together with an existence theorem. JEAN [6] gives another approach
based on a cross-section method. It is the later we shall expose here.

At this point we must introduce the Poincaré mapping :

$$\mathscr{C} : \quad y \in \mathbb{R}^n \longrightarrow q(T,0,y) \in \mathbb{R}^n \qquad\qquad (2)$$

where $q(T,0,y)$ is the value at the time T of the solution of (1) which
has $(0,y)$ as initial conditions (T being the period of equation (1)).

It is easy to see that an invariant torus of solutions to (1) is
equivalent to the existence of an invariant closed curve for the Poincaré mapping (2). JEAN [6] uses what he calls a "thick" cross section
method to study the existence of such an invariant closed curve. We
shall attempt here to give an idea of this method which bears some re-
semblance with the cross section method in dynamical systems. Successive
iterates of a given point by the Poincaré mapping may be considered as
lying on a smooth curve. The method consists in finding amongst this
family of curves, a closed one. Considering a portion of space $\mathscr{S}$ enclosed between two hyperplanes S and $\mathscr{C}$S , the second being the Poincaré
image of the first, its intersection with a given curve in the family
is composed of segments of curve. Let A be such a segment ; there exists
a segment of curve B which is the first segment met in $\mathscr{S}$ after running
from A along the curve (see Fig. 1).

A mapping Φ is thus defined which maps
such arcs A into their first proximate
B. A precise mathematical definition of
Φ is found in [6].

If the mapping Φ thus defined has a
fixed point then there is a closed invariant curve for the Poincaré mapping and
the fixed point is the part of the closed
invariant curve which is in $\mathscr{S}$. JEAN
shows that under certain conditions one
is assured that Φ has a fixed point ;
from a computationnal point of view
fixed points of Φ are too difficult to
attain and would involve too heavy a
computation. The mapping Φ is therefore
approximated by a simpler mapping ψ
which to a given point x in S maps the
point where an interpollating curve of

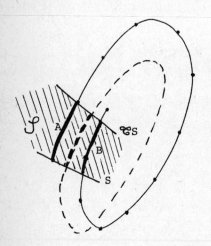

FIG. 1

the Poincaré iterates issued from x, intersects S . This mapping ψ is of course determined in an implicit manner and therefore one does not use Newton's method to find its fixed points. The derivative of ψ is approached by finite differences. The algorithm used is the following :

$$
\left[
\begin{array}{l}
- x^o \in S \subset \mathbb{R}^{n-1} \quad \text{given} \\
- x^{k+1} = x^k - (D_k - I)^{-1} (\psi(x^k) - x^k)
\end{array}
\right.
\tag{3}
$$

where I is the identity in $\mathbb{R}^{n-1}$ and D_k an (n-1) order matrix which coefficients are

$$
d_{ij}^k = \frac{\psi_i(x^k + he_j) - \psi_i(x^k)}{h}
$$

(e_j is the jth vector of an orthonormal basis of S).

For more details on the "thick" cross section method and a justification of the approximation of Φ by ψ see [6] and [7].

III- NUMERICAL RESULTS,

This algorith was tested on an example of two second order differential equations modelizing a coupled circuit of two electrical oscillators with a saturated self :

$$
\left.
\begin{array}{l}
\dot{y}_1 = y_3 \\[4pt]
\dot{y}_2 = y_4 \\[4pt]
\dot{y}_3 = - \omega_o^2 y_1 + K\omega_o^2 y_2 - 2q\omega_o (1 + 8a_1 y_1^2) y_3 - \frac{8}{3}\omega_o^2 (a_1 y_1^3 - Ka_2 y_2^3) + \\[4pt]
\qquad\qquad\qquad\qquad 2\omega\omega_o \; E \cos \omega t \\[4pt]
\dot{y}_4 = - \omega_o^2 y_2 + K\omega_o^2 y_1 - 2q\omega_o (1 + 8a_2 y_2^2) y_4 - \frac{8}{3}\omega_o^2 (a_2 y_2^3 - Ka_1 y_1^3)
\end{array}
\right\}
\tag{4}
$$

BOUC-IOOSS-DEFILIPPI [8] had shown that for the parameter value $\lambda = 220 \times \frac{\omega}{\omega_o} = 772.72$ the periodic solution to (4) bifurcates into an invariant torus of solutions. We therefore took up this example and starting at the parameter value $\lambda = 773$ used algorithm (3) to compute a fixed moint of ψ, that is a closed invariant curve for the Poincaré mapping $\mathscr{C}$. The algorithm converged very rapidly, and was used for successively greater values of the parameter, the bifurcation branch was thus explored. The eigen-values of the matrix D^k are calculated so as to have an idea of the stability of the fixed points determined by (3). Around the parameter value $\lambda=776.31$ the spectral radius of D^k becomes greater than one which may indicate a loss of stability at this point. However for yet greater values of the parameter the algorithm converges and so enables us to attain unstable invariant closed curves.

The above results being difficult to visualise a certain number of Poincaré iterates issued from the fixed point of ψ determined by (3) for successive values of λ are plotted, the closed invariant curves appear more clearly on the figures shown in § IV.

IV- SUCCESSIVE BIFURCATIONS OF THE INVARIANT TORUS.

The first two components, y_1 and y_2, of the Poincaré iterates are plotted here. One may observe that as the parameter value increases and

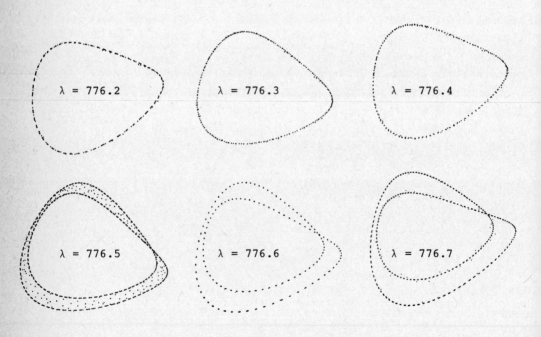

$\lambda = 776.2$ $\lambda = 776.3$ $\lambda = 776.4$

$\lambda = 776.5$ $\lambda = 776.6$ $\lambda = 776.7$

FIG. 2

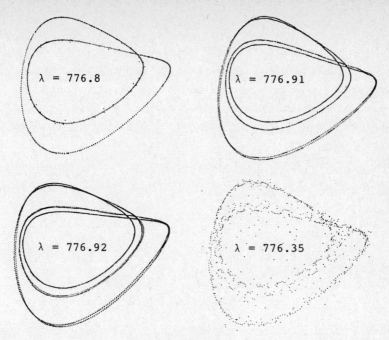

FIG.3

becomes greater than 776.31 the instability of the closed curve becomes apparent. It is interesting to note that for example for the parameter value λ=776.5 the closed curve found by algorithm (3) is unstable, the Poincaré iterates do not stay on the curve but are attracted by a new stable closed curve that one qualifies as double. This state of things remains until the parameter reaches the value 776.9 where the "double" curve becomes itself unstable and the Poincaré iterates are attracted by a "quadruple" curve. At parameter value 776.92 the points are then attracted by an "octuple" curve. The following enlargements show more clearly this dedoubling phenomena.

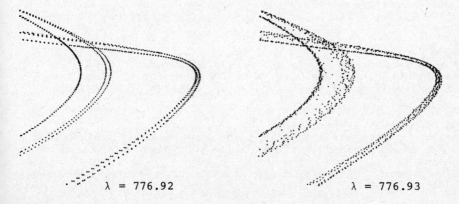

FIG.4

V- CONCLUSION.

One is of course tempted to view these results in the light of
Feigenbaum's [9] universal theory in nonlinear systems. The values
of the parameter for which the curves dedouble, were sought for with
a little more precision. Unfortunately it becomes rapidly too difficult to differentiate a 16-uple curve from a 32-uple curve. Because
of this merely the first three values of $\delta_n = \dfrac{\lambda_{n+1} - \lambda_n}{\lambda_{n+2} - \lambda_{n+1}}$ were cal-

culated,

$$\delta_o = 8.19 \quad , \quad \delta_1 = 7.71 \quad , \quad \delta_3 = 5.18$$

REFERENCES

[1] MOSER, J.
On the construction of almost periodic solutions for ordinary
differential equations.
*Proc. Int. Conf. on Functional Analysis and Related Topics,
pp. 60-67, Tokyo (1969).*

[2] MOSER, J.
Stable and random motions in dynamical systems.
Annals of Mathematics Studies, Princeton University Press (1973).

[3] CARWRIGHT, M.L.
Almost periodic flows and solutions of differential equations.
Proc. Lond. Math. Soc., 3, 355-380 (1967).

[4] BOGOLYUBOV, N. ; MITROPOL'SKII, Yu.
Les méthodes asymptotiques en théorie des oscillations non
linéaires, Moscou 1955.
Traduction en langue française : Gauthier-Villars, Paris (1962).

[5] THOULOUZE-PRATT, Elaine
Existence Theorem of an invariant torus of solutions to a
periodic differential system.
*Nonlinear Analysis, Theory, Methods & Applications, 5, 195-202
(1981).*

[6] JEAN, M.
Sur la méthode des sections pour la recherche de certaines
solutions presque périodiques de systèmes forcés périodiquement.
*Int. Journal of Nonlinear Mechanics, 15, 367-376, Pergamon
Press (1980).*

[7] THOULOUZE-PRATT, Elaine ; JEAN, M.
Analyse numérique du comportement d'une solution presque pério-
dique d'une équation différentielle périodique par une méthode
des sections.
*Soumis pour publication à Int. Journal of Nonlinear Mechanics,
Sept. 1981.*

[8]   BOUC, R. ; DEFILIPPI, M. ; IOOSS, G.
      On a problem of forced nonlinear oscillations. Numerical exam-
      ple of bifurcation into an invariant torus.
      *Nonlinear Analysis, Theory, Methods & Applications, 2, 211-224,
      (1978).*

[9]   FEIGENBAUM, Mitchell J.
      Quantitative Universality for a Class of Nonlinear Transfor-
      mations.
      Journal of Statistical Physics, 19, 25-52 (1978).

CHAPTER 4

Stochastic modelling of rhythms

EVOLUTIVE SPECTRAL ANALYSIS BY AUTOREGRESSIVE PROCESS OF ISOTOPIC CLIMATIC DATA FROM ANTARCTICA

BY

AIT OUAHMAN A.
GLANGEAUD F.
BENOIST J.-P.

RESUME - *ANALYSE SPECTRALE EVOLUTIVE PAR MODELE AUTOREGRESSIF DE DONNEES CLIMATIQUES ISOTOPIQUES RECUEILLIES EN ANTARCTIQUE*

L'échelle de temps est un des problèmes importants posés pour l'interprétation des données climatiques isotopiques. Pour un carottage de 906 m réalisé à Dôme C (Antarctique), l'analyse spectrale évolutive par modèle autoregressif semble montrer qu'au cours de la période glaciaire ($\approx$ 15 000 ans BP à $\approx$ 30 000 ans BP) l'accumulation était égale à 75 % de la valeur actuelle. Ce résultat confirme la chronologie provisoire (1). En admettant une accumulation de 3,7 cm an^{-1} équivalent en glace pour l'Holocène (jusqu'à $\approx$ 11 000 ans BP) on montre l'existence de trois périodes (2 500 ans, 1 330 ans et 830 ans). Ces résultats pourraient donc, s'ils sont confirmés, fournir une base aux chronologies obtenues par une démarche sensiblement équivalente pour un carottage à Camp Century (Groenland) (2) et à la Station Byrd (Antarctique) (3).

ABSTRACT

The time scale is one of the problems when studying climatic isotopic series. For a 906 meters deep ice core from Dome C (Antarctica), evolutive spectral analysis with an autoregressive model suggests that the accumulation rate during the last glacial age ($\approx$ 15,000 years BP to $\approx$ 30,000 years BP) is 75 % of the present value. This confirms the previously determined time scale (1). Assuming the accumulation rate is about 3.7 cm yr^{-1} of ice equivalent for the Holocene, the data contains three periodicities (2,500 years, 1,330 years and 830 years). If these results are confirmed, they could ensure, a posteriori the chronologies found using a similar approach for ice cores from Camp Century (Greenland) (2) and Byrd Station (Antarctica) (3).

Climatic changes are of particular importance to man's supply system. To put present changes in a proper perspective, information on

a much longer time scale is required. Furthermore, the changes are not
necessarily synchronous nor uniform in amplitude or even in direction
and improved knowledge and understanding of climatic variations requires a
global data base with sufficient regional resolution. As the instrumental
record on Antarctica does not go beyond the last 25 years, proxy data such
as that given by isotopic composition of snow layers must be studied (4).

Many factors other than the atmospheric condensation temperature
may influence the mean δ composition of the deposited cold snow layers
(4). These factors, which are not directly related to local temperature,
cause a "noise" which covers the climatic information (5) (6).

Another problem in dating snow layers is that of time scale. We
are often faced with several chronologies and no objective criterion to
choose between them. Evolutive spectral analysis would be an efficient
means of making this choise.

An isotopic series from Camp Century (Greenland) has already
been analysed by classical Fourier analysis (2). The results show a frequency
varying quite regularily from 2,100 years for the top to 4,000 at the bottom
of the ice core. To improve the chronology, this periodicity was assumed
to be equal to the 2,400 year periodicity in the modulations of C^{14}
abundance. As will be seen, our approach is quite different.

I - DATA

During the 1977-78 Antarctic field season a 906 m deep ice core
was drilled at Dome C (74°49'S, 124°10'E, elevation 3240 m, present mean
annual temperature - 53,5 °C) (7).

I-1- Ice core sampling :

In order to keep the number of samples within a reasonnable limit
three sample lengths were used :

maximum depth	approximative age of max. depth	sample length	approximate sample time-span
50 m	1,000 yrs	0.35 to 0.5 m	≃ 10 yrs
400 m	10,000 yrs	1.86 to 2.56 m	≃ 70 yrs
905 m	30,000 yrs	3.2 to 3.85 m	≃ 140 yrs

In all, the core was cut into 484 contignous samples.

The deuterium values were determined by mass spectrometry and are
expressed in δ D % versus SMOW (Standard Mean Oceanic Water with a D/H ratio
equal to 155.76 10^{-6}) (8). The standard deviation is $\pm$ 0.5 % and therefore

all the data can be used. The measured value is the average over the sample length. This process represents sampling after integration with a variable sampling rate. The measured values are plotted in Fig. 1.

I-2- Time scale :

From 0 to about 230 meters, snow layer density increases from 0.34 gr cm^{-3} to 0.917 gr cm^{-3} (density of ice). Discontinuous densities measured along the core were fitted by a continuous density - depth profile. The real depth was transformed to meters of ice equivalent. For ice core dating various methods are avalaible (9) : measurements of radiative decay, periodic changes of various parameters and specific horizons dated from other sources. A preliminary time scale can be calculated from the simplest ice flow model(10). This model has many limitations (11) but it can be applied with reasonable confidence to the Dome C area (1).

The age of ice (t.yr) with depth can be computed using :

$$t = \frac{H}{\lambda} \ Ln \ \frac{H}{H - z} \qquad (1)$$

where λ is the accumulation rate, H the total ice thickness (3,400 m) and z the depth, all expressed in meters of ice equivalent.

The unknown accumulation rate can be determined using climatic features appearing in Dome C ice core and dated with the C^{14} method applied to southern hemisphere marine cores (Indian ocean). Taking into account that the amount of vapour decreases with temperature, the following rates have been given (1) : (3.7 $\pm$ 0.04) cm yr^{-1} of ice equivalent for the Holocene (about 11,000 years) and (2.78 $\pm$ 0.04) cm yr^{-1} for the last glacial age (15,000 years B.P. to $\simeq$ 30,000 years B.P.). Over the transition period the accumulation rate decreases regularly. According to these values, the bottom of the core is about 32,000 years old.

Assuming a variable accumulation rate, the study of crystal size gives an age of 53,000 years for the bottom of the core (12).

The microparticle concentrations indicate that the accumulation rate has remained constant over the time period covered by the Dome C core (13). According to this study, the age of ice at the core bottom is between 22,000 yr and 30,000 yr. Taking λ = 3.7 cm yr^{-1} of ice equivalent, equation 1 gives 27,000 years for the bottom age . This value lies between those mentioned above.

It is therefore necessary to determine whether or not the accumulation rate has changed and if so by how much. In doing so, one of the assumptions made in (2) will be used if climatic data countains periodicities, these periodicities are continuous and stable. Using the method of evolutive spectral analysis, described later, we shall test two dating models : a time scale with constant accumulation rate ($\lambda = 3.7$ cm yr^{-1} of ice equivalent), referred to as model 1 and model 2 with variable accumulation rate.

II - DATA INTERPOLATION AND FILTERING

Whatever the time scale, the data is heterogeneous because of the three different sampling rates and missing data. Such data cannot be processed directly using data processing methods which need a regular sampling rate.

First of all, linear interpolation with constant sampling intervals less than the original maximum sampling rate was applied to the data. It was checked that error could be neglected at low frequencies.

Fig. 1 shows the original data. It contains long periodicities (> ≈ 5,000 years) as well as the shorter periodicities which have to be analysed. The amplitude difference between these two kinds of fluctuations necessitates the elimination of lower frequencies by filtering. A non recursive filter with three transition points was used to eliminate the low frequencies (14 - 15).

Linear interpolation introduces spurious high frequencies. Because of the three sampling rates, the data must be homogenized. According to the Shannon's sampling theorem, only periodicities longer than $2.T_{max}$ (T_{max} is the maximum sampling rate in the original data) are significant. A time smoothing was made by convolution with a triangular window with a width of $2 T_{max}$. The data processed in this manner will be used as an input to the evolutive spectral analysis.

III - EVOLUTIVE SPECTRAL ANALYSIS USING AN AUTOREGRESSIVE PROCESS

Data can contain various components of variable frequency and amplitude with time. Such data can be represented by 3 dimensional surface giving the energetic distribution as a function of time t and frequency f. The projection of the crest-lines of this surface gives the frequency-time relationships.

Two types of process exist, those for which the components are frequency modulated and those with stable frequencies (16). According to the assumption stated in the first part of this paper, isotopic data belongs to the second type.

III-1- Principle of the autoregressive process :

Classical Fourier analysis processes the data as a whole and is very sensitive to sample errors. It therefore cannot be applied to this climatic series because its unstationnarity.

As already shown (17), spectral analysis using an autoregressive process is highly suited to the analysis of short sequences. The evolutive spectral analysis of isotopic data is only possible with such a method.

In the estimation of spectral power density by an autoregressive model, data is identified with the synthetic output of a filter with a white noise input (18).

An AR process can be expressed as :

$$y_n = \sum_{i=1}^{p} \hat{a}_i \, y_{n-i} + e_n \qquad (2)$$

where a_i represents the coefficients of the filter, p the order of the process and e_n a mean averaged noise with a variance σ^2.

The spectral power density is expressed as :

$$S\,(\nu) = \frac{2\,\sigma^2\,\Delta t}{\left|1 - \sum_{n=1}^{p} a_i \exp\,(-\,j\,2\pi\,n\,\nu\,\Delta t)\right|^2} \qquad (3)$$

Burg (19) introduced the notion of forward and backward prediction. In the forward prediction the point n is predicted from the p previous data in the signal. In the backward prediction the p following points are used to predict the value y_n so the total prediction error is :

$$P_T = \frac{1}{2}(P_f + P_b) \qquad (4)$$

with

$$P_f = \frac{1}{N-p} \sum_{N=N-p}^{N} \left(y_n - \sum_{i=1}^{p} \hat{a}_i \, y_{n-i}\right)^2$$

$$P_b = \frac{1}{N-p} \sum_{n=N}^{N+p} \left(y_n - \sum_{i=1}^{p} \hat{a}_i \, y_{n+i}\right)^2$$

III-2- Choise criterion :

The use of an AR process is based on the following considerations (20) : its definition is very simple, the estimation of the coefficient is obtained by a simple matrix inversion and the A.R. process gives the eigen modes of the studied process. This is very important for our study, where the objective is to detect the components which will be over the elementary analysis sequence the eigen modes of the signal. An AR process is less sensitive to the quality of the estimated correlation function and to the underestimation of process order than Pisarenko's model (21) (22) (23).

III-3- Parameters estimation :

To perform an evolutive spectral analysis, two sorts of methods are avalaible : global methods (for which the complete computation is reiterated for each contiguous sequence of N samples) and recursive methods (for which the parameters are updated taking into account new acquisitions). Recrusive methods require less computer time.

Burg's estimator is non-biaised and defined non-negative, however, it is underoptimal because error power is only minimised using the last coefficient. For short sequences, this estimator is highly sensitive to the initial phase and the splitting of frequency peaks can occur (23).

The optimal solution (in terms of least squares) is given by the covariance method (23). The differenciation of the prediction error with respect to all coefficients of the model gives the linear system

$$\underline{\underline{R}}_N \cdot \underline{A} = \underline{S} \qquad (5)$$

$\underline{A} = a_j$ coefficient of AR filter

$\underline{\underline{R}}_N = R_{ik}$ covariance matrix

$$R_{ik} = \left[\sum_{i=p+1}^{N} y_{i-j}\, y_{i-k} + \sum_{i=1}^{N-p} y_{i+j}\, y_{i+k} \right] \qquad \begin{array}{l} \text{i line subscript} \\ \text{j column subscript} \end{array}$$

$\underline{S}$ = covariance vector

$$\underline{S}^T = [s_j] = \sum_{i=p+1}^{N} y_{i-j}\, y_i + \sum_{i=1}^{N-p} y_{i+j}\, y_i$$

In time recursive methods a recurrence allows the computation of $\underline{R}_N$, $\underline{R}_N^{-1}$ and $\underline{S}_N$ for each step from their values in the previous step.

If the process is stationary, the knowledge of a new sample-point ensures the accurracy of parameter estimations and the length N of the estimation memory will therefore be increased.

The computation of the recurrence is performed with the recursive least squares algorithm. A detailed description can be found in (24 - 25).

III-4- Derivation of the order of the AR process and the size of the estimation memory :

The order p of an AR process depends on the noise to signal ratio and on the number of components to be studied. A signal with m simple frequencies (i.e. constant frequency and amplitude) is correctly described by a 2 m order AR process. The optimal order to analyse an N-sample sequence is given by the F.P.E. (Final Prediction Error) criterion or by the maximum likelihood criterion and is always inferior to N/2 (26).

The estimation memory size N is always greater than the longest periodicity in the data. The memory size is optimum when equal to the length over which the process is locally stationnary. This is calculated, for each iteration, by the evolutive program.

IV - ISOTOPIC DATA ANALYSIS RESULTS

Signal filtering was performed with a Plurimat-S and the evolutive spectra computed with a Norsk data computer. The computer memory size limits the range of analysis to 256 samples for time, 128 samples for frequency and limits the study to six simultaneous frequencies.

The spectrum estimated by the Fourier transform or by the maximum enthropy method is used to determine the frequency-band for the analysis. The data is filtered to eliminate frequencies outside of the studied range.

Model	T_{max}	Memory size 49 samples	Cut-off frequencies and corresponding periodicities	
1	27,266 yrs	5,194 yrs	$2.62 \ 10^{-4} \ yr^{-1}$ (3810 yrs)	$1.96 \ 10^{-3} \ yr^{-1}$ (510 yrs)
2	31,988 yrs	6,122 yrs	$2.25 \ 10^{-4} \ yr^{-1}$ (4440 yrs)	$1.85 \ 10^{-3} \ yr^{-1}$ (540 yrs)

Table 1 - Characteristics of the signals

IV-1- Order estimation :

The MEM, together with the FPE criterion, gives the AR process order. As there are no dating modifications for the Holocene (fig. 1), the order was estimated to be p = 12 using this period alone. This working method can be used to follow the modifications induced by changing the time scale.

IV-2- Simulation results (24) :

Before examining results from isotopic data processing. Various numerical simulations must be presented as they shed light on the interpretation of the results.

The simulation results depend on the initial phase of the signal and the same AR process sampled with two different rates can therefore give two different results.

An unstable frequency can disturb the adjacent frequencies and leads to branching as shown in fig. 2a.

If a signal with simple frequencies has various sampling rates, the results can be as shown in fig. 2b.

If the data is filtered with an abrupt cut-off filter, frequencies corresponding to this abrupt cut-off will be present.

Results for isotopic data processing are given in fig. 3 (model with constant accumulation) and in fig. 4.

IV-3- Spectral analysis results :

In fig. 3 and 4, all the features obtained from numerical simulations can be seen. The frequency numbered 4 in the two figures corresponds to the filter cut-off frequency and does not need to be considered. The circled areas correspond to branching zones where unstable frequencies interfere. The initial phase influence can be seen by comparing results from the two models in the first part of the Holocene (the data differs only in the analysis sampling rate).

In fig. 3, there are three zones with stable periodicities :

2,500 yrs from 2,600 to 8,250 years B.P.
2,060 yrs from 18,900 to 24,600 years B.P.
625 yrs from 17,700 to 24,600 years B.P.

In fig. 4, the results are :

2,500 yrs from 2,950 to 7,500 years B.P.
2,500 yrs from 18,100 to 29,000 years B.P.
825 yrs from 19,000 to 29,000 years B.P.

These zones are shaded in the figures.

In fig. 4, the 2,500 year periodicity (referenced 1) remains stable over the first part of the Holocene and the last part of the glacial age. Its relative instability during the intermediate stage of analysis, when the estimation memory N incorporated an increasing amount of transition age data, will be examined below.

If the frequency is stable, the modification of accumulation rate (and as consequence the sampling-rate) would give a $2500/0.75 = 1880$ year periodicity for model 1. The periodicity determined for the last part of the glacial age is 2,060 years. This value agrees well, with the theoretical value (1,880 years) taking into account a 10 % uncertainty for the accumulation rate.

With the same modification, the 825 years becomes 619 years, a value in very good agreement with the 625 year periodicity found in the first model.

Three relatively stable periodicities were considered in the first part of the Holocene for model 1 : 2,500 years, 1,250 years and 825 years. These frequencies are numbered 1,2 and 3 respectively in fig. 3. If the glacial age accumulation is 75 % of the Holocene value, these periodicities must be 1,875 years, 937 years and 619 years respectively. The theoretical results are represent by horizontal continuous lines. The result is nearly perfect for the 825 yr periodicity, in good agreement for the 2,500 yr periodicity and incorrect for the 1,250 yr periodicity.

Taking the same periodicities for the Holocene in model 2 and assuming that they are stable with this dating, these periodicities would theoretically give three horizontal lines (numbered 1, 2, 3 in fig. 4).

Very good results are obtained for the 2,500 years periodicity.

The second frequency is not present and is replaced by a less stable ≈ 1,330 year periodicity. This can be explained by a modification in phase or by combination of frequencies. The 825 year frequency appears only in the last part of the glacial age and the small stable area in the Holocene age cannot be retained as it is less than the estimation memory size.

In the intermediate area (from 8,400 to 17,600 years B.P.) the sampling rate is unsatisfactory as shown by the increasing instability and interference at all frequencies (fig. 3). In spite of the preceding results concerning model 2 (fig. 4), the stability of frequencies is very poor in the intermediate area. Two factors may have affected the results : the instantaneous variation in the accumulation rate taken for the transition dating or the relationship itself may erroneous. A steeper variation of accumulation rate with smooth branching without discontinuities is suggested by the three results. As will be pointed out below, many other factors may have influenced the dating over the climatic transition.

IV-4- Discussion of results :

All these results suggest that the accumulation has varied but it remains to be seen whether the age of 53,000 years assumed in (12) is valid. Assuming that 3.7 cm yr^{-1} of ice equivalent is a reasonable value for the Holocene accumulation rate, a rate of about 1 cm yr^{1} of ice equivalent must be considered for the glacial period to reach an age of 53,000 years for the bottom of the core. As previously demonstrated, the 2,500 year periodicity in model 1 would drop to ≈ 900 years for the glacial period. Such a drop is not evident in fig. 3 and 4. To explain the results given in (12), it is possible that the accumulation rate is erroneous and differs for the Holocene period from those previously assumed. This hypothesis seems to be invalid and recent studies (see 29 for a review) show that for the last 2,000 years the mean accumulation is 4 cm yr^{-1} of ice equivalent. This value is not significantly different from (3.7 ± 0.4) cm yr^{-1} . Further evidence is given by C^{14} dating (1). Another assumption can be made to explain the 53,000 year value. The ice viscosity may have been modified during the cold period. This assumption is supported by studies of ice cores from Devon Island (28).

It should be remembered that our study has many limiting factors. As pointed out in (11), the depth to time transformation has many limitations and this transformation is the basis of the two models tested. Changes in ice sheet altitude and ice viscosity are not taken into account and have probably disturbed the ice flow over the climatic transition.

Taking into account the accumulation rate inaccuracy and the result instability, the periodicities are 2,500 $\pm$ 250 years, 1,330 $\pm$ 150 yrs and 830 $\pm$ 100 yrs.

The 2,500 year periodicity seems to be the most significant and represents up to 20 % of the variance of the HF signal from $2.62 \ 10^{-4} \ yr^{-1}$ to $1.96 \ 10^{-3} \ yr^{-1}$. This frequency range corresponds to 510 yr to 3800 yr periodicities. The two others are less significant, 7 % for 830 yrs and 5 % for 1,330 yrs.

In (30), it is shown that climatic variation exists over all time ranges and suggests the 2,500 year periodicity. Our 2,500 year periodicity determined without any reference to the modulations of atmospheric C^{14} abundance, confirms, a posteriori, the Camp Century ice core chronology (2) value taken as 2,400 years. In fact these modulations are now well documented (31 - 32) and the possibility of solar activity variations exists (32 - 33). However the relationship between these variations and the earth's climate is far from being accepted by the scientific world (34 - 35 - 36). Our results confirm those from the Byrd ice core in which a 2,400 year periodicity was found over the first 20,000 years.

Taking into account all these results, the 32,000 year age of the Dome C ice core bottom seems to be the most probable value.

CONCLUSION

An original method for evolutive spectral analysis was applied to a climatic isotopic series considered to be a non-stationnary AR process, in order to test two corresponding time scales. Although the absolute age of the bottom of the core cannot be determined using this method, it seems possible to confirm the value of 0.75 for the change in the accumulation rate as previously assumed (1).

In the studied bandwith, three stable periodicities are shown by the isotopic data : (2500 $\pm$ 250) yrs, (1,330 $\pm$ 150) yrs and (830 $\pm$ 100) yrs. The stable and continuous 2,500 year periodicity seems to be the most significant and represents 20 % of the H. F. signal. This periodicity, calculated

285

without any reference to modulations of C^{14} abundance, confirms the chronologies of the Camp Century ice core (2) and of the Byrd ice core for the
first 20,000 years.

Many factors limit this study. First of all this method needs
further work on the choice of order and memory for the A.R. process
identification when the data is non-stationnary. The influence of filtering
and homogeneization has to be considered. A doubt remains on the frequency
of 2,500 years because it could be also a cut-off effect. Other computation
and simulations will be performed to check the significance of this periodicity.

The two models tested are based on the same dynamic assumptions and it
would be very useful to apply this method to dynamic models that take into
account ice viscosity variations.

AIT OUAHMAN A.   (1)*
GLANGEAUD F.   (1)
BENOIST J.-P.   (2)

(1)   Centre d'Etudes des Phénomènes Aléatoires et Géophysiques
       Equipe associée au CNRS n°93
       B. P. 46
       38400 SAINT MARTIN D'HERES (France)

(2)   Laboratoire de Glaciologie et Géophysique de l'Environnement
       Laboratoire propre du CNRS
       2, rue Très Cloitres
       38031 GRENOBLE CEDEX (France)

(*)   Presently at Université Caddi Ayyad
                     Marrakech
                     Maroc

References

(1) LORIUS C., MERLIVAT L., JOUZEL J., POURCHET M., 1979.
A 30 000 yr isotope climatic record from Antarctic ice. Nature,
280   644-648.

(2) DANSGAARD W., JOHNSEN S.J., CLAUSEN H.B. and LANGWAY C.C.Jr,
1971. The late cenozoïc glacial ages. Karl K Turebian, Editor
copyright (c) 1971 by Yale University.

(3)JOHNSEN S.J.,DANSGAARD W., CLAUSEN H..B. and LANGWAY C.C.,
1972. Oxygen isotope profiles through the Antarctic and Greenland
ice sheets, Nature, 235 : 429.

(4)DANSGAARD W., JOHNSEN S.J., CLAUSEN H.B., GUNDESTRUP N.,
1973. Stable isotope glaciology. Meddelelser om Grønland, Bd 197,
N°2 : 1-53

(5) ROBIN G de Q., 1981. Climate into ice : the isotopic record in polar ice
sheets. IAHS., Pub. N°131 : 207-216.

(6) ROBIN G. de Q. : to be published. In Cambridge monograph on isotopic
and temperature profiles in polar ice sheets. Cambridge University
Press.

(7) LORIUS C., DONNOU D., 1978. Campagne en Antarctique, Nov. 1977-
Février 1978. Courrier du CNRS 30 : 6-17.

(8)JOUZEL J., MERLIVAT L., LORIUS C. and POURCHET M., 1981.
A 30 000 yr climatic record : main results deduced from oxygen 18
and deuterium profiles from Dome C (Antarctica). Presented at
Symposium on variations in the global water budget, 10-15 august 81,
Oxford U K .

(9) HAMMER C.U., CLAUSEN H.B., DANSGAARD W., GUNDESTRUP N., JOHNSEN S.J. and REEH N, 1978. Dating of Greenland ice cores by flow models, isotopes, volcanic debris and continental dust. Journal of Glaciology, Vol. 20 , N°82.

(10) NYE J.F., 1957. The distribution of stress and velocity in glaciers and ice sheets. Proceedings of the Royal Society, Serie A, Vol. 239, N°1216 : 113-133.

(11) LLIBOUTRY L., 1965. Traité de Glaciologie, Masson et Cie, Paris, Vol. 2 : 578.

(12) DUVAL P., LORIUS C., 1980. Crystal size and climatic record down to the last ice age from Antarctic ice. Earth and Planetary Sciences Letters, Vol. 48 : 59-64.

(13) THOMPSON L.G., MOSLEY-THOMPSON E., PETIT J.R., 1981. Glaciological interpretation of microparticle concentrations from the french 905 m Dome C Antarctica core. IAHS, Pub. N°131 : 227-234.

(14) RABINER L.R., GOLD B. and Mc CONEGAL C.A., 1970. An approach to the approximation problem from non recursive digital filters. IEE Transactions on audio and electroacoustics, Vol. AV 18, N°2 : 83-105.

(15) AIT OUAHMAN A., 1981. Caractérisation des signaux climatiques isotopiques : séries obtenues par carottage en Antarctique. Thèse de 3e cycle préparée à l'Institut National Polytechnique de Grenoble (soutenue le 16 juillet 1981)

(16) GENDRIN R. and de VILLEDARY C., 1979. Unambiguous determination of fine structures in multicomponent time varying signals. Annales des Télécommunications, Vol. 34, N°3-4.

(17) ULRYCH T.J., 1972. Maximum Entropy Power Spectrum of Truncated Sinusoïds. Journal of Geophysical Research, Vol. 77, N°8, 1396-1400.

(18) ULRYCH T.J., SMYLIE D.E., JENSEN O.G. and CLARKE G.K.E. 1973. Predictive filtering and smoothing of short records by using maximum entropy. Journal of Geophysical Research, Vol. 78, N°23.

(19) BURG J.P., 1968. A new analysis for time series data. Paper presented at Advanced Study Institute on Signal Processing, Nato Enstide, Netherlands.

(20) GUEGEN G., 1979. Apport de la modélisation en traitement du signal, GRETSI, Nice, mai 1979, pp. 77/1-77/11.

(21) PISARENKO V.F., 1973. The retrieval of Harmonics from a covariance function. Geophysical Journal of the Royal Astronomical Society, Vol. 33 : 347-366.

(22) LACOUME J.L., 1979. Différentes approches de l'analyse spectrale. Annales des Télécommunications, Vol. E 35 N°3-4.

(23) ULRYCH T.J. and CLAYTON R.W., 1976. Time series modelling and and maximum entropy. Physics of the earth and Planetary Interiors, Vol. 12 : 188-200.

(24) FARGETTON H., 1979. Frequences instantanées de signaux multicomposantes. Thèse de Docteur Ingénieur préparée à l'Institut National Polytechnique de Grenoble (soutenue le 21 décembre 1979).

(25) FARGETTON H., GENDIN R. and LACOUME J.L., 1980. Adaptive methods for special analysis of time varying signals. Signal Processing : theory and applications, Kunt M. and de Coulau F. Ed. Math Holland Puls and Eurasip.

289

(26)ULRYCH T.J., and BISHOP T.M., 1975. Maximum entropy analysis and autoregressive decomposition. Reviews of Geophysics and Space Physics, Vol. 13, N°1 : 183-200.

(27) AKAIKE , 1974. A new look at the statistical model identification IEE Transactions of Automised Control, Vol AC-19, N°6, décembre 1974.

(28) KOERNER R.M. and FISCHER D., 1979. Discontinuous flow towards the bed of the Devon Island ice cap as evidenced by oxygen isotope, microparticles concentration and ice texture variations between two surface to bedrock cores in Symposium on glacier beds, Ottawa, August 1978. Journal of Glaciology, Vol. 23, N°89.

(29) BENOIST J.P., JOUZEL J., LORIUS C., MERLIVAT L. and POURCHET M. To be published in Proceedings of the third International Symposium on Antarctic Glaciology , Columbus, september 1981.

(30) PALTRIDGE G., 1979. The problem with climate prediction, New Scientist, 19avril 1979, p. 194-195.

(31)SUESS H.E., 1980. Solar activity, cosmic ray produced Carbon 14 and the terrestrial climate. Proceedings of the international conference on sun and climate organised in Toulouse, septembre 1980.

(32)SUESS H.E., 1980. Radio carbon geophysics. Endeavour New Series, Vol. 4, N°3, Pergamon Press.

(33) RAISBECK G.M. And YIAN F., 1980. [10] Be as a potential probe of solar variability influence on climate. Proceedings of the international conference on sun and climate organised in Toulouse , September 1980.

(34) EDDY J.A., 1977. Climate and the changing sun. Climatic change, Vol. 1 : 173-190.

(35) WIGLEY T.M.L., 1980. Sun-Climate Links, Nature, Vol. 288 p. 317-319.
(36) WHILLIAMS L.D., WIGLEY T.M.J. and KELLY P.M., 1980. Climatic trends at high northern latitudes during the last 4000 yrs compared with C^{14} fluctuations. Proceedings of the Int. Conference on Sun and Climate organised in Toulouse, september 1980.

FIGURE CAPTIONS

Figure 1 - D/H ratio. The time scale on the right is the one referred to
model 2 and is expressed in years Before Present (B.P.). The three
arrows indicate climatic features which have also been identified
in deep sea cores and which have been dated by the C^{14} method.
(1)   Holocene (hot period) from 0 to 10,800 yrs B.P.
(2)   Climatic transition from 10,800 to 15,000 yrs B.P.
(3)   Glacial age from 15,000 to 32,000 yrs B.P.

Figure 2 - Numerical solution results.
2-a) Branching between two disturb frequencies
2-b) Sample frequencies with varying sampling rate

Figure 3 - Results of evolutive spectral analysis for isotopic data with
constant accumulation (model 1). The area between the two continuous
lines corresponds to the climatic transition, and between the two
dotted lines, to the area affected by the estimation memory size.
The shaded areas show the stable periodicity. The circled areas
exhibit interference between two frequencies. The circled numbers
refer to those in fig. 4.

Figure 4 - Results of evolutive spectral analysis for isotopic data with
variable accumulation (model 2). The area between the two continuous
lines corresponds to the climatic transition, and between the two
dotted lines, to the area affected by the estimation memory size.
The shaded areas show the stable periodicity. The circled areas
exhibit interference between two frequencies. The circled numbers
refer to those in fig. 3.

δ D ‰

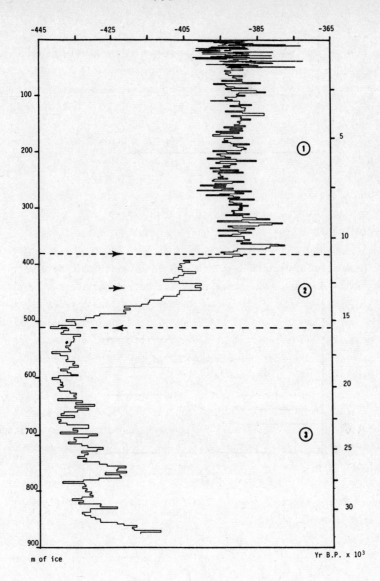

m of ice

Yr B.P. x 10³

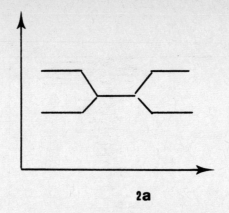

2a

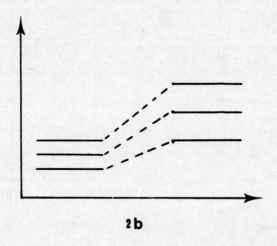

2b

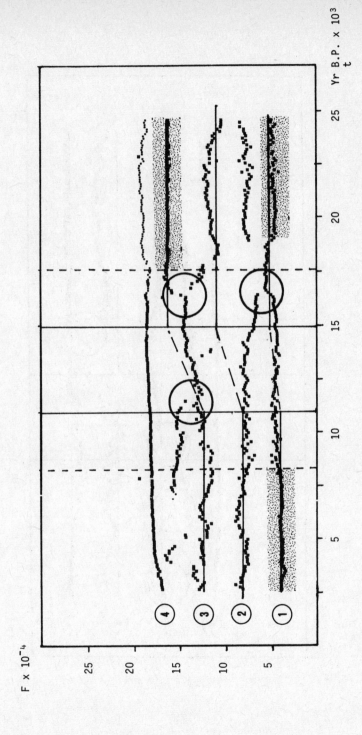

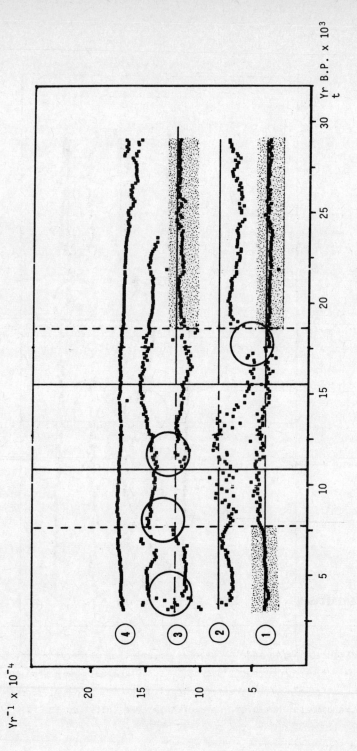

OPTIMAL RANDOMNESS IN FORAGING MOVEMENT :

A CENTRAL PLACE MODEL

P. Bovet

Institut de Neurophysiologie et Psychophysiologie

CNRS - INP 9

BP 71, 13277 Marseille Cedex 9

The present theoretical model clearly comes within the framework of "optimal foraging theory", even though it was initially conceived independently. A complete review of the theory can be found, for instance, in the paper by Pyke, Pulliam and Charnov (1977). We shall mainly be dealing here, however, with that part of the theory which concerns optimal patterns of movement.

In the framework of the optimal foraging theory, one particular point should be emphasized : the importance of the random element in this kind of model. Actually, many models of animal movement are probabilistic (Table 1).

Table 1. Examples of probabilistic models of animal movements.

Authors	Reference	Behaviour	Animals
WILKINSON	1952	Homing	Sea birds
SAILA & SHAPPY	1963	Migration	Salmon
ROHLF & DAVENPORT	1969	Cinesis & taxis	- general -
LEVIN, KERSTER & NIEDZLEC	1971	Foraging	Pollinators
KITCHING	1971	Dispersal	- general -
CODY	1974	Foraging	Flocks of birds
PYKE	1978	Harvesting	- general -
WEHNER & SRINIVASAN	1981	Homing	Ant

The use of probabilistic models obviously means that patterns of movement are matched by some sort of random process. But it is striking that, even when the predictions of probabilistic models fit the data closely, authors have not stressed the part played by randomness. Moreover, some of them even insist on the fact that this movement is not random. This is the case for instance with Levin *et al.* (1971) and Wehner and Srinivasan (1981).

Of course, there is a problem of definition at the outset. As Batschelet (1965) has pointed out, biologists often use the term : "random distribution", to mean : "uniform random distribution". In the study of spatial movement, uniform distribution corresponds to what physicists call isotropic movement. Let us call it : Brownian movement.

It should be stressed however, that "non-uniform" random distribution is quite frequent in biology. Let us take Mendel's laws, for instance. In the case of the mono-hybridism of peas, we know that the phenotypes of the second generation are distributed according to the following probabilities : .75 for long-stem peas, and .25 for short-stem peas. But nobody would contest the fact that the process is random.

Let us now return to the field of animal behaviour. In my opinion, whatever the name given to it, the random element present in models of patterns of movement must be brought out because it is responsible for the main properties of these models. I have suggested elsewhere (Bovet, 1979) that random behaviour may be efficient in some cases. In the field of patterns of movement, randomness represents a very economical means of ensuring important biological functions such as : diffusion, dispersal, exhaustive exploration, and so on. This explains why this paper is entitled "optimal randomness" instead of "optimal directionality". Admittedly, "optimal directionality in central place foraging" or "optimal diffusion in central place foraging" would have been rather more truthful headings ; for, as in the work published by Cody (1974) and by Pyke (1978), the problem here is to find by simulation the optimal directionality of patterns of movement that maximises the area covered by a foraging bout of a given length. An equivalent problem is that of finding the optimal directionality that will minimize the length of the foraging bout for a given area covered.

The model presented here differs from those of Cody and Pyke in that it splits the foraging bout into a search path and a home path. The former is typically a harvesting path, according to the definition given to harvesting by Pyke (1978) ; whereas the second is strictly home oriented.

A distinction is thus made in my model between two different mechanisms involved in the bout : the one occurring before encountering the prey, and the other after having caught the prey. These two parts of a foraging bout are naturally charged to the same energy budget. This implies that the cost of the home path determines the characteristics of the search path.

The model can thus be called a central place foraging model, according to the definition given by Orians and Pearson (1979), and used by Kramer and Nowell (1980) and by Killeen et al. (1981).

There is a further difference to be noted between my model and those developed by Cody and Pyke. In all three cases, the foraging path is modelled on a sequence of linear segments and changes of direction. But in Cody's and Pyke's models, only four directions are available in the simulation process, whereas in my model, all possible directions are available to the extent of the number of decimal figures available on the computer.

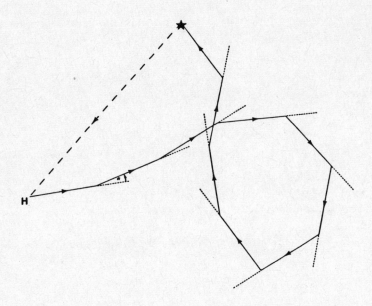

Figure 1. Example of foraging bout produced by simulation.

Figure 1 shows an eleven-step foraging path that can be produced by my central place model. I have actually been working with foraging paths of several hundred steps, and this example is given only as a simplified illustration.

The search path is entirely defined by the random distribution of the changes of direction α. For this purpose, we have been using a normal distribution, with a mean equal to zero and a standard deviation equal to σ

But because we are working with a circle, this leads to the wrapped normal distribution (Batschelet, 1965).

The random path can be transformed into a random surface by means of a simple geometrical construction based on a rectangle and a circle at each step (Fig. 2).

It should be noted that in the theoretical results presented below the length of each step is a constant, equal to the width of the search path.

$$a = b$$

In the more general case that I have studied, however, the step length is proportional to the path width. Relating the length and the width of the step is important, because, according to the sensorial capacities of an animal, this could help us to find one criterion with which to analyse concrete data.

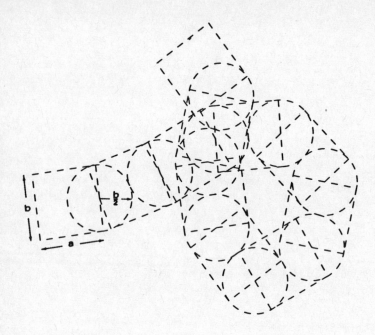

Figure 2. Surface construction corresponding to the foraging bout of Fig. 1.
a = step length ; b = path width.

This leads to a given surface, and the problem is to determine the area of this surface, without re-counting any place that has been already explored (Fig. 3).

This is done by simulation, using a 400 x 400 grid. This allows considerable precision in estimating the area explored.

Let us now consider that the width of the path - which is here equal to the length of each step - is our unit of measurement. Thus, given a certain standard deviation σ in the changes of direction, and a certain area S to be covered, we let a random process run until the given area S has been covered. The process is then stopped, and the total length T is computed. By definition :

T = the length of the search path + the length of the straight home path.

This simulation was run 500 times for each value of σ, and then the average value of T was computed.

Figure 4 shows the results for some values of the area S to be covered. These show a very clear minimum in the total distance T to be travelled, which corresponds to an

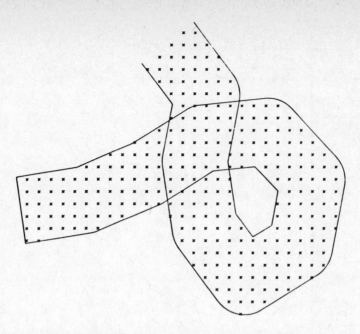

Figure 3. Estimation of the area corresponding to the surface of Fig. 2.

optimal value of the standard deviation σ. This means that for any given search area, there is an optimum directionality.

Figures 5, 6 and 7 present some examples of random foraging bouts which correspond to various directionalities. The bout in Fig. 5 is theoretically too directional. The search path may result in a home path that is too long. The bout in Fig. 6 is theoretically optimum. The expected total length is minimum. And the bout in Fig. 7 shows a directionality that is a bit too small, which results in walking for a long time before covering the whole area to be searched.

On the basis of the results of the simulation, the optimum value of the standard deviation can be approximately expressed as follows :

$$\sigma_{opt.} = 1.367 - 0.143 \ln S$$

We would point out that we do not use the same index of directionality as Pyke (1974), who uses the mean vector component : mean cos α. We have found, however, that these two indexes can easily be related using the following expression :

$$\text{mean cos } \alpha = e^{-\frac{\sigma^2}{2}}$$

Once we have carried out this transformation, it is striking that our results are very close to those of Pyke, who, as I mentioned, does not take into account the

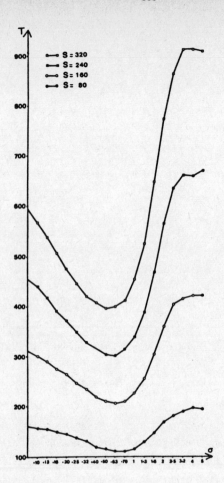

- Figure 4 . Expected length of a foraging bout with respect to its directionality.
T = total length (search path + home path) ; S = covered area (search path only) ;
σ = standard-deviation of the distribution of rotations (search path).

return distance, but works with a bounded foraging area.

In summary, our model is applicable to animals which : first, forage only by harvesting ; and second, return home after having caught a certain amount of prey.

Incidentally, this model seems to be particularly suitable for the study of insect
foraging behaviour. We are now trying to apply it to the foraging paths of an African
ant (*Smithistruma emarginata*) being studied by DEJEAN (1980).

My model provides a good tool for analyzing this sort of data. In particular, the
model provides some help in the choice of the scale with which the natural path
should be segmented.

301

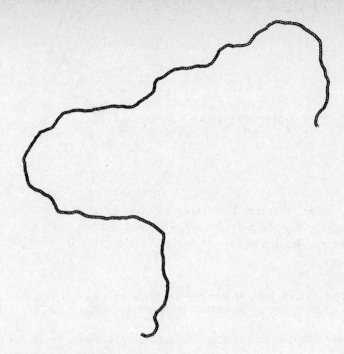

Figure 5. Example of foraging bout with:

$$a = b = 1, \sigma = 0.25, S = 320, T = 320 + 114.2 = 434.2$$

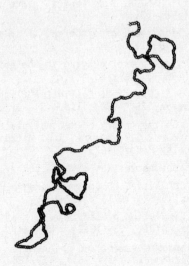

Figure 6. Example of foraging bout with:

$$a = b = 1, \sigma = 0.63, S = 320, T = 322 + 81.7 = 403.7$$

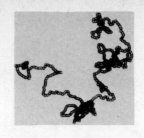

Figure 7. Example of foraging bout with :

$$a = b = 1, \sigma = 1, S = 320, T = 394 + 37.8 = 431.8$$

I would like to thank Professor C. Flament and René Lozzi for their advice throughout this work, Danièle Bellan for her help in writing the computer programs, and Deborah Hicks and Jessica Blanc for their collaboration in debugging my english language.

References.

BATSCHELET, E. Statistical methods for the analysis of problems in animal orientation and certain biological rhythms. Monograph of American Institute of Biological Sciences, 1965, 57 pp.

BOVET, P. La valeur adaptative des comportements aléatoires. L'Année Psychologique, 79 (1979), 505-525.

CODY, M.-L. Optimization in ecology. Science, 183 (1974), 1156-1164.

DEJEAN, A. Etude comparée du comportement de prédation d'une fourmi primitive (Odontomachus troglodytes) et de trois fourmis de la tribu des Dacetini (Strumygenys rufobrunea, Serrastruma serrula, Smithistruma emarginata). Bulletin de la Société Française pour l'Etude du Comportement Animal, 2 (1980), 43-63.

KILLEEN, P. R. ; SMITH, J.P. ; HANJON, S.J. Central place foraging in Rattus norvegicus. Anim. Behav., 29 (1981), 64-70.

KITCHING, R. A simple simulation model of dispersal of animals among units of discreta habitat. Oecologia, 7 (1971) : 95-116.

KRAMER, D.L. ; NOWELL, W. Central place foraging in the eastern chipmunk, Tamias striatus. Anim. Behav., 28 (1980), 772-778.

LEVIN, D.A. ; KERSTER, H.W. ; NIEDZLEK, M. Pollinator flight directionality and its effect on pollen flow. Evolution, 25 (1971), 113-118.

ORIANS, G.H. ; PEARSON, N.E. On the theory of central place foraging. In : Analysis of Ecological Systems , D.J. Horn, G.R. Stairs, R.D. Mitchel, eds., pp. 155-177, Colombus : Ohio State University Press, 1979.

PYKE, G.H. Are animals efficient harvesters ? Anim. Behav., 26 (1978), 241-250.

PYKE, G.H.; PULLIAM, H.R. ; CHARNOV, E.L. Optimal foraging : a selective review of theory and tests. Q. Rev. Biol., 52 (1977) : 137-154.

ROHLF, F.J. ; DAVENPORT, D. Simulation of simple models of animal behaviour with a digital computer. J. of Theor. Biol., 23 (1969), 400-424.

SAILA, S.B. ; SHAPPY, R.A. Random movement and orientation in Salmon migration. J. Cons. perm. int. exp. Mer, (Danemark), 28 (1963), 153-166.

WILKINSON, D.H. The random element in bird navigation. J. Exp. Biol., 29 (1952), 532-560.

WEHNER, R. ; SRINIVASAN, M.V. Searching behaviour of desert Ants, genus Cataglyphis (Formicidae, Hymenoptera). Journal of Comparative Physiology, 142 (1981), 315-338.

A MODEL FOR WEATHER CYCLES BASED ON DAILY RAINFALL OCCURRENCE

E. Galloy (1), A. Le Breton (2), S. Martin (1)

Summary.

The weather cycles corresponding to the succession of dry and wet days, during a
given time of the year in a given meteorological station, are modeled by use of an
alternating renewal process based on shifted negative binomial distributions for the
lengths of spells. For three French stations and different times, the model is found
to fit data well with respect to persistences, averages and variances of numbers of
dry or wet days.

1. Introduction.

This paper is devoted to modeling weather cycles corresponding to the succession of
dry an wet days in a given climatological station for a given time π (month or set
of months) of the year. A dry (resp. wet) day is a day in which less (resp. more)
than a certain fixed threshold α mm of precipitation was recorded ($\alpha = 1$ in the
following applications). A dry (resp. wet) spell is a sequence of consecutive dry
(resp. wet) days between two wet (resp. dry) days.

In order to represent the weather cycles under consideration, we can use, for a
preliminary statistical description of the rhythm, a discrete time boolean stochastic
process : precisely we can define a family of binary random variables (ε_n ; n = 1,...
N) where

ε_n = 1 if the nth day of the time π is dry,
ε_n = 0 if the nth day of the time π is wet,
with n = 1,...,N and N the length of π . Then, to every model for the process (ε_n ;
n = 1, ..., N) corresponds a statistical model for the concerned weather-cycles.
Different approaches for describing the succession of days with respect to rainfall
occurrence have been used in the litterature (see e.g. [1], [2], [3], [4]). In the
present work we consider a model in the form of an alternating renewal process
(A.R.P.) ; this means that in particular we assume the phenomenon is periodic in the
mean and the underlying period T is the sum of the average duration of a dry spell
and that of a wet spell, these averages being homogeneous from one weather cycle to
another. Since in a previous study [5] we have shown that shifted negative binomial
(S.N.B.) distributions are able to represent satisfactorily the development of dry
or wet spells with respect to persistences, we choose an A.R.P. model which is based

(1). E.R. 30, CNRS, B.P. 53, 38041 Grenoble–Cédex, France
(2). Laboratoire I.M.A.G., B.P. 53 X, 38041 Grenoble–Cédex, France

on S.N.B. distributions for the lengths of spells.

Part 2 of the paper is devoted to the description and the analysis of the model, an interpretation of the parameters is proposed and some probabilistic characteristics of interest are provided ; moreover the statistical problem of fitting the model to observed data is discussed. In part 3 of the paper the model is used for describing the phenomenon at three weather stations in France for the different months of the year. Part 4 is a conclusion.

2. The basic model.

We assume that for the time π the development of a weather spell beginning in that time does not depend on the developments of the previous spells. We also assume that the phenomenon unfolds homogeneously all along π. Then, if we set that the length of a dry or wet spell is a random variable, the succession of the days from the first day of π is described by a stochastic process with two possible states. Moreover the distribution of the future, given the observation of a first dry (resp. wet) day at some day in π , is completely determined by the set of distributions $(p^1_n ; n \geqslant 1)$ and $(p^0_n ; n \geqslant 1)$ for the length of a dry spell and a wet spell respectively (given that it begins on π). When distributions $(p^i_n ; n \geqslant 1)$, $i = 0,1$ are fixed, the distribution of the process on π is fully defined by the set of the probabilities p_1 and p_0 that the first day of π is dry or wet and the distributions $(a^i_n ; n \geqslant 1)$, $i = 0,1$, where $(a^1_n ; n \geqslant 1)$ (resp. $(a^0_n ; n \geqslant 1)$)is the distribution of the length on π of a dry (resp. wet) spell given that it may have begun before π.

2.1. Structure and parameters of the model.

Let us denote by $\varepsilon_0, \varepsilon_1, ..,\varepsilon_n,...$ the successive states of the considered process from the day preceding the beginning of π, with the convention that $\varepsilon_n = 1$ (resp. 0) if the nth day is dry (resp. wet) and that an event of the type $[\varepsilon_n = i + 1]$ is $[\varepsilon_n = (i+1) \bmod 2]$ i.e. $[\varepsilon_n = 1]$ if $i = 0$ and $[\varepsilon_n = 0]$ if $i = 1$. Then, if P is the underlying probability one has :

$$p_1 = P [\varepsilon_1 = 1] ; \quad p_0 = P[\varepsilon_1 = 0] = 1 - p_1$$

$$a^i_n = P [\varepsilon_{n+1} = i + 1, \varepsilon_n = ... = \varepsilon_1 = i / \varepsilon_1 = i] ; i = 0,1 ; n = 1,2,...$$

$$p^i_n = P [\varepsilon_{n+1} = i + 1, \varepsilon_n = ... = \varepsilon_1 = i, \varepsilon_0 = i + 1] ; i = 0,1 ; n=1,2,$$

and the process $(\varepsilon_n ; n \geqslant 1)$ is a delayed A.R.P. describing the succession of dry and wet days until the end of the last spell which begins on π.

In order to reflect the assumption of homogeneity of the phenomenon on π, we are led to assume that the process $(\varepsilon_n ; n > 1)$ is stationary i.e. is a pure equilibrium A.R.P. . This means (cf. for example [4]) that we set, for $i = 0,1$:

$$p_i = \frac{\mu^i}{\mu^0 + \mu^1} \; ; \; a_n^i = \frac{1}{\mu^i} \sum_{k \geq n} p_k^i \; , \; n = 1, 2..., $$

where μ^i is the mean of the distribution $(p_n^i \; ; \; n \geq 1)$. If P_i (resp. A_i) stands for the generating function of $(p_n^i \; , \; n \geq 1)$ (resp. $(a_n^i \; , \; n \geq 1)$, $i = 0,1$, the equalities for $(a_n^i \; ; \; n \geq 1)$ are equivalent to

$$A_i(t) = \frac{1}{\mu i} \frac{t}{1-t} (1 - P_i(t)) \; ; \; i = 0,1$$

In the following we assume that distributions $(p_n^i \; ; \; n \geq 1)$, $i = 0,1$ are S.N.B. distributions i.e. for some $h_i > 0$ and $d_i > 0$, $i = 0,1$

$$p_n^i = P_n(h_i, d_i)$$

$$= \binom{h_i/d_i + n-2}{n-1} (\frac{1}{1+d_i})^{h_i/d_i} (\frac{d_i}{1+d_i})^{n-1} \; ; \; n \geq 1,$$

or equivalently

$$P_i(t) = t \left[(1 + d_i) - d_i t \right]^{-h_i/d_i} \; ; \; i = 0,1 .$$

So the model is parametrized by h_1, d_1, h_0, d_0 ; these parameters can be interpreted as follows :

. h_1 (resp. h_0) is the mean value of the length of a dry (resp. wet) spell after its first day given that it begins on π i.e.

$$\mu^i = h_i + 1, \; i = 0,1$$

. $h_1 (d_1 + 1)$ (resp. $h_0 (d_0 + 1)$ is the variance of that length.

. $h_1 + h_0 + 2$ (resp. $h_1 (d_1 + 1) + h_0 (d_0 + 1)$)is the mean value (resp. the variance) of length of a weather cycle.

. $\frac{d_1}{h_1}$ (resp. $\frac{d_0}{h_0}$) is related to the nature of the persistence of the dryness (resp. wetness). If $\tilde{p}_n^1$ (resp. $\tilde{p}_n^0$) is the persistence of the dryness (resp. wetness) at the nth day for a dry (resp. wet) spell beginning in π i.e.

$$\tilde{p}_n^i = \frac{\sum_{k \geq n+1} p_k^i}{\sum_{k \geq n} p_k^i}$$

then (cf. [5]) for $\frac{d_i}{h_i} < 1$ (resp. > 1) one has $\lim \nearrow (resp. \searrow) \; \tilde{p}_n^i = \frac{d_i}{d_i+1}$ and for $\frac{d_i}{h_i} = 1$ one has $\tilde{p}_n^i = \frac{d_i}{d_i+1}$, $n = 1, 2...$

2.2. Some probabilistic characteristics in the model .

Adapting techniques used by COX and MILLER [6] , [7] in the case of continuous time renewal processes it is possible (cf. [4]) to compute the probability that exactly m days among the N days of π are dry i.e.

$$Q_N(m) = P\left[\sum_{k=1}^{N}\varepsilon_k = m\right]$$

For example the following holds :

$$Q_n(n) = \frac{\mu^1}{\mu^0 + \mu^1}\sum_{k \geqslant n} a_k^1$$

$$= \frac{1}{\mu^0 + \mu^1}\sum_{k \geqslant 1} k\, p_{n+k-1}^1$$

Moreover one can compute the mean and the variance of the number of dry days on π. One has

$$m_{1,N} = E\left\{\sum_{k=1}^{N}\varepsilon_k\right\} = N\frac{\mu^1}{\mu^0 + \mu^1}.$$

and

$$\sigma_{1,N}^2 = \text{var}\left\{\sum_{k=1}^{N}\varepsilon_k\right\}$$

$$= N.\text{var}(\varepsilon_1) + 2\sum_{k<1}\text{Cov}(\varepsilon_k, \varepsilon_1)$$

where

$$\text{var}(\varepsilon_1) = \frac{\mu^1\,\mu^0}{(\mu^0 + \mu^1)^2}$$

while

$$\text{Cov}(\varepsilon_k, \varepsilon_1) = P\left[\varepsilon_k = \varepsilon_1 = 1\right] - \left(\frac{\mu^1}{\mu^0 + \mu^1}\right)^2$$

$$= P\left[\varepsilon_1 = \varepsilon_{1-k+1} = 1\right] - \left(\frac{\mu^1}{\mu^0 + \mu^1}\right)^2$$

Then it follows that :

$$\sigma_{1,N}^2 = N.\frac{\mu^1\,\mu^0}{(\mu^0 + \mu)^2} + 2\sum_{h=1}^{N-1}(N-h)\left\{P\left[\varepsilon_1 = \varepsilon_{h+1} = 1\right] - \left(\frac{\mu^1}{\mu^0 + \mu^1}\right)^2\right\}$$

with

$$P\left[\varepsilon_1 = \varepsilon_{h+1} = 1\right] = \frac{\mu^1}{\mu^0 + \mu^1}\cdot w_h$$

where $w_h = P\left[\varepsilon_{h+1} = 1 / \varepsilon_1 = 1\right]$; $h = 1, 2 \ldots$

One can show that if W is the function defined by

$$W(s) = \sum_{l=0}^{\infty} w_l\, s^l$$

then

$$W(s) = \frac{1}{1-s}\left\{1 - \frac{s}{\mu^1(1-s)}\cdot\frac{(1-P_0(s))(1-P_1(s))}{1-P_0(s).P_1(s)}\right\}$$

This provides a means to compute probabilities w_l , $l = 0, 1, \ldots$ and therefore the exact variance σ^2_N . Taking into account the fact that, if

$$\psi_N = E \left\{ \left(\sum_{k=1}^{N} \varepsilon_k \right) \left(\sum_{k=1}^{N} \varepsilon_k + 1 \right) \right\}$$

$$= \sigma^2_{1,N} + N^2 \left(\frac{\mu^1}{\mu^0 + \mu^1} \right)^2 + N \frac{\mu^1}{\mu^0 + \mu^1}$$

and

$$\phi(s) = \sum_{N \geq 1} \psi_N s^N$$

then one has

$$\phi(s) = \frac{2 \mu^1}{\mu^0 + \mu^1} \cdot \frac{s}{(1-s)^2} W(s),$$

it is possible to obtain (cf. [4]) the following approximation of $\sigma_{1,N}^2$ for large N :

$$\sigma_{1,N}^2 = \frac{(\mu^1)^2 \mu_2^0 + (\mu^0)^2 \mu_2^1}{(\mu^1 + \mu^0)^3} \cdot N + \frac{(\mu^1 \mu_2^0 - \mu^0 \mu_2^1)^2}{2(\mu^1 + \mu^0)^4}$$

$$- \frac{(\mu^1)^2 \mu_3^0 + (\mu^0)^2 \mu_3^1}{3(\mu^1 + \mu^0)^3} + \frac{2\mu^1 \mu^0 + (\mu^1 \mu^0)^2}{6(\mu^1 + \mu^0)^2} + \sigma(1) ,$$

where, for $i = 0, 1$, μ_2^i (resp. μ_3^i) is the variance (resp. the third central moment) of the distribution $(p_n^i, n \geq 1)$.
In the case of S.N.B. distributions one has :

$$\mu^i = h_i + 1 \; ; \; \mu_2^i = h_i (d_i + 1)$$

$$\mu_3^i = h_i (h_i + d_i)(h_i + 2d_i + 3) - 3\mu^i \mu_2^i - (\mu^i)^3 + 3\mu_2^i + 3(\mu^i)^2 - 2\mu^i.$$

2.3. Fitting the model to data

Under the assumption that the years during which data have been recorded are homogeneous, the observations on the different times π of these years are considered as "independent trajectories" governed by one of the possible process distributions described in § 2.1. So, the estimation of the parameters h_1 and d_1 (resp. h_0 and d_0) can be based on some independent sample $x_1^1, \ldots, x_1^{k_1}$ (resp. $x_0^1, \ldots x_0^{k0}$) of the lengths of dry (resp. wet) spells which have begun on π. The likelihood method leads to estimate h_i by

$$\hat{h}_i = \bar{x}_i - 1$$

where $\bar{x}_i$ is the empirical mean of $(x_i^1, \ldots, x_i^{k_i})$ but it doesn't provide an easily computable estimate for d_i. The method of moments gives the estimates

$$\hat{h}_i = \bar{x}_i - 1$$

and

$$\hat{d}_i = \frac{s_i^2}{(\bar{x}_i - 1)} - 1$$

where s_i^2 is the empirical variance of $(x_i^1, \dots x_i^{ki})$.

In order to evaluate how the model fits the data, one can compare the theoretical persistences, probabilities for lengths, means and variances for numbers of dry days (computed by means of formulas in § 2.1. and § 2.2. for the estimated values of the parameters) to the corresponding observed empirical quantities.

3. Fit of the model to the data at Strasbourg, La Rochelle and Montélimar (France).

The model described in § 2 is used for modeling the phenomenon of rainfall occurrence at Strasbourg (48°33'N, 7°37'E), La Rochelle (46°11'N, 1°11'W) and Montélimar (44°35'N, 4°44'E) for the different months of the year ; these stations have been chosen, among 31 for which persistences have been modelled by S.N.B. distributions (cf. [8]), because of their different seasonal characteristics.

3.1. Description of the data.

The basic data are series of amounts of precipitation recorded in three French weather stations during the recent years 1949-1977 ([9] , [10]). A Fortran program is used to count systematically the sequences of consecutive days in which the amount is between two levels I_1, I_2 . These sequences are assigned to the time (month or set of months) containing their first day. In order to count dry (resp. wet) spells the levels have been fixed to $I_1 = 0$ and $I_2 = 1$ mm (resp. $I_1 = 1$ mm and I_2 very large).

In table 1, we give, as examples, the observed numbers of wet and dry sequences beginning during January for the three stations.

3.2. Results about persistences.

In table 2, for each month and each station, the estimated values of parameters h_1, d_{1/h_1} , h_0, d_{0/h_0} are given. On figure 1, one can see that the seasonal variation of these parameters is quite different from one station to another. It is also different from the case of dry sequences to that of wet sequences.

Figures 2, 3 and 4 provide the means to compare on a logarithmic scale for a given station and a given month, the observed frequences of dry sequences longer than n days and the corresponding probabilities computed in our model (A.R.P. + S.N.B.) and in a fitted Markov model of order 2. The three chosen examples correspond to different types of evolution of the persistence during the development of a spell. For October at Montélimar (fig. 2), the persistence decreases $(d_{1/h_1} = 0.76)$; the Markov model is not adapted. For May at Montélimar (fig. 3) the persistence is approximately constant $(d_{1/h_1} = 1,06)$ and the two models are satisfactory. For December at Strasbourg (fig. 4) the persistence increases $(d_{1/h_1} = 1.98)$ and our model provides the

Table 1

Numbers of sequences	Strasbourg		La Rochelle		Montélimar	
	dry	wet	dry	wet	dry	wet
1	28	68	57	76	23	59
2	24	30	30	40	14	27
3	10	17	15	10	9	11
4	11	3	6	11	8	4
5	9	3	8	4	10	4
6	5	2	3	2	6	2
7	4	1	7	2	4	1
8	4		5	1	5	
9	8		5		4	
10	3		2	2	2	
11	6		2	1	2	
12	1		1		1	
13	2				1	
14	1		2	1	2	
15			1		3	
16	1		1			
17	3		1			
18			1			
19					3	
20			1		1	
21	1				1	
22	2					
23			1			
24	1					
25					1	
26						
27	1					
28						
29						
30						
31					1	
35					1	
38	1					
56					1	
Total numbers of observed sequences	126	124	149	150	103	108

Observed numbers of sequences starting on January

Table 2

		J	F	M	A	M	Jn	Jt	A	S	O	N	D
STRASBOURG	h_1	4.76	4.29	3.77	3.35	2.60	2.84	2.83	3.05	4.44	4.34	4.12	3.90
	d_1/h_1	1.43	1.49	1.34	1.16	1.31	2.51	1.07	1.35	1.81	1.05	2.28	1.98
	h_0	0.81	1.04	0.69	0.78	0.83	0.99	0.80	0.95	0.90	0.92	0.92	0.90
	d_0/h_0	0.92	1.00	1.17	0.89	0.63	0.76	0.85	0.79	1.11	1.14	1.06	1.75
LA ROCHELLE	h_1	2.82	4.58	3.35	3.93	4.35	5.80	5.85	5.19	3.53	4.44	3.80	3.07
	d_1/h_1	1.85	1.84	1.77	1.60	1.68	0.99	1.09	1.16	1.09	1.05	1.66	2.16
	h_0	1.19	1.81	1.17	0.78	0.95	0.81	0.59	1.06	1.08	1.70	2.15	1.58
	d_0/h_0	2.12	1.59	0.74	0.88	0.57	1.07	1.73	0.77	1.76	1.76	1.55	1.72
MONTELIMAR	h_1	5.65	5.44	5.02	5.62	4.53	5.26	8.81	5.12	5.72	5.59	3.84	5.32
	d_1/h_1	1.87	1.92	1.42	1.25	1.06	1.11	0.90	1.12	0.72	0.76	1.92	1.25
	h_0	0.86	0.98	1.22	0.72	0.93	0.62	0.43	0.49	0.82	0.98	0.89	0.78
	d_0/h_0	1.05	0.82	0.71	1.22	0.91	0.92	0.80	0.67	0.99	0.66	0.63	0.72

Estimated values of the parameters h and d/h

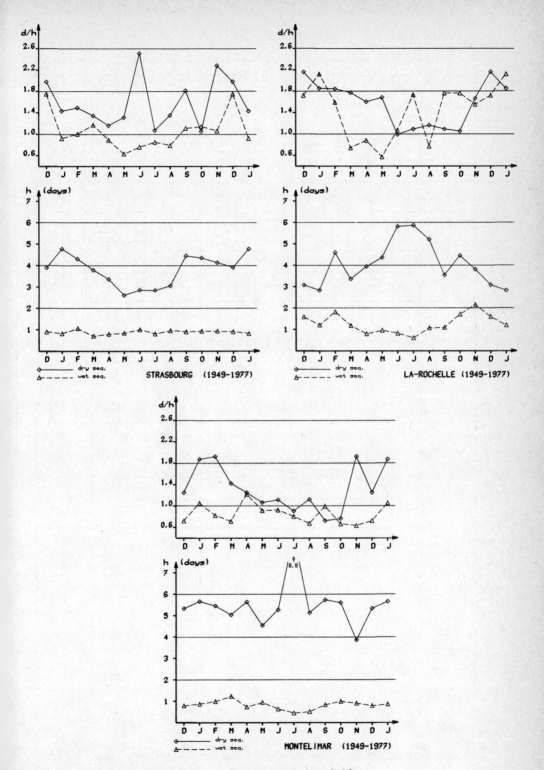

Fig. 1 – Seasonal evolution of the parameters h and d/h

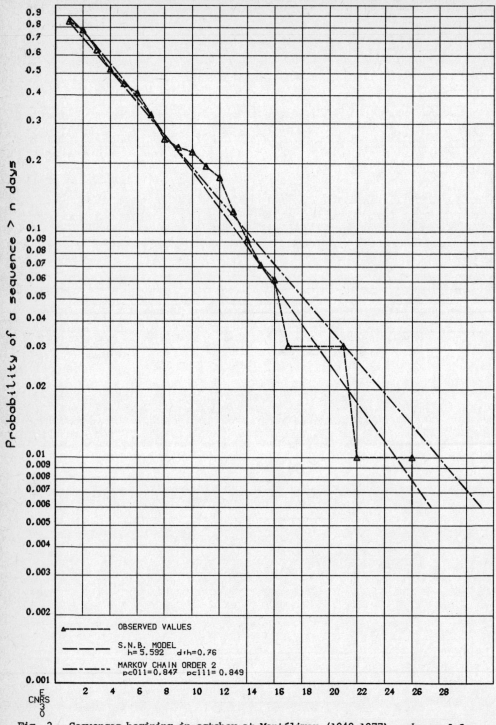

Fig. 2 – Sequences begining in october at Montélimar (1949–1977) : observed frequences and computed probabilities of a dry sequence longer than n days.

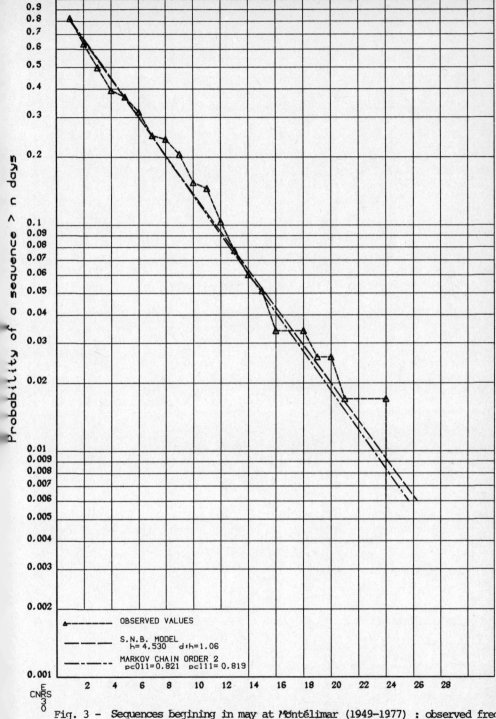

Fig. 3 – Sequences begining in may at Montélimar (1949–1977) : observed frequences and computed probabilities of a dry sequence longer than n days.

314

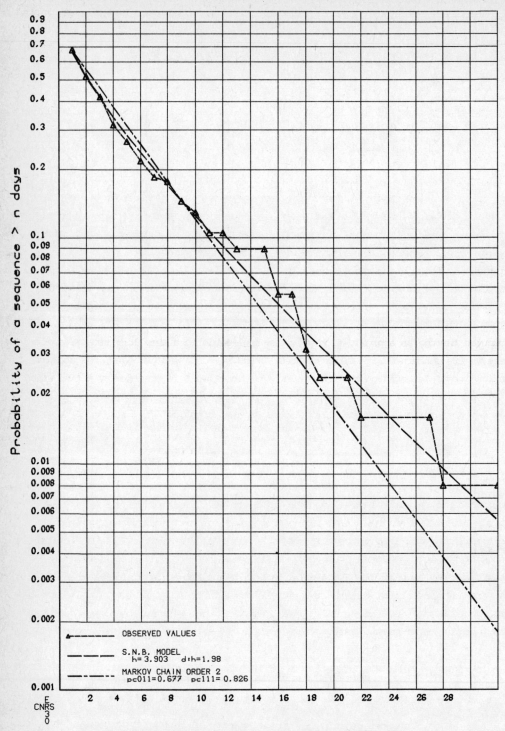

Fig. 4 - Sequences begining in december at Strasbourg (1949-1977) : observed frequenc
and computed probabilities of a dry sequence longer than n days.

best fitting.

3.3. Results about averages and variances of numbers of dry days.

It is clear that the averages m_1, m_0 and the variances σ_1^2, σ_0^2 , of the numbers of dry
and wet days on a given month are related by

$$m_0 = \text{(number of days in the month)} - m_1$$

and

$$\sigma_0^2 = \sigma_1^2 .$$

So we provide only the values for the case of dry days.

In table 3 and figure 5, for each month and each station the observed mean and
standard deviation are compared with the corresponding m_1 and σ_1 computed from the
fitted A.R.P. model by use of the exact value for m_1 and of the approximation for
σ_1 (cf. § 2.2.). Except for February at La Rochelle the model fits the means well
(maximal difference about one day) ; the seasonal variations of the mean are well
represented by the A.R.P. model. Concerning the standard deviation, the seasonal
evolution is also well described by the model but the computed values are not so
close to those observed. This fact may be explained as follows : on one hand σ_1 is
computed through an approximation which is applicable to a very long time π, and
here we are concerned with times of about 30 days ; on the other hand, the approximation itself is based on the assumption that the time π is preceded by a time with
similar characteristics, and here, as we have seen before, some consecutive months
may be characterized by quite different parameters h and d.

4. Conclusion.

In the present paper we have used a model in the form of an alternating renewal
process based on shifted negative binomial distributions in order to describe weather cycles corresponding to the succession of dry and wet sequences for the different months of the year at Strasbourg, La Rochelle and Montélimar. Because of its
good fitting to experimental data, though it is based on simplifying assumptions,
this model may be helpfully suggestive regarding the mechanism of the weather at
the considered stations (and in many others where it is appropriate [11]). It provides a statistical description of the weather rhythm on which may be based a study of
its possible relation with other phenomena (in the spirit of papers [12] and [13]).

Table 3

		STRASBOURG		LA ROCHELLE		MONTELIMAR	
		computed	observed	computed	observed	computed	observed
J	m_1	23.6	23.2	19.7	19.7	24.2	24.2
	σ_1	3.4	3.4	4.4	4.3	3.7	3.5
F	m_1	20.4	20.5	18.8	16.8	21.6	21.6
	σ_1	3.6	4.4	4.9	5.9	3.7	3.8
M	m_1	22.9	23.4	20.7	21.7	22.7	23.6
	σ_1	3.2	3.4	4.0	4.3	3.9	3.9
A	m_1	21.3	21.6	22.0	22.1	23.8	23.7
	σ_1	3.1	3.5	3.4	3.4	3.1	2.6
M	m_1	20.6	20.3	22.8	22.2	23.0	23.1
	σ_1	3.2	3.3	3.7	3.6	3.3	3.4
Jn	m_1	19.8	19.6	23.7	23.8	23.8	23.3
	σ_1	4.0	4.1	3.0	2.9	2.8	3.1
Jt	m_1	21.1	21.2	25.2	25.2	27.1	26.9
	σ_1	3.1	3.8	2.9	2.7	2.2	2.4
A	m_1	20.9	20.9	23.3	23.3	24.9	25.3
	σ_1	3.5	3.8	3.5	4.3	2.6	2.6
S	m_1	22.2	21.4	20.6	20.9	23.6	23.4
	σ_1	3.7	4.1	3.7	3.9	2.8	3.1
O	m_1	22.8	23.8	20.7	21.5	23.8	24.4
	σ_1	3.4	4.2	4.6	5.1	3.0	3.8
N	m_1	21.8	21.2	18.1	17.1	21.6	21.2
	σ_1	4.0	4.0	5.2	5.5	3.7	2.9
D	m_1	22.3	22.8	19.0	19.4	24.2	23.7
	σ_1	4.0	4.1	4.9	4.9	3.3	2.9

Observed and computed averages and standard deviations of the numbers of dry days.

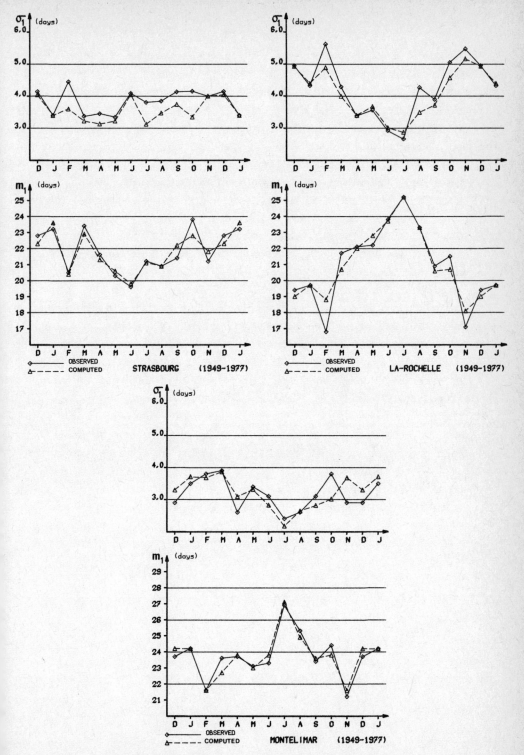

Fig. 5 – Seasonal evolution of the means and standard deviations of the number of dry days.

References

[1] . GABRIEL, K.R. and NEUMANN, J. "On a distribution of weather cycles by lenghts", Quart. J.R. met. Soc., 83, 1957, 375-380.

[2] . GABRIEL, K.R. and NEUMANN, J. "A Markov chain model for rainfall occurrence", Quart. J.R. met. Soc., 88, 1962, 90-95.

[3] . GREEN, J.R. "A Model for rainfall occurrence", Journal of the Royal Stat. Soc., Series B, 26, 1964, 345-353.

[4] . BUISHAND, T.A., Stochastic modelling of daily rainfall sequences, Ph. D. Thesis 77-3, Agricultural Univ. Wageningen, The Netherlands, 1977.

[5] . LE BRETON, A. and MARTIN, S. "Un modèle pour l'étude des séquences climatologiques", Séminaire de statistique, Laboratoire I.M.A.G., 1979, 3-34.

[6] . COX, D.R., Renewal theory, Methuen and Co., London, 1962.

[7] . COX, D.R., and LEWIS, P.A.W., The theory of stochastic processes, Methuen and Co., London, 1965.

[8] . GALLOY, E., Contribution à l'étude de la sécheresse ; Modélisation des séquences climatologiques sur un réseau de stations couvrant l'ensemble de la France, Ph. D. Thesis, Univ. Scientif. et Médicale de Grenoble, to appear.

[9] . Bulletin annuel du service météorologique de la métropole et de l'Afrique du Nord, Direction de la Météorologie Nationale, Paris, 1955-1962.

[10] . Résumé mensuel du temps en France, Direction de la Météorologie Nationale, Paris, 1960-1977.

[11] . GALLOY, E., LE BRETON, A., and MARTIN. S., Un modèle de processus pour l'étude de la succession des jours secs et humides ; Application à un réseau de stations couvrant l'ensemble de la France. Rapport de Recherche, Laboratoire I.M.A.G., to appear.

[12] . THOMAS, R., this volume.

[13] . BACONNIER, P., BENCHETRIT, G., DEMONGEOT, J. and PHAM, T.D., this volume.

A STATISTICAL APPROACH TO
DIFFERENCE-DELAY EQUATION MODELLING IN ECOLOGY -
TWO CASE STUDIES

by

K. S. Lim and H. Tong

Department of Mathematics
University of Manchester
Institute of Science and Technology
Manchester, U.K.

Abstract

In the field of ecology, the importance of delay equations is
well recognised. In the field of time series analysis, a new
class of non-linear models has been developed by Tong which
exploits explicitly the notion of a delay and a threshold.
In this paper, we demonstrate, with real ecological data, how
the former may be used to motivate the latter, which in turn
verifies the appropriateness of the former. It is this inter-
course between statistics and ecology which explains the
success of this new class of models in its practical applications
to some ecological data.

Key words:- DIFFERENCE-DELAY EQUATION; THRESHOLD AUTOREGRESSION;
             CANADIAN LYNX; CANADIAN MINK AND MUSKRAT.

INTRODUCTION

Delay equations, in both discrete and continuous time, are the basic models for animal populations in which the density dependent regulatory mechanisms operate with some finite time delay. These models are capable of explaining the cyclic nature of many observed populations, because they can give rise to a stable limit cycle when the delay is in excess of the 'natural' period. Hutchinson (1948) was probably the first in recognising the importance of the delay. Specifically, he proposed the now classic logistic-delay equation

$$\frac{dx(t)}{dt} = x(t) \ (a-bx(t-T)),$$

where x(t) is the population density at time t and T denotes the delay. Authors who have recently emphasised the significance of the delay include, among many others, May (1980), Maynard-Smith((1974) and Levin and May (1976).

The above authors have given detailed discussions of the biological implications of the delay equations. However, the practical problem of fitting these models to data as well as the data-analytic interpretations of these models does not seem to be so well documented in the biological journals. Recently, Tong has developed a new class of non-linear time series models, the threshold autoregressive models, which exploits explicitly the notion of a delay (see Tong and Lim, 1980, for a comprehensive discussion). In biological terms, the methodology developed for the identification and fitting of threshold models may be used as a statistical implementation of delay systems.

Our discussion will be entirely in discrete time since we are going to use annual data for our illustrations. Details of the theory and fitting procedure of threshold models are omitted since they may be found in Tong and Lim (1980). We would emphasise that the entropy maximisation principle due to Akaike (1977) plays a rather important role in our approach. We concentrate on two case studies.

CANADIAN LYNX DATA

The Mackenzie River Series of annual Canadian lynx trappings for the years
1871-1934 is now classic. Much statistical work has been reported on the literature
and they are mainly linear. We refer in particular to Part 4 of Volume 140 of the
Journal of the Royal Statistical Society Series A. We have reproduced the data plot
on a logarithmic scale (base 10).in Figure 1.

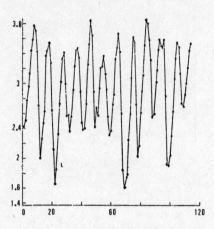

FIG. 1: The Canadian Lynx Data

(Listing of the data may be found on P.430 of the above-mentioned journal). Let x_t
denote the population size at time t (t = 1,2,...), logarithmically transformed to
base 10.

We now list what we believe to be important empirical evidence as follows:-

(1)   The ascension periods tend to exceed the descension periods substantially;

ascent period:	7	6	6	5	5	6	6	6
descent period:		4	4	4	4	3	4	4	3

6(5-8)   6   5
4(6-3)   4

TABLE 1: Ascent and descent periods of lynx data

(2) Given that the population size, x_{t-j}, was approximately below 3 (on the logarithmic scale), the population size x_t tends to be increasing. The reverse is true when x_{t-j} was approximately above 3. In short, there is a turning point at around 3. In addition, there is an apparent systematic shift to the left in the location of the turning point as j increases from 2 to 5 (marked circles). When j is equal to 1, no obvious turning point is detected.

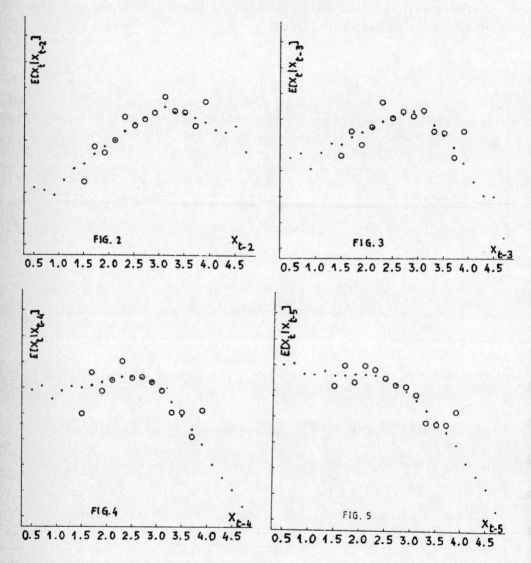

FIGS. 2 to 5: Regression function of lynx data 'o' and simulation '+'

(3) The scatter diagrams of (x_t, x_{t-j}), $j = 1, \ldots, 6$, consist of spirals which, with
      j increasing, show a systematic change of orientation (Figs. 6 to 11). Speci-
      fically, it starts with predominantly anti-clockwise spirals at $j = 1$ and changes
      to predominantly clockwise spirals at $j = 6$. A complete spiral tends to take
      9 or 10 years. The regions of inaccessibility (which are especially obvious at
      $j = 1$ and 2) are particularly interesting because they may be interpreted as
      portraying a stochastically perturbed limit cycle, which is related to the
      'crater-like' structure to be mentioned in (6).

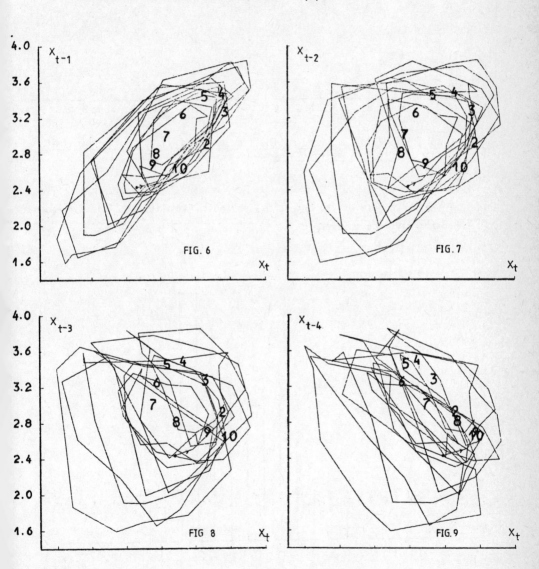

FIG. 6

FIG. 7

FIG 8

FIG. 9

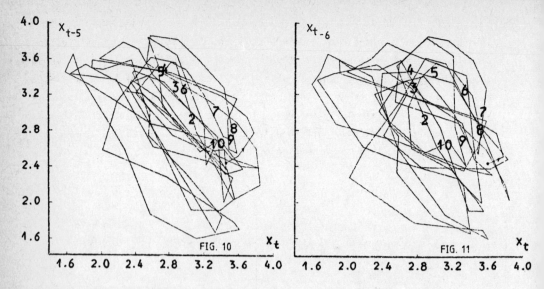

FIGS. 6 to 11: Scatter diagrams of the lynx data (1821-1934) with the limit
cycle of SETAR (2;8,3)

(4) The marginal histogram of the data shows obvious bimodality with the anti-mode
at approximately 3 (Figure 12A).

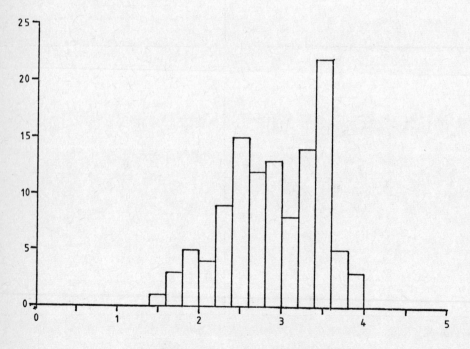

FIG. 12A: Histogram of lynx data

325

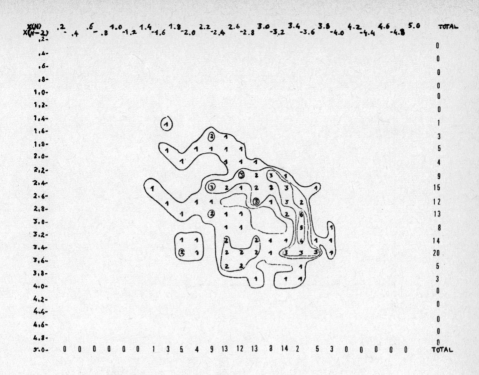

FIG. 12B: Bivariate histogram of lynx data (X_t, X_{t-2})

(5) The power spectrum estimate using a window method clearly reveals the existence
of higher harmonics to the fundamental period of approximately 9½ years. This
implies that the periodic structure of the data is non-cosinusoidal (see Figure
13). Of course, this point is related to point (1). Also, the modulus of the
bispectral density function shows two prominent peaks (Figure 14) and the argument
of the same is clearly non-zero. (Table 2B). The latter implies that the data
are time-irreversible, i.e. x_t and x_{-t} have different probabilistic structure.
(For a detailed discussion of the physical meaning of a bispectrum, see, e.g.
Hasselman, Munk and MacDonald, 1963).

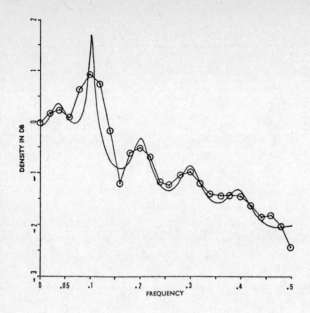

FIG. 13: Spectral density function - ⊙-, estimate using the
Blackman-Tukey window, ——, estimate from AR model fitting

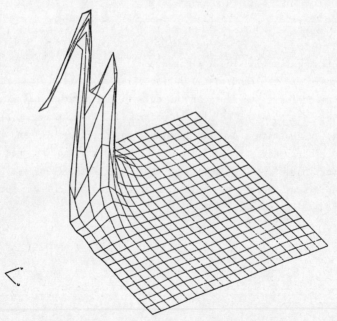

FIG. 14: Bispectral density function estimate (log lynx data) - modulus

ω_2	0.00	.05	.10	.15	.20	.25	.30	.35	.40	.45	.50	.55	.60	.65
1.00	.00													
.95	-.00	-.39	-.60											
.90	.00	-.43	-.73	-1.08	-1.61									
.85	-.00	-.53	-.88	-1.22	-1.69	-2.32	-3.05							
.80	-.00	-.72	-1.18	-1.51	-1.90	-2.42	-3.07	2.63	2.20					
.75	-.00	-.98	-1.56	-1.85	-2.13	-2.54	-3.09	2.62	2.18	1.80	1.31			
.70	-.00	-1.20	-1.84	-2.18	-2.35	-2.64	-3.10	2.62	2.14	1.75	1.31	.78	.49	
.65	-.00	-1.42	-2.30	-2.52	-2.58	-2.76	-3.11	2.64	2.11	1.70	1.33	.91	.58	.42
.60	-3.14	2.28	2.75	-2.03	-2.86	-2.92	3.12	2.69	2.14	1.68	1.35	1.10	.81	
.55	-3.14	2.05	1.82	2.15	2.86	3.09	2.99	2.69	2.23	1.71	1.36	1.22		
.50	-3.14	2.10	1.69	1.64	1.83	2.48	2.68	2.58	2.31	1.88	1.49			
.45	-3.14	2.16	1.67	1.51	1.56	1.84	2.22	2.36	2.32	2.15				
.40	-3.14	2.01	1.58	1.40	1.38	1.51	1.81	2.11	2.26					
.35	-3.14	1.80	1.43	1.27	1.20	1.25	1.47	1.81						
.30	-3.14	2.04	1.46	1.25	1.15	1.10	1.19							
.25	-3.14	2.50	1.72	1.36	1.21	1.12								
.20	-3.14	2.77	2.17	1.60	1.33									
.15	3.14	2.88	2.55	2.07										
.10	3.14	2.94	2.77											
.05	3.14	3.02												
+0.00	0.00													

ω_1: 0.00, .05, .10, .15, .20, .25, .30, .35, .40, .45, .50, .55, .60, .65

(in units of π)

TABLE 2A: Estimated bispectral argument (Threshold Model)

(6) The bivariate histograms of (x_t, x_{t-j}), $j = 1,\ldots,6$, show particularly interesting non-Gaussianity of the data structure. Notice especially the 'crater-like' structure (see Figs. 15 to 20 and 12B, and c.f. Figs. 6.to 11).

DATA (1821-1934)

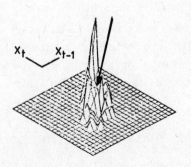

FIG. 15

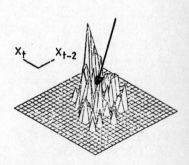

FIG. 16

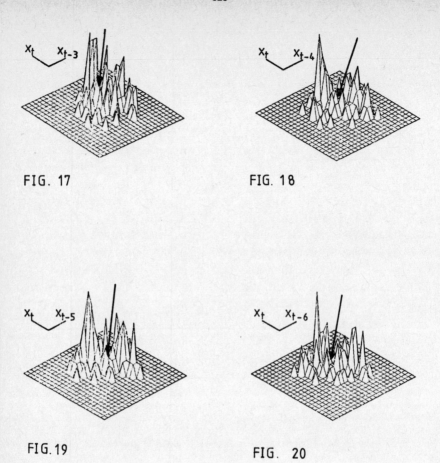

FIG. 17   FIG. 18

FIG. 19   FIG. 20

FIGS. 15 to 20:   Bivariate histograms of (X_t, X_{t-k}), $k = 1, 2, \ldots, 6$

We take the view that no statistical/ecological model to this data set may be considered satisfactory if it fails to incorporate, in one way or another, the above features.

In the (self-exciting) threshold autoregressive model, SETAR, we are about to propose for the lynx data, the so-called delay parameter and the threshold parameter play a rather crucial role in that they are responsible for the non-linearity of the model. These parameters may be based on the following well-known ecological consider-ations:-

1. There often exists a delayed regulation in an ecosystem due to (see, e.g., Maynard-Smith, 1974):

(i)   development time, T, taken for the young (or an egg) to develop into an adult. In the lynx case, it is known that it reaches sexual maturity at <u>two</u> years;

(ii)   discrete breeding seasons. A species may breed only at a specific time. In the lynx case, it is known that births usually take place in March-April.

2. <u>Competition</u> for resources of the habitat provides a <u>self-regulation</u> (see, e.g., Solomon, 1969). The animal may become more aggressive when its population density rises above a <u>certain level</u>, and this change is, sometimes at least, associated with a decline in the net rate of reproduction. The population can undergo qualitative changes at high density, and these changes can continue for some generations after the density has 'crashed' again to lower levels.

The following SETAR model has been fitted by Tong and Lim (1980) to the lynx data of 1821-1934. The model was originally identified on <u>purely</u> statistical grounds. (Coefficients are now rounded to two decimal places).

$$
x_t = \begin{cases}
\begin{aligned}
& 0.52 + 1.04\, x_{t-1} - 0.18\, x_{t-2} + 0.18\, x_{t-3} - 0.43\, x_{t-4} \\
& (0.37) \quad (0.11) \qquad (0.17) \qquad\quad (0.17) \qquad\quad (0.17) \\[4pt]
& + 0.35\, x_{t-5} - 0.30\, x_{t-6} + 0.22\, x_{t-7} + \varepsilon_t^{(1)} \quad \text{if } x_{t-2} \le 3.12, \\
& \;\;(0.17) \qquad\;\; (0.19) \qquad\;\; (0.17) \\[10pt]
& 2.66 + 1.42\, x_{t-1} - 1.16\, x_{t-2} - 0.11\, x_{t-3} + \varepsilon_t^{(2)} \quad \text{if } x_{t-2} > 3.12, \\
& (0.50)
\end{aligned}
\end{cases}
$$

where var $\varepsilon_t^{(1)}$ = 0.0255 and var $\varepsilon_t^{(2)}$ = 0.0516. Standard errors of the parameter estimates are given in parentheses. Notice that the delay parameter is 2 and the threshold parameter is 3.12. Our model is, in fact, a difference-delay equation which is piece-wise linear and involves higher lags. Tong (1981) has shown that, from the standpoint of Bayesian statistics, a piece-wise approach is quite natural and has an intimate connection with catastrophe theory. The autocorrelation function of the fitted residuals (Figure 21) suggests that the fit is adequate from the point of view of "fitting the model in order to reduce the data to white noise".

330

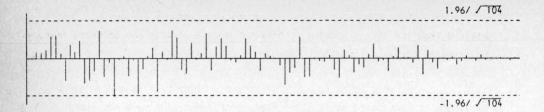

FIG. 21: Autocorrelation function of normalized fitted residuals
from SETAR (2;8,3)

It is particularly interesting to see that the statistical identified delay
parameter of 2 years turns out to be so closely related to the development time.
The threshold parameter of 3.12 may be interpreted as the threshold separating two
different modes of reproduction. Although this model seems to conform well to ecological considerations, does it capture the empirical features discussed at the
beginning of this section?

(1') The systematic part of model (2) shows a periodic function with an ascension
period of 6 years and a descension period of 3 years (Figure 22). This agrees
well with the observed feature mentioned in (1). It is also interesting to
report that, during the stage of statistical identification, we have observed
that no potential model with a delay parameter equal to one year turns out to
admit a limit cycle. (For further details, we refer to an unpublished doctoral
thesis by K. S. Lim, 1981, UMIST). This observation reinforces our earlier
comment in connection with the role played by the development time. At the
colloquium, Tong conjectured that, with d fixed at 1, no piece-wise linear
recursion can lead to a periodic solution with period ≥ 9. If true, this
conjecture would have interesting biological and physical implications.

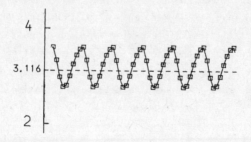

FIG. 22: Systematic part of SETAR (2;8,3)

(2') Figures 2 to 5 (marked crosses) show that the regression functions of x_t on x_{t-j} obtained from the fitted model (2) show good agreement with the observed features mentioned in (2). The turning points and their systematic shift are clearly visible. The agreement is equally good when $j = 1$ (see Lim's doctoral thesis).

(3') The systematic part of model (2) corresponds to the cycles marked by the numerals 2, 3, 4, 5, 6, 7, 8, 9 and 10 in that order in Figs. 6 to 11. The general shape and orientation agree well with those observed in (3).

(4') The marginal distribution of the fitted model does not exhibit bimodality. However, bimodality does develop when the noise variances are reduced by a factor of 9 (Table 3). The locations of the two modes and the anti-model are then in reasonable agreement with those observed in (4). However, the left modal value is slightly greater than the right modal value for the fitted model. Further noise variance reduction reveals an interesting region of inaccessibility as shown in Tables 4 and 5 (c.f. Fig. 12B).

TABLE 3 (reduction factor = 9)

Z(N) / X(N-2)	1.8 1.6	2.2 -2.0	2.6 -2.4	-2.8	3.0 -3.2	3.4 -3.6	3.8 -4.0	4.2						TOTAL
1.8-														0
2.0-			2											2
2.2-			2	49	43	13	2							109
2.4-			3	48	396	307	95	3						852
2.6-			25	155	256	687	581	288	4					1996
2.8-			11	146	349	112	224	734	251					1827
3.0-		1	26	181	312	99	10	152	737	23				1541
3.2-		1	35	221	373	166	113	406	606	25				1946
3.4-			5	54	286	426	501	358	48	1				1676
3.6-					1	12	17	14	5					49
3.8-														0
TOTAL	0	0	2	109	852	1997	1827	1540	1946	1676	49	0	0	9998

TABLE 4 (reduction factor = 25)

Z(N) / X(N-2)	1.8 1.6	2.2 -2.0	2.6 -2.4	-2.8	3.0 -3.2	3.4 -3.6	3.8 -4.0	4.2						TOTAL
2.0-														0
2.2-				15	12	3								30
2.4-				2	18	399	281	37	2					739
2.6-				6	123	291	812	674	274	2				2182
2.8-				1	145	469	71	152	775	310				1923
3.0-				9	157	295	66		82	774	7			1390
3.2-				12	257	475	111	60	394	650	5			1964
3.4-					25	238	575	462	435	21	1			1757
3.6-							4	4	4	1				13
3.8-														0
4.0-														0
TOTAL	0	0	0	30	740	2183	1924	1389	1963	1757	13	0	0	9998

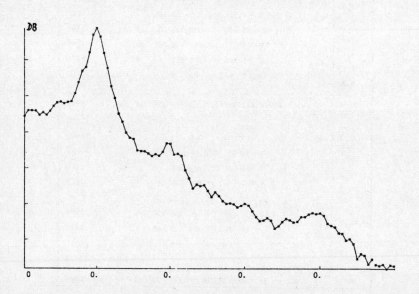

2.4-									0
2.6-				11111110	1111				3332
2.8-				1111		1111			2222
3.0-									0
3.2-				1111		1111			2212
3.4-					1111	1111			2222
3.6-									0
3.8-									
TOTAL	0	0	0	0	033332221	022222222	0	0	0	9998

TABLE 5
(reduction factor = ∞)

TABLES 3 to 5: Bivariate distribution with reducing noise variance

(5') Figs. 23 and 24 and Table 2A show good agreement with Figs. 13 and 14 and Table 2B respectively. This implies that the fitted SETAR model has succeeded in accounting for the time irreversibility exhibited by the data to quite a large extent. It is also interesting to mention that on replacing the ε-terms in equation (2) by periodic functions with periods 7, 8, 9, 10 and 11 years respectively, beats are observed except for the two 'heteroperiods' of 9 and 10 years with which a synchronisation is observed. It seems plausible to suggest that, rather than keeping a precise non-integral period of approximately $9\frac{1}{2}$ years as is sometimes suggested, the species may well have a more flexible period which is either 9 years or 10 years (see Pemberton and Tong, 1981).

FIG. 23: Spectral density through SETAR (2;8,3)

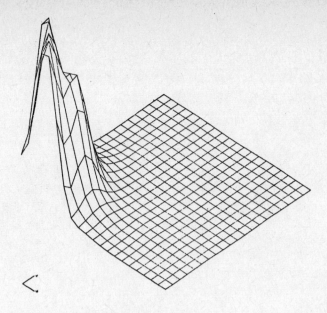

FIG. 24: Bispectral density function estimate through SETAR (2;8,3) - Modulus

ω_2	0.00	.05	.10	.15	.20	.25	.30	.35	.40	.45	.50	.55	.60	.65
1.00	-.00													
.95	-.00	-.62	-1.28											
.90	.00	.33	-1.08	-1.63	-1.96									
.85	-.00	1.22	.37	-1.43	-1.95	-2.37	-2.88							
.80	-.00	1.27	.98	-.91	-1.78	-2.35	-2.89	2.80	2.26					
.75	-.00	1.15	1.29	-1.05	-1.65	-2.19	-2.86	2.78	2.22	1.71	.97			
.70	-.00	1.02	1.59	2.83	-2.12	-2.20	-2.78	2.74	2.15	1.58	.85	.52	·.58	
.65	-.00	.84	1.66	2.49	-3.09	-2.73	-2.92	2.67	2.10	1.61	.92	.50	.58	.58
.60	-.00	.72	1.49	2.26	2.79	3.07	3.07	2.60	2.05	1.74	1.52	1.30	.73	
.55	-3.14	1.22	1.50	1.77	2.30	2.77	2.88	2.60	2.02	1.71	1.70	1.99		
.50	-3.14	2.50	1.83	1.67	1.67	2.05	2.56	2.54	2.07	1.62	1.55			
.45	-3.14	2.87	2.09	1.80	1.69	1.68	1.97	2.31	2.19	1.81				
.40	-3.14	2.71	2.06	1.82	1.75	1.75	1.84	2.11	2.24					
.35	-3.14	1.78	1.65	1.62	1.62	1.68	1.82	1.99						
.30	-3.14	2.38	1.60	1.54	1.50	1.50	1.63							
.25	-3.14	2.91	1.96	1.60	1.53	1.48								
.20	-3.14	2.96	2.57	1.83	1.60									
.15	3.14	2.91	2.77	2.42										
.10	3.14	2.89	2.79											
.05	3.14	2.99												
ω_2 ↑ 0.00	0.00													
ω_1	0.00	.05	.10	.15	.20	.25	.30	.35	.40	.45	.50	.55	.60	.65

(in units of π)

TABLE 2B: Estimated bispectral argument (log lynx data)

(6') Figs. 25 to 30 show good agreement with the general non-Gaussian shapes observed in (6). Crater-like structure is clearly visible. (For reasons of economy, we have not included figures which are 90° rotations of Figs. 25 to 30, but they are obtainable from the authors on request.

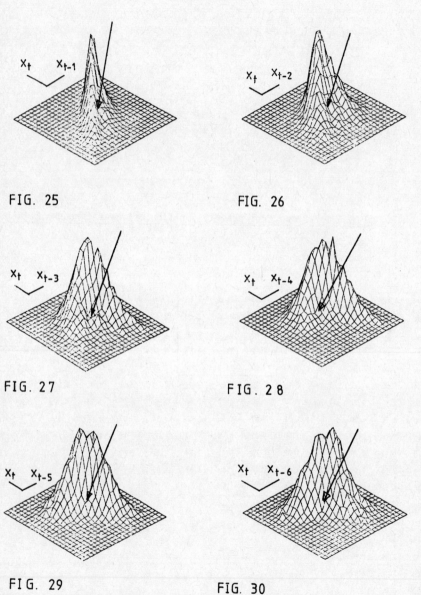

SETAR (2;8,3)

FIGS. 25 to 30: Bivariate histograms of (X_t, X_{t-k}), $k = 1,2,..,6$

We may now conclude that ecological arguments have provided the relevant motivation for the difference-delay equation model (2), which, in turn, has verified the appropriateness of the ecological arguments through this model's ability in capturing a large number of observational features. We would remark that this class of models is also very useful for short and long range forecasts (see Tong and Wu, 1981).

CANADIAN MINK AND MUSKRAT DATA

This classic data set (see Figure 31) is extracted from Jones (1914), who compiled his data using the Hudson Bay Company record of 1848-1911. In the last example we studied a single species. It seems interesting to study the feasibility of the threshold models, appropriately extended, for the analysis of a predator-prey ecosystem. It is known that the mink is an important predator of the muskrat and there is an approximate ten-year cycle.

(i)

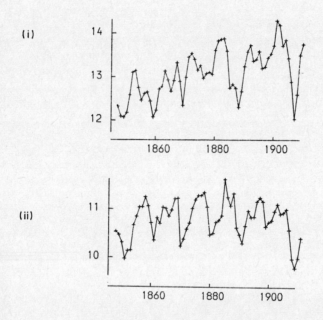

(ii)

FIG. 31: Muskrat (i) and Mink (ii) data

The cycles for the mink, like those for the lynx, tend to be negatively skew and those for the muskrat tend to be positively skew. There is also an observed lead-lag relation of approximately two years between the two species, which tends to be non-uniform with respect to the maxima and the minima, with the former tending to take longer.

To facilitate statistical model fitting, the logarithmically transformed muskrat data are usually differenced once. (See, e.g., Jenkins, 1975, Chan and Wallis, 1978, Ghaddar and Tong, 1981). Also, models in these references involve lagged terms up to and including t-4. The following (closed-loop) threshold autoregressive model, TARSC, has been suggested by Tong and Lim (1980), in which x_t denotes the natural logarithm of the number of minks, and y_t denotes the first difference of the natural logarithms of the number of muskrats. Again, standard errors of parameter estimates are included in parentheses and the estimates have now been rounded to two decimal places.

$$
x_t = \begin{cases}
\begin{aligned}
&8.16 + 0.34\ x_{t-1} + 0.45\ y_{t-1} + 0.07\ x_{t-2} - 0.07\ y_{t-2} \\
&(2.17)\quad (0.16)\qquad\ (0.15)\qquad\ \ (0.18)\qquad\ \ (0.19) \\[6pt]
&-0.41\ x_{t-3} + 0.54\ y_{t-3} + 0.22\ x_{t-4} + \varepsilon_t^{(1)}\quad \text{if } y_{t-5} < -0.04, \\
&(0.22)\qquad\ \ (0.17)\qquad\ \ (0.20) \\[12pt]
&5.41 + 0.53\ x_{t-1} + 0.47\ y_{t-1} + 0.36\ x_{t-2} - 0.28\ y_{t-2} \\
&(2.74)\ (0.16)\qquad\ (0.16)\qquad\ \ (0.23)\qquad\ \ (0.15) \\[6pt]
&-0.22\ x_{t-3} + 0.20\ y_{t-3} - 0.16\ x_{t-4} + \varepsilon_t^{(2)}\quad \text{if } y_{t-5} > -0.04, \\
&(0.18)\qquad\ \ (0.17)\qquad\ \ (0.21)
\end{aligned}
\end{cases}
\tag{3a}
$$

where var $\varepsilon_t^{(1)}$ = 0.0369, var $\varepsilon_t^{(2)}$ = 0.0234.

$$
y_t = \begin{cases}
\begin{aligned}
&2.90 - 0.02\ y_{t-1} - 0.70\ x_{t-1} - 0.30\ y_{t-2} + 0.43\ x_{t-2} \\
&(1.71)\ (0.15)\qquad\ (0.14)\qquad\ \ (0.14)\qquad\ \ (0.16) \\[6pt]
&0.05\ y_{t-3} + \eta_t^{(1)}\qquad\qquad \text{if } x_{t-5} < 10.96, \\
&(0.13) \\[12pt]
&5.85 + 0.30\ y_{t-1} - 0.54\ x_{t-1} - 0.13\ y_{t-2} + \eta_t^{(2)}\quad \text{if } x_{t-5} > 10.96, \\
&(1.43\quad (0.14)\qquad\ (0.13)\qquad\ \ (0.14)
\end{aligned}
\end{cases}
\tag{3b}
$$

where var $\eta_t^{(1)}$ = 0.0385, var $\eta_t^{(2)}$ = 0.0841.

The usual diagnostic check suggests that the fitted residuals are acceptably white. However, from the statistical viewpoint, the model (3) could be considered slightly over-parametrised although, similarly to linear models, only terms up to lag t-4 are used. It is therefore important to check whether the fitted model has captured any of the obvious data-analytic features.

The delay parameter of 5 years is not easy to interpret biologically because the muskrat data have been differenced. However, the systematic parts of the fitted model for x_t and 'integrated' y_t are shown in Figure 32, which agree well with the general trend of the observed features of the data.

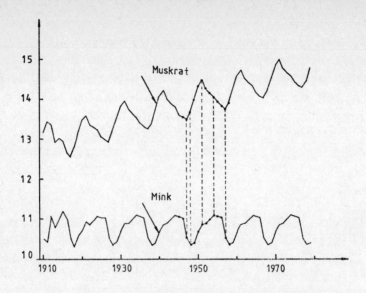

FIG. 32: Systematic part of mink-muskrat model

Specifically, the linear growth of the (log) muskrat data and its positively skew cycles of 10-year period are in reasonable agreement with the data features. Similarly, the negatively skew cycles of 10-year period for the (log) minks are also in good agreement with the observed period. It is particularly interesting to note that the maxima of the (log) muskrat cycles lead those of the (log) mink cycles by 3 years, while the lead for the minima is only 1 year.

The fitting period terminates at year 1909. The forecast values of 1910 and 1911 seem to compare well with the observed (see Table 6).

Mink

Year	Data	Prediction
1910	9.9891	10.5014
1911	10.4045	10.4328

Muskrat

Year	Data	Prediction
1910	13.5267	13.1449
1911	13.7784	14.2015

TABLE 6: One-step-ahead predictions of mink and muskrat

Although only two-point forecasts are available due to the shortness of the data
length, they do add to one's confidence in suggesting that the model is not unreasonable.

In view of the shortness of the data length, bivariate histograms and regression
functions are probably not very informative. Nevertheless, just to give the general
feel of the model we have given in Figs. 33 to 40 the regression functions of the mink
data (marked circles) and the fitted model (marked crosses). The systematic variation
of the regression functions of the fitted model, with increasing lag, seems to give
a meaningful 'smoothing' of those of the observed data. Table 7 gives some relevant
statistics.

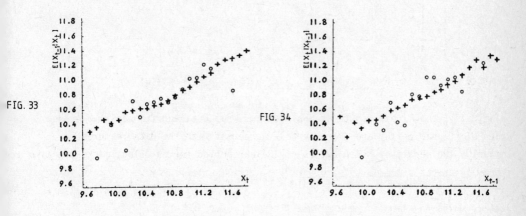

FIG. 33   FIG. 34

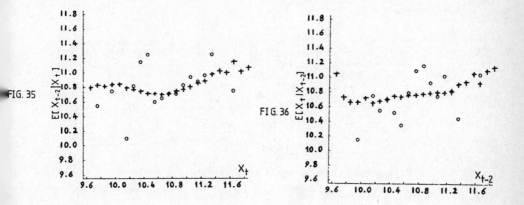

FIG. 35   FIG. 36

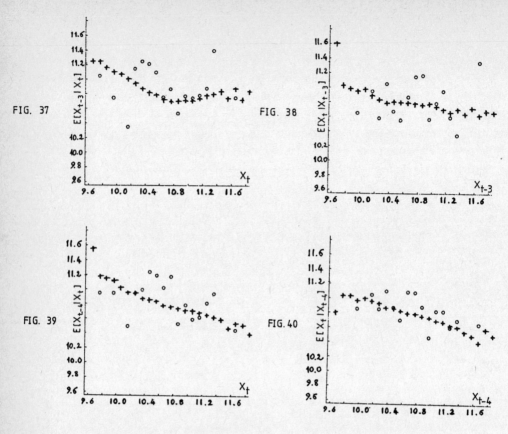

FIGS. 33 to 40: Regression function of mink data 'o' and simulation '+'

	Mink		Difference of Muskrat	
	Data	Simulated Data	Data	Simulated Data
Mean	10.8020	10.7722	0.0049	-0.0080
Variance	0.1492	0.1137	0.1245	0.1236

TABLE 7: Some statistics for the comparison of model with data
(model values are based on a 10,000-point simulation)

    Tables 8 and 9 give respectively the data bivariate histogram and the model bivariate histogram of (x_t, x_{t-1}). Tables 10, 11 and 12 give the model bivariate histograms of (x_t, x_{t-1}) with the noise variance reduced by a factor of 9, 81 and respectively. The general shapes seem to develop in the right direction, with most of the probability content lying above the 135° diagonal. (More details may be found in Lim's thesis).

341

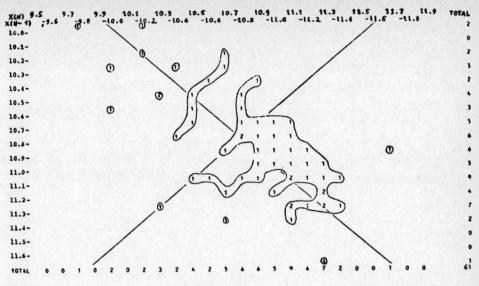

TABLE 8: (X_t, X_{t-1}) Distribution of Mink data (1849-1909)

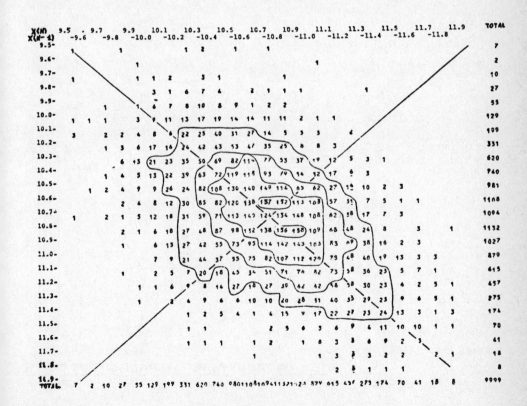

TABLE 9: (X_t, X_{t-1}) distribution of X_t from TARSC

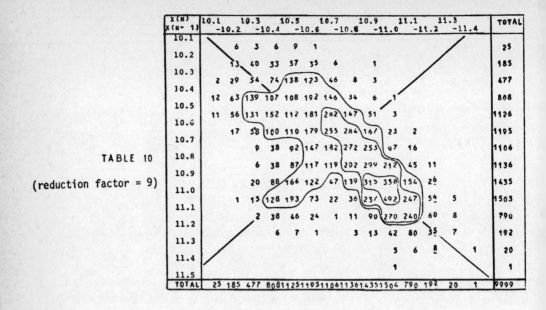

TABLE 10

(reduction factor = 9)

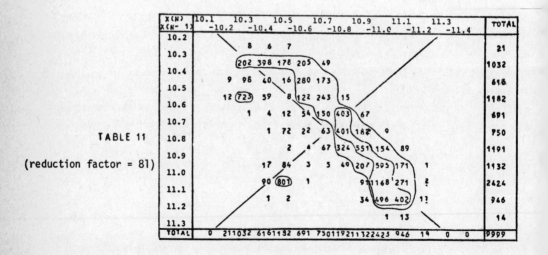

TABLE 11

(reduction factor = 81)

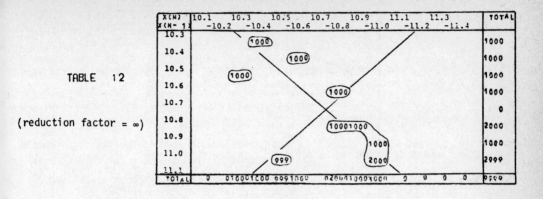

TABLE 12

(reduction factor = ∞)

TABLES 10 to 12: (X_t, X_{t-1}) distribution of X_t with reducing noise variances

In spite of the shortness of the data length, our difference-delay equation model seems to yield meaningful results. Thus, difference-delay equation models do offer exciting prospects for the analysis of predator-prey ecosystems. We would also point out that, so far as we are aware, no other bivariate non-linear time series models fitted to real ecological data have been reported in the literature.

CONCLUSION

In the field of time series analysis, linear theory has dominated the subject for the last fifty years or so. However, it is clear that linear modelling of the data studied in this paper cannot offer much structure and is ad hoc. To gain a deeper understanding of these data, as well as their associated ecosystems, an interplay between statistics and biology is crucial and the evidence shown in our present study has demonstrated that the class of threshold time series models, which are non-linear, can make a positive contribution in this respect.

REFERENCES

AKAIKE, H. (1977) "On entropy maximization principle", Proc. Symp. Appl. of Statist. ed. P. R. Krishnaiah, pp. 27-41, Amsterdam: North-Holland.

CHAN, W. Y. T. and WALLIS, K. F. (1978) "Multiple time series modelling: another look at the mink-muskrat interaction", Applied Statistics 27: 168-175.

GHADDAR, D. K. and TONG, H. (1981) "Data transformation and self-exciting threshold autoregression", to appear in Applied Statistics.

HASSELMAN, K., MUNK, W. and MACDONALD, G. (1963) "Bispectrum of ocean waves", Time Series Analysis, ed. M. Rosenblatt, pp. 125-139, New York: Wiley.

HUTCHINSON, G. E. (1948) "Circular causal systems in ecology", Annals of New York Academy of Sciences 50: 221-246.

JENKINS, G. M. (1975) "The interaction between the muskrat and mink cycles in North Canada", Proceedings ofthe 8th International Biometric Conference (Contanta, Romania, August 1974). (L.C.A. Corsten and T. Postelnia, eds.)

JONES, J. W. (1914) "Fur-farming in Canada (2nd ed.)" Commission of Conservation, Ottawa, Canada.

LEVIN, S. A. and MAY, R. M. (1976) "A note on difference-delay equations", Theoretical Population Biology 9: 178-187.

MAY, R. M. (1980) "Non-linear phenomena in ecology and epidemiology", Annals of The New York Academy of Sciences 357, 267-281.

MAYNARD-SMITH, J. (1974) "Models in Ecology", Cambridge University Press, Cambridge, U.K.

PEMBERTON, J. and TONG, H. (1981) "Threshold autoregression and some frequency-domain characteristics", to appear in "Handbook of Statistics", ed. K. R. Krishnaiah, Amsterdam: North-Holland.

TONG, H. and LIM, K. S. (1980) "Threshold autoregression, limit cycles and cyclical data (with discussion)", Journal of Royal Statistical Society (B), 42: 245-292

TONG, H. and WU, Z. M. (1981) "Multi-step-ahead forecasting of cyclical data by threshold autoregression", invited paper presented at 4th International Time Series Meeting, 22-26 June, 1981, Valencia, Spain. Proceedings to be published by North-Holland (ed. O. D. Anderson).

IDENTIFICATION AND MODELLING TECHNIQUES FOR BIOLOGICAL RHYTHMS

W. Malbecq[*] and J. De Prins
Université Libre de Bruxelles, Belgium
* Boursier I.R.S.I.A.

Introduction

We are interested in statistical methods of detection and vali-
dation of rhythms in biomedical sciences, particularly in the field
of chronobiology. Subsequently we define as signal every observed
variable as function of time. This means that, with this definition,
the signal is including as well noise fluctuations as the (supposed)
deterministic signal. Our approach is mainly empirical: knowing
the data, we try to build one or more models, to estimate their
coefficients and to test the underlying hypotheses. This last point
is very important for statistical inference and we show, with the
help of some examples, that the most classical hypotheses (independence, normality,...) are not always respected in practice.

To establish models, methods of spectral analysis may be useful.
We may consider that they belong roughly to a couple of categories:
the methods using deterministic functions and the ones based on
theory of stochastic processes. It justifies more or less that, in
a model, we consider the signal as given by the summation of deterministic functions and stochastic processes. We shall look at
experiments where the signal remains relatively stable. This means,
for instance, that an observed rhythm does not show any important
abrupt changes of amplitude or period. This condition allows us
to assume wide sense stationarity of the model.

1 Overview of some models

In order to analyze biological data and to describe them by mathematical parameters we use mainly spectral analysis models.

1.1 Fourier model

This technique is well adapted to strictly periodic signals, i.e.

$$\varphi(t) = \varphi(t+kP) \qquad k = \pm 1, \pm 2, \ldots$$
$$P = period$$

Due to this, $\varphi(t)$ may be represented by a Fourier series:

$$\varphi(t) = A_o + \sum_{j=1}^{\infty}(A_j COS jwt + B_j SIN jwt) \qquad w = 2\pi/P$$

In practice, for our models, there will be a finite number of terms
(M) due to the limitations of the sampling. It is important to
realize that this model, as every mathematical model, gives an
approximative description of the phenomenon. As a matter of fact,

the biological signals are not strictly periodic. This representation does not explain the biological fact and it is just a handy mathematical trick.

Usually, the estimation of the coefficients is based on regression theory. In that case, a true deterministic signal is considered and some noise is superimposed to it. The last one explains the differences between the data and the model.

$$y_i = A_o + \underbrace{\sum_{j=1}^{L}(A_j COSjwt_i + B_j SINjwt_i)}_{\text{deterministic part}} + \underbrace{\varepsilon_i}_{\text{noise}} \quad i=1,\ldots,N$$

where t_i is the ith observation time.
ε_i is the noise at time t_i.
L is the number of harmonics selected by the user.

The most common hypotheses are the following:

$$\varepsilon_i \sim \mathcal{N}(0,\sigma^2) \quad \text{Gaussian distribution}$$
$$E[\varepsilon_i \cdot \varepsilon_j] = \delta_{ij}\sigma^2 \quad \text{uncorrelated residuals}$$

Under this Gaussian white noise assumption, it is easy to show that the estimation by means of least squares is optimal (WILKS 1962). The estimates $(\hat{A}_o,\hat{A}_j,\hat{B}_j ; j\neq1,\ldots,L)$ are obtained by minimizing the sum of squares of residuals i.e.:

$$A_o = \hat{A}_o$$
$$\text{and } A_j = \hat{A}_j \quad B_j = \hat{B}_j \quad \text{minimize} \sum_{i=1}^{N}(y_i - A_o - \sum_{j=1}^{L}(A_j COSjwt_i + B_j SINjwt_i))^2$$

If the selected model is correct, the estimates are unbiased and their covariance matrix is optimal (determinant minimal = efficiency). Moreover some hypotheses $(A_j^2+B_j^2=0,\ldots)$ may be tested by means of Student and Fisher distributions.

The difficult part will be the selection of the significative harmonics and the good choice of their number $(2L+1 \leqslant N)$ in order to distinguish signal from noise.

This method is very useful when the period P of the signal is well known (if periodicities appear clearly).

Another point of view is to evaluate the discrete Fourier transform (D.F.T.) of the data. This method can be applied to data which are regularly spaced over the observation interval and it is useful in the case of deterministic signals. Indeed there is a one to one correspondance between the set of data and the set of the Fourier coefficients $\tilde{A}_o,\tilde{A}_j,\tilde{B}_j$:

$$\tilde{A}_o = \frac{1}{N}\sum_{i=1}^{N} y_i$$
$$\tilde{A}_j = \frac{2}{N}\sum_{i=1}^{N} y_i \cos\frac{2\pi(i-1)j}{N}$$
$$\tilde{B}_j = \frac{2}{N}\sum_{i=1}^{N} y_i \sin\frac{2\pi(i-1)j}{N} \quad 0<j<\frac{N}{2} \text{ and } j \text{ is integer}$$

and $\widetilde{A}_{\frac{N}{2}} = \frac{1}{N} \sum_{i=1}^{N} (-1)^{(i-1)} y_i$ if N is even

$$y_i = \widetilde{A}_o + \sum_{0<j<\frac{N}{2}} \left[\widetilde{A}_j \cos\frac{2\pi}{N}j(i-1) + \widetilde{B}_j \sin\frac{2\pi}{N}j(i-1) \right] + (-1)^{(i-1)} \widetilde{A}_{\frac{N}{2}}$$

if N is even

In this case, we obtain estimations for the spectral lines at frequencies $2\pi j/N$ $(0<j<N/2$, and at π if N is even). We do not consider random part for the signal. This kind of analysis is well adapted when we try to detect periodicities in a set of data where they do not appear clearly.

To close this section, let us remark that the least squares and the D.F.T. estimations for the same Fourier coefficients are equivalent when the data are regularly spaced over an integer number of periods P.

1.2 Autoregressive methods

These more recent techniques are mainly based on the adjustment of a purely stochastic process. All the regularities of the phenomenon are described in terms of correlations. The knowledge of the process parameters induces the knowledge of its spectrum and its correlation function.

For example, in the case of regularly spaced data, the autoregressive numerical filter is:

$$y_t = \sum_{j=1}^{p} \alpha_j\, y_{t-j} + \varepsilon_t$$

for a process with mean 0
ε_t is a Gaussian white noise with mean 0 and variance σ_ε^2.

It means that the set of data is supposed to be produced by linear filtering of a white noise. The main problem is the estimation of the filter coefficients α_j $(j=1,\ldots,p)$.

Having such estimations $\hat{\alpha}_j$ of α_j and $\hat{\sigma}_\varepsilon^2$ of σ_ε^2, the power spectrum is:

$$\hat{f}(w) = \frac{\hat{\sigma}_\varepsilon^2}{|1 - \sum_{j=1}^{p} \hat{\alpha}_j z^{-j}|^2 2\pi}$$ $z = e^{2\pi i \nu}$

with $\Delta t = 1$
and $\nu \in [-.5 ; .5]$

Many estimation methods are available. The first is based on the maximum entropy principle i.e. finding f(w) in order to maximize

$$\int_{-\pi}^{\pi} \log f(w)\, dw$$

under p constraints

$$\int_{-\pi}^{\pi} f(w)\, e^{ij w}\, dw = \gamma(j)$$ where $\gamma(j)$ j=1,...,p are the p first preassigned autocovariances of the process.

This technique is equivalent to the estimation of α_j by means of the Yule Walker equations. Other estimation methods may be used: the least squares (uni- or bidirectional), the maximum likelihood, ... The last one gives the best estimators but the amount of calculation is often very important.

This autoregressive approach seems to be well adapted to noise analysis because any stationary process may be described by an A.R.
model. For example, LINKENS (1979) has given some applications of
this approach in biology. But, in practice, it is not sure that
this representation (with finite number of coefficients) is adequate (GUTOWSKI et al. 1978).

After all, one of the most important facts is the choice of the
order of the model. If it is too small the spectrum will be incom-
plete, in the other case the spectrum will describe a particular
series which is not general enough. The most used criterions are
the Final Prediction Error (F.P.E.) and the Akaike Information
Criterion (A.I.C.) (AKAIKE 1970).

2 Testing the model and robust methods

In both cases, estimation methods will give values for the parameters. But before using them for interpretation of the phenomenon,
it is very important to control whether the hypotheses, mainly
independence and normality, are fulfilled and, if necessary, to
use robust methods.

2.1 Correlations

A critical hypothesis in regression theory is the one of independence of the errors. To test it, we have to look at the estimated
residuals ($\hat{\epsilon}_i$). Two kinds of procedures may be used: the nonparametric tests and the parametric ones.

Nonparametric tests are often easy to apply and they are independent of any distribution assumption. For example, we may use the
sign test, the run test, the length of runs test,...

Used carefully, parametric tests give information too: for
instance, white noise assumption may be tested by means of sampling
correlations. For these the 95% approximate confidence limits are
$(-2/\sqrt{N}, 2/\sqrt{N})$ for a normal white noise (CHATFIELD 1976).

When significative correlations are detected, three solutions are
possible:
 -to take more parameters for the regression model thinking it was
  not complete.
 -to decimate the series (CORNELISSEN et al. 1980).
 -to modify the white noise hypotheses and to consider ARMA processes for the residues.

Example. We show data of human rectal temperature (LEVINE et al.
1979). They are recorded automatically every twelve minuts during
a few weeks. Let us look at one day. The first adjustment is made
with a single sine function (fig.1). Under the white noise hypothesis the number of runs has a probability =.95 to vary between
51 and 71. In our case, we have ·8 runs which implies the presence
of significative correlations. When we take a model with five
harmonics, the number of runs is increased but is still falling
outside the interval (28) (fig.2). This solution is not quite
satisfactory in this case.

We have to underline that correlations have great influence upon
the distribution of the estimators, especially upon the variance.
That is why the confidence limits are deeply modified and so is

the level of the test. When we adopt the solution of the correlated
noise model, new problems have to be solved: estimation, choice of
order of the process,...

Several estimation methods may be used: the least squares (MALBECQ
and DE PRINS 1981) and the maximum likelihood. This last one is
much more time consuming. Recently an algorithm for the evaluation
of the likelihood function was proposed by HARVEY and PHILLIPS
(1979). It is based on state space representation and Kalman filter.

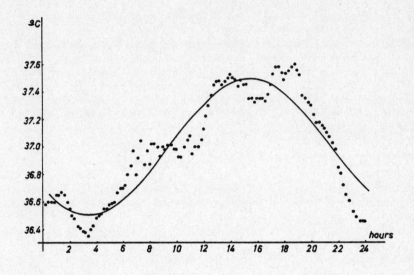

Figure 1

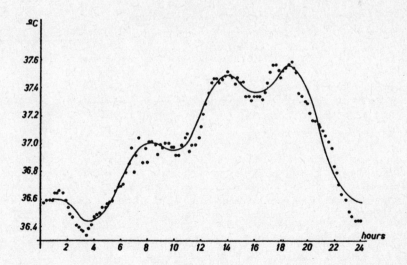

Figure 2

2.2 Normality

This assumption is very important too. First, if the data correspond to a non Gaussian case, the estimators are no longer optimal.
Moreover the least squares are very sensitive to outliers (ANDREWS
et al. 1972). The non respect of this hypothesis may be produced
by a perturbation of the normal distribution, a larger kurtosis
of the underlying distribution, etc...

In regression theory many methods were proposed recently. These
estimation techniques are called robust for they resist to the
non respect of normal assumption. They are mainly based on a ponde-
ration of the extreme observations.

As example, let us show an experiment done by BIRKELAND in which
some melatonin data are very far from the mean function. This divergence is probably due to short spontaneous   awakings of the
subject. Although these points are not erroneous measurement, they
are not representative of the situation during the whole sampling
period. We may consider them as a typical perturbation of a
Gaussian distribution. (fig.3).

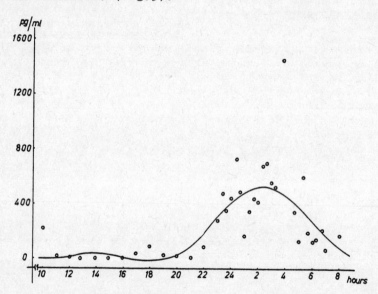

Figure 3

One of the most used techniques was proposed by HUBER (1964). It
is an alternative to least squares.
In the least squares case we minimize $\sum_{i=1}^{N} \varepsilon_i^2$

In the robust case we minimize $\sum_{i=1}^{N} \rho(\varepsilon_i)$

where $\rho(\varepsilon) = \varepsilon^2$ if $|\varepsilon| < ks$

$\rho(\varepsilon) = ks(2|\varepsilon| - ks)$ if $|\varepsilon| > ks$

and   s is a robust estimation of the standard
deviation.

These techniques present some drawbacks. The residuals have to be independent. There is often a parameter to select; in the example k can take different values $(1, 1.5, 2, ...)$. The optimal choice depends on the distribution of the residues, which is unknown.

In fact a robust method is a compromise between the gain of efficiency when the data are non Gaussian and its loss when the assumption of normality is correct. Let us remark that, in practice, the search for the kind of distribution is very difficult because we have to look at the tails of the distribution. The only thing we can do is to evaluate some parameters: the skewness, the kurtosis, quotients of quantiles,...

For the study of stochastic processes it seems to be more difficult to find robust methods. At this time only a few solutions were proposed in the statistical literature. KLEINER et al. proposed two robust algorithms in the case of autoregressive spectral analysis. They are mainly based on the Huber's metric described before. On the other hand, MARTIN (1980) proposed a robust version of the maximum likelihood. It is based on a robust Kalman filter.

3 Unequidistant data

In practice sometimes, owing to circumstances, the sampling is not regular. Two kinds of sampling schemes may occur: missing points in a regular sheme and a quite irregular one. The distribution of the times of measure has to remain more or less uniform because otherwise, a large gap wil make the problem ill-conditioned and the classical methods cannot be applied. For stochastic models JONES (1980) has proposed algorithms to estimate parameters. The first is adapted to regular sampling shemes with missing data while the other works for totally unequidistant data. In the second case, the autoregressive process is no longer discrete but becomes continuous:

$$X^{(p)}(t) = \sum_{j=1}^{p} \alpha_j X^{(p-j)}(t) + \mathcal{E}(t)$$

where $X^{(k)}(t)$ is the kth derivative of $X(t)$.

The evaluation of the likelihood function is based on Kalman filter and state space representation.

Conclusions

We have underlined some of the many problems which may occur in the modelling of rhythms in biology. They are related to spectral analysis of time series. Usually we shall start with a simple model for example the cosinor (NELSON et al. 1979). Testing the assumptions of this simple model will usually show us that we have to improve it. On the one hand, the amount of calculation will become more and more important while, at the other hand, different types of improvements will generally lead us to a multiplicity of non rejectable models. Some people may be disturbed by this multiplicity: we believe that, if several models are plausible, one should consider them all and study how their respective solutions vary. Sometimes, a satisfactory agreement among the various solutions may induce confidence.

Let us emphasize three points
-At this time, some of the problems are not completely solved.
For instance, the robustness in stochastic models: there are a
few algorithms and even the definition of robustness is not well
established. Many research work must be provided in this field.
-Data analysis belongs to an interactive process. One has to analyze data from several points of view. On the bases of those
results, one will still try other procedures until one feels to
have a good "picture" of the studied experience (SNYDER 1973).
-An empirical or theoretical model may be used if it is based on
tested assumptions. This means that, with the help of our data,
we are unable to reject the implicit or explicit hypotheses of
the model. Moreover it means that we are using the best statistical procedures.

References

AKAIKE, H. (1970), Statistical Predictor Identification. Ann.
Inst. Stat. Math., 22, 203-217.
ANDREWS, D.F., BICKEL, P.J., HAMPEL, F.R., HUBER, P.J., ROGERS,
W.H., TUKEY, J.W. (1972), Robust Estimates of Location.
Princeton University Press.
CHATFIELD, C. (1976), The Analysis of Time Series, Theory and
Practice. Chapman and Hall.
CORNELISSEN, G., HALBERG, E., BINGHAM, C., HALBERG, F. (1980),
Circadian Rythm in Automatically-Recorded Human Rectal and
Axillary Temperature and Wrist Activity and the Derivation
of Ultra-Conservative Confidence Ellipses for the Single Co-
sine in the Case of Positively Correlated Data.Chronobiologia,
VII, 2, 276.
GUTOWSKI, P.R., ROBINSON, E.A., TREITEL, S. (1978), Spectral
Estimation, Fact or Fiction. IEEE Trans. on Geoscience Electr.,
GE-16, nº2 .
HARVEY, C.C., PHILLIPS, G.D. (1979), Maximum Likelihood Estimation
of Regression on Models with Autoregressive-Moving Average
Disturbances. Biometrika, 66, 1, 49-58.
HUBER, P.J. (1964), Robust Estimation of Location Parameter. Ann.
Math. Stat., 35, 73-101.
JONES, R.H. (1980), Maximum Likelihood Fitting of ARMA Models to
Time Series with Missing Observations. Technometrics, 22, 3,
389-395.
JONES, R.H. (1980), Fitting a Continuous Time Autoregression to
Discrete Data. In Applied Time Series Analysis II, ed. by
D.F. Findley. New-York: Academic Press.
KLEINER, B., MARTIN, R.D. (1979), Robust Estimation of Power
Spectra. J.R. Statist. Soc. B, 41, nº3, 313-351.
LEVINE, H., HALBERG, F., HILLMAN, D.C., FANNING, R., CORNELISSEN,
G., DE PRINS, J. (1979), Alteration of Circadian Core Tempe-
rature Rhythm and Values Outside Habitual Idiochronodesm as
a Result of Laryngitis and Transmeridian Flight. Chronobiologia
VI, 2, 127.

LINKENS, D.A. (1979), Covariance Prediction Error Filter (CPEF)
    Tracking of Time Varying Biomedical Rhythms. J. Interdiscipl.
    Cycle Res., 10, 4, 273-295.
MALBECQ, W., DE PRINS, J. (1981), Application of Maximum Entropy
    Methods to Cosinor Analysis. J. Interdiscipl. Cycle Res., 12,
    2, 97-107.
MARTIN, R.D. (1980), Robust Methods for Time Series. Private
    Communication.
NELSON, W., TONG, Y.L., LEE, J.K., HALBERG, F. (1979), Methods
    Cosinor-Rhythmometry. Chronobiologia, VI, 4, 305-323.
SNYDER, M. (1973), Interactive Data Analysis and Nonparametric
    Statistics. Proceedings of APL Congress 73, Copenhagen. Ed.
    Gjerløv, Helms, Nielsen, North-Holland Publishing Company
    Amsterdam-London; American Elsevier Publishing Co., Inc. New-
    York. 483-487.
WILKS, S. (1962), Mathematical Statistics, Wiley.

CHAOTIC CURVES

Michel MENDÈS FRANCE

-:-:-:-

§.0.1. - Introduction

The purpose of this article is to propose two methods for measuring the quantity
of chaos of a plane curve. We would like to be able to analyze the difference between
the two curves (a) and (b) shown in Figure 1.

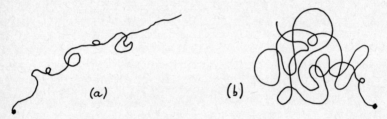

(a)   (b)

Figure 1

In part one, we present the notion of <u>entropy</u> with reference to physics. Low
entropy corresponds to predictibility and great regularity (curve (a)). High entropy on the contrary describes chaos and randomness (curve (b)).

The second part of this article is devoted to <u>dimension</u> theory. Following one of
B. Mandelbrot's basic ideas, we shall define the dimension of a plane curve :
a one dimensional curve has a tendency to regularity as curve (a) whereas, on the
contrary, a two dimensional curve wanders about the plane (or a portion of the plane)
as if it were going to fill in a two dimensional set (curve (b)). Non-integer dimensions are of course possible and correspond to curves which are in between
determinism and chaos. It was a surprise to me to discover that our approach to
dimension is closely linked to Bovet's study of animals in search of their prey discussed in this book [1].

Both concepts entropy and dimension are quite obviously related and we shall see in particular that a 0 entropy curve is indeed one dimensional as one might guess.

Our last paragraph is concerned with a different approach to dimension, namely Poincaré's biological dimension. We shall try to convince the reader that the number of dimensions (either ours or Poincaré's) depends not only on the "observed object", but also on the "observer". Our conclusion could be that intelligence (of the observer) lowers the dimension (of the observed).

Part I : Entropy

§ . I. 1. - Wheeler's model of the electron

In his Nobel prize address, Feynman [5] describes Wheeler's attempt to explain why all electrons are alike. There is only one electron and this electron takes on the shape of a long oriented curve known as a "world line" in the four dimensional space-time Universe. When actually observing electrons at time $t = t_o$, what we see is the intersection points of the curve and of the constant time hyperplane $t = t_o$.

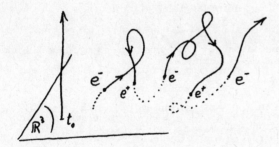

Figure 2

As time flows, the hyperplane moves upwards and the electrons describe certain trajectories. An intersection point can be either an electron e^- if the curve is oriented in the positive t direction as it cuts the hyperplane or a positron e^+ otherwise (a positron is an anti-electron). As the hyperplane goes upwards, some e^- and some e^+ may collide and thus disappear. Conversely, a couple e^-, e^+ may appear.

This model is not considered a serious one, yet, it shows that a curve is a system of moving particles. A system of particles has a certain entropy. It follows that by averaging the entropy over the time, we should be able to define the entropy of the curve. In the following paragraphs we actually show how to define and compute such an entropy.

§ . I. 2. - Entropy of N particles

From information theory, we can define the entropy of N particles to be log N . Suppose that N = N(t) depends on t . Suppose furthermore that N(t) has an average, say

$$\overline{N} = \lim_{T \to \infty} \frac{1}{T} \int_0^T N(t) \, dt.$$

(Other averages may be preferable, especially if the set we average on is compact. This depends on the context.) By definition, the entropy of the global system is

$$H = \log \, (\text{average of } N(t)).$$

(rather than the average of log N(t)).

§ . I. 3. - Entropy of finite curves

Let Ω be the set of plane curves of finite length. We are interested in the shape of curves so we shall identify two curves Γ and Γ' as soon as there exist trans- lations, rotations, reflections, homotheties or any combinations of these transfor- mations which send one curve onto the other. For example, all finite straight seg- ments must be identified.

A curve Γ (or its class) is called a "world line". An infinite straight line D wich intersects Γ is called an "instant" (think of Wheeler's model. Here, time is not directed and is not even unidimensional : each intersecting line D is a different instant).

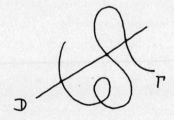

Figure 3

The state of Γ at instant D is the set $\Gamma \cap D$ of intersecting points (particles in Wheeler's model). Let $N(D)$ be the number of elements of $\Gamma \cap D$. We define the average of $N(D)$ as follows.

In the (x, y)-Cartesian plane, D is characterized by its equation

$$x \cos \theta + y \sin \theta - \rho = 0 \qquad (\rho \geq 0, \ 0 \leq \theta < 2\pi)$$

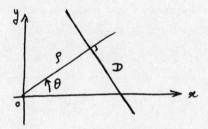

Figure 4

so that in the (ρ, θ)-plane, D is represented by a point. The measure dD in the (ρ, θ)-plane is the usual two-dimensional Lebesgue measure $dD = d\rho \, d\theta$. The average of $N(D)$ is then

$$\overline{N} = \int_{D \cap \Gamma \neq \emptyset} N(D) \, dD \ / \int_{D \cap \Gamma \neq \emptyset} dD \ .$$

By definition, the entropy of the finite curve Γ is $H(\Gamma) = \log \overline{N}$. A well known result of H. Steinhaus (see Santaló [10]) states that

$$\overline{N} = 2 \, \frac{\text{length } \Gamma}{\text{length } \partial K} = 2 \, \frac{|\Gamma|}{|\partial K|}$$

where ∂K is the boundary of the convex hull K of Γ.

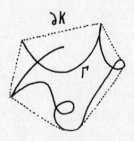

Figure 5

Hence the entropy of the finite curve Γ is

$$H(\Gamma) = \log \frac{2|\Gamma|}{|\partial K|} \quad . \tag{1}$$

Notice that $H(\Gamma)$ does not depend on the particular representative Γ of the class Γ, and so is independent of the unit with which we measure lengths.

We could have taken formula (1) as the definition of the entropy of Γ. Our approach seems however more appropriate in that it gives some evidence why formula (1) is an entropy.

Straight segments are the only finite curves to have entropy 0. Any other curve has strictly positive entropy. An algebraic curve (or a portion of) of degree ν has entropy at most $\log \nu$ (indeed, $N(D) \leq \nu$ so that $\overline{N} \leq \nu$). The entropy of a closed convex curve is $\log 2$.

§.I.4. - Entropy of infinite curves

Let Γ be a curve of infinite length (Γ may be either bounded or unbounded in the plane). Let $s \geq 0$. We denote by Γ_s the beginning portion of Γ of length s ; $|\Gamma_s| = s$. By definition, the entropy of Γ is

$$h(\Gamma) = \lim_{s \to \infty} \frac{H(\Gamma_s)}{\log s} \quad .$$

(If the limit does not exist, we define the upper entropy $\overline{h}(\Gamma)$ and the lower entropy $\underline{h}(\Gamma)$ by replacing the symbol lim repsectively by lim sup and lim inf .)

The entropy $h(\Gamma)$ (as well as $\overline{h}(\Gamma)$ and $\underline{h}(\Gamma)$) is independent of the particular representative of Γ in its class.

Quite obviously, $0 \leq h(\Gamma) \leq 1$. Given any $\alpha \in [0,1]$, there exists an infinite curve Γ such that $h(\Gamma) = \alpha$. We now give some examples. If Γ is an infinite straight line, or any infinite curve which tends to infinity "rapidly" (think of the exponential spiral $\rho = e^\theta$), then $h(\Gamma) = 0$. An unbounded algebraic curve has entropy 0 (indeed, $H(\Gamma_s) \leq \log(\text{degree } \Gamma)$). On the other hand, if Γ is very chaotic, then $h(\Gamma) = 1$. If Γ has infinite length but stays bounded in the plane, $h(\Gamma) = 1$. Notice also that spirals such as $\rho = \log \theta$ have entropy 1. This should not surprise the reader. Spirals are associated both with order (a shell is best described by an exponential spiral : see T.A. Cook [2], D'Arcy Thompson [3], P. Stevens [11]) and with disorder(think of spiral patterns in turbulent fluids. See Figure 11). It could be interesting to study the shape of turbulent spirals and to compare it with the logarithm spiral $\rho = \log \theta$ (According to tradition, $\rho = e^{\theta}$ is called a logarithm spiral ! In our article, we definitely abandon this quaint tradition and refer to exponential spiral when speaking of $\rho = a^{\theta}$ and to logarithm spiral when speaking of $\rho = c \log \theta$).

§ . I. 5. - Where number theory enters the picture

We now wish to illustrate our definitions by number theoretic curves. Let $u = (u_n)$ be a sequence of real numbers. Consider the exponential sum

$$z_N = \sum_{n=0}^{N-1} \exp 2i\pi u_n .$$

In the complex plane, the ratio z_N/N represents the center of gravity of the N points $\exp 2i\pi u_o$, ... $\exp 2i\pi u_{N-1}$ on the unit circle. The original sequence (u_n) is said to be uniformly distributed (mod 1) if the center of gravity z_N/N approaches 0 as N goes to infinity (the usual definition is more restrictive).

In the complex plane, plot the points $z_o = 0$, z_1 , z_2 , ... Joining the points z_{N-1} to z_N for all $N \geq 1$, we thus obtain an infinite polygon $\Gamma[u]$ which depends on the sequence $u = (u_n)$. $\Gamma[u]$ may be thought of as a walk on the complex plane, with steps of equal lengths.

It is easy to show that if

$$\sum_{n=0}^{N-1} \exp 2i\pi u_n = O(N^{\alpha}), \qquad \alpha < 1$$

then

$$\underline{h}(\Gamma[u]) \geq 1-\alpha$$

which proves that the better the sequence u is uniformly distributed, the higher the entropy of $\Gamma[u]$. In other words, good uniform distribution implies chaos.

The following pictures show the polygon $\Gamma[u]$ for classical arithmetic sequences (see [4]), where we have represented the 200 first sides in Figure 6 and 4 000 sides in Figures 7, 8, 9 and 10.

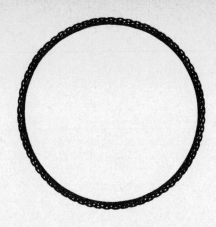

FIGURE 6. The curve $\Gamma_{200}(\sqrt{17}\,n)$

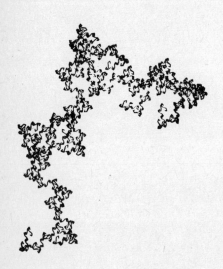

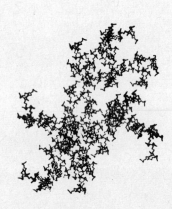

FIGURE 7. The curve $\Gamma_{4000}((\sqrt{2}\,n^2))$.

FIGURE 8. The curve $\Gamma_{4000}((e\,n^2))$

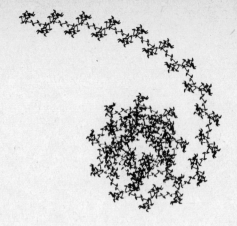

FIGURE 9. The curve $\Gamma_{4000}((\pi n^2))$.

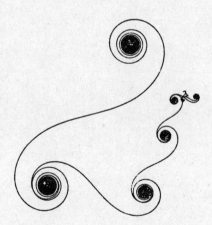

FIGURE 10. The curve $\Gamma_{4000}(((n+1)\log(n+1)))$.

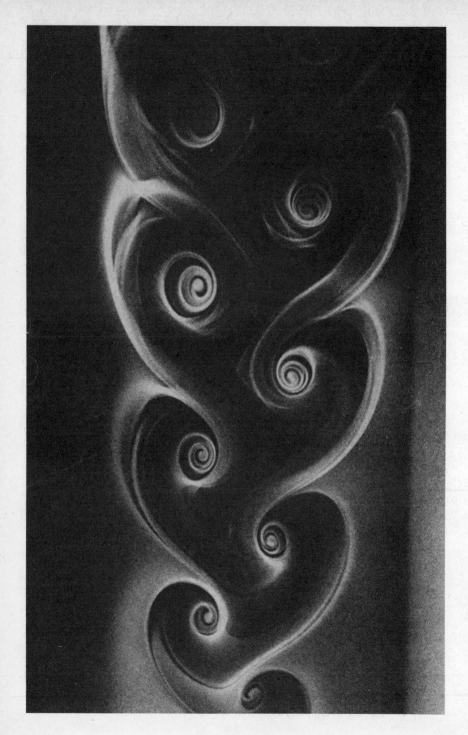

Figure 11

The sequence (αn) in Figure 6 is quite regular even though it has maximal entropy (remember that a bounded infinite curve has entropy 1). More interesting are the sequence $(\sqrt{2}\ n^2)$, $(e\ n^2)$ and (πn^2). The last one is particularily remarkable. The repetitive "local" pattern seems to be related to the approximate equality

$$\pi = \frac{355}{113} \ .$$

The curve $\Gamma((n \log n))$ is reminiscent of turbulence as shown on Figure 11.

The topics discussed in the previous paragraphs can be extended to higher dimensions. Γ would be a p-dimensional variety in $\mathbb{R}^n$ $(p \leq n)$ and an instant D would be a hyperplane. The $(p-1)$-dimensional measure $\mu_{p-1}(\Gamma \cap D)$ is then to be averaged and

$$H(\Gamma) = \log[\text{average } \mu_{p-1}(D \cap \Gamma)]\dots$$

(Compare with Pebusque [8], this volume.)

Part II : Dimension

§ . II. 1. - The wandering carterpillar

Imagine a carterpillar eating a leaf. The carterpillar will meander about the leaf leaving a path of width δ where the leaf is eaten.

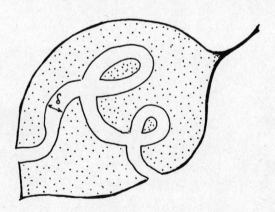

Figure 12

When the path will have filled the entire surface of the leaf, the leaf will be completely eaten up, and at that stage we can consider that the carterpillar has travelled
on a two dimensional curve. Had the carterpillar not visited the whole area of the
leaf, we would have measured the dimension of its path by the approximate formula

$$\text{dim} = \frac{\log (\text{Area visited})}{\log (\text{perimeter of the leaf})} \ .$$

If the leaf is convex, if δ is small compared to the size of the leaf, then this ratio
is indeed comprised between 1 and 2 and can take any value between these two
extremes. The higher the dimension, the more complex the curve is. Dimension 1
corresponds to regularity and dimension 2 to unpredictability.

In the following paragraph we shall give a precise definition of the dimension of
a curve and we shall then study its mathematical properties as well as some
"zoological" implications.

§ . II. 2. - Dimension of an unbounded curve

Let Σ be a half plane and let Γ be its boundary. Consider an origin 0 and a
circle C_ρ centered on 0 , with radius ρ

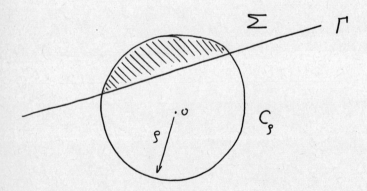

Figure 13

An easy computation shows that as ρ tends to infinity,

$$\text{length} (\Gamma \cap C_\rho) \sim 2\rho$$
$$\text{area} (\Sigma \cap C_\rho) \sim \frac{1}{2} \pi \rho^2 \ .$$

The exponents 1 and 2 of ρ correspond to the usual dimensions of the line Γ and of the surface Σ. This simple observation leads us to redefine dimension.

Let Γ be any unbounded curve (not necessarily straight as before). We could define

$$\dim(\Gamma) = \lim_{\rho \to \infty} \frac{\log\left[\text{length }(\Gamma \cap C_\rho)\right]}{\log \rho} \, .$$

Unfortunately, this definition is easily criticized : a very wandering curve would have a dimension larger than 2. This is unreasonable since all subsets of the plane should have dimensions less than 2 or equal to 2.

We thus modify our definition. Let $\delta > 0$ be given and consider

$$\Gamma(\delta) = \{p \in \mathbb{R}^2 \, / \, \text{distance }(p, \Gamma) < \delta \} \, .$$

$\Gamma(\delta)$ is a "magnified" curve as in Figure 12. By definition

$$\dim(\Gamma) = \lim_{\delta \to 0} \lim_{\rho \to \infty} \frac{\log\left[\text{area }(\Gamma(\delta) \cap C_\rho)\right]}{\log \rho} \, .$$

This dimension has all the required properties. For example,

$$1 \leq \dim(\Gamma) \leq 2$$

and $\dim(\Gamma)$ does not depend on the unit used to measure distances. (It may happen that $\lim$ does not exist. We would then define upper and lower dimensions. See [4] and [7].)

A straight line and a regular curve tending to infinity are one-dimensional. A chaotic unbounded curve is two-dimensional. The complexity of a curve is thus measured by its dimension. This is one instance of a general idea beautifully illustrated in B. Mandelbrot's book [6].

There actually is a simple relationship between the entropy $h(\Gamma)$ and $\dim(\Gamma)$:

$$1 \leq \dim(\Gamma) \leq \frac{1}{1-h(\Gamma)} \, .$$

This shows that if Γ is deterministic (i.e. has entropy 0), then Γ is one-dimensional. The converse is false : the curve $y = \sin(e^x)$ has maximal entropy (namely 1) and minimal dimension (namely 1).

In this volume, Bovet [1] discusses the path followed by harvesting animals
in search of their unseen prey. Having but little knowledge of the whereabouts of
the prey, on harvesting, animals try to cover a maximal area and thus, like our
hypothetical wandering canterpillar, the curve it follows will have a dimension which
is close to 2. It is interesting to notice that on the contrary, an intelligent being
who knows where the prey is hiding, will go directly to it following a straight line
(one-dimensional). Hence this idea that the dimension of the trace of an animal
measures its "intelligence" : the smaller the dimension is, the more advanced the
animal is. Intelligence lowers the dimension.

The link between intelligence and dimension also appears in an altogether different context which we would like to present now.

§ . II. 3. - Poincaré biological dimension

In [9], H. Poincaré discusses the concept of dimension in terms of muscular
work. Suppose we wish to locate an object. In principle this could be done using one
eye in the following way. First we look from left to right (say) and stop when we
meet the vertical plane which contains both us and the object. We then lower or lift
the direction of the eye,   until the eye is exactly in the direction of the object.
Finally the contraction of the cristallin informs us of its distance. Poincaré claims
that we have made three independent efforts left-right, up-down, near-far before
we actually had located the object. He thus concludes that we live in a three dimensional space.

This approach to dimension is somewhat naive because among other things, we
do not know what the meaning of independence is. Yet it does prove something.
Suppose that our brain was formed of two disconnected parts. Imagine now that I
wanted to locate an object using both of my eyes. Each eye independently would give
me three pieces of information. I would then live in a 6-dimensional world !
As it happens, our brain is not split into two disconnected halves and the left half
communicates with the rigth half. The ability to synthetize our information and to understand that the 6 visual pieces of information are not independent is precisely
a prerogative of our intelligence. Once again we are led to the idea that intelligence
collapses dimensions...

REFERENCES

[1] P. BOVET, Optimal randomness in foraging movement : a central place model, This volume.

[2] T.A. COOK, Curves of life, Dover 1979.

[3] D'ARCY THOMPSON, On growth and form ; abridged edition edited by J.T. Bonner, Cambridge University Press 1969.

[4] F.M. DEKKING, M. MENDÈS FRANCE, Uniform distribution modulo one : a geometrical viewpoint ; Jour. reine angewelt Mathemat. (to appear).

[5] R. FEYNMAN, Nobel prize lecture, 1966.

[6] B.B. MANDELBROT, Fractals, form, chance and dimension ; Freeman, San Francisco 1977.

[7] M. MENDÈS FRANCE, G. TENENBAUM, Dimension des courbes planes, papiers pliés et suites de Rudin-Shapiro, Bull. Soc. Math. France, 109 (1981), 207-215.

[8] M.J. PEBUSQUE, Mise en évidence d'un rythme circadien... This volume.

[9] H. POINCARÉ, La Science et l'Hypothèse, Flammarion 1968.

[10] L. SANTALÓ, Integral geometry and geometric probability ; Encyclopedia of Mathematics, Addison Wesley 1976.

[11] P.S. STEVENS, Patterns in Nature ; Little, Brown and Co.

Michel MENDÈS FRANCE
Laboratoire associé au C.N.R.S. n° 226
U.E.R. de Mathématiques et d'Informatique
Université de Bordeaux I
F 33405 TALENCE CEDEX

TIME SERIES ANALYSIS AND BIOLOGY

by

PHAM DINH TUAN

Laboratoire IMAG
Université de Grenoble
B.P. 53 X, 38041 Grenoble-Cédex, France

Abstract

The paper surveys principal methods of time series analysis in view of applications in biology. The main emphasis is the detection and measurement of rhythms. Methods of smoothing, regression, spectral estimation, periodogram analysis, complex demodulation, autoregressive model fitting, ..., among others are discussed.

§1. - Introduction.

Time Series Analysis is an area of Statistics which concerns many different disciplines : Acoustic, Biology, Econometric, Geology, Control..., only to mention a few. The purpose of this paper is to make available to biologists usual methods of time Series Analysis, in view of applications to biological series. The main concern is the study of rhythms. Other applications, mainly the analysis of the electroencephalogram (EEG) or the electrocardiogram (ECG) are only brieftly mentioned.

The analysis of biological series are not without difficulties. A review of these can be found in Sulberger (1970, 1973). The problem arises from (i) the length of the series is usually short since limited by experimental constraints (life time of the observed subjects, duration of an assay...) and long records might be nonstationary, (ii) the sampling points could be unequispaced or missing (due to sleep period, for exemple) and (iii) usually only a tranverse sample of several short series from different subjects is available, but little is known about their comparability.

Time series techniques are mostly asymptotic techniques. They perform well for long series but one should be cautions in applying them to short series. Still, unless the series are very short, they could provide valuable informations. Also, long biological or biomedical series do exists, though rare (Solberger, 1970). For short series, some specific procedures have been proposed, but they usually require rather strong model assumptions. For series with unequispaced or missing sample points, there exists procedures to deal with them, in the domain of spectral analysis (Jones, 1971, Haggan, 1977). For transverse sample, one can adopt one of two following attitude : either one believes that the different series arise from identical and well synchronised mecanisms, in this case one can treat the series as a multivariate sample, otherwise, one would analyse each short series seperately.

One can roughly group time series techniques into three classes : (i) elementary techniques such as smoothing, trend and cyclicial component estimation, regression, (ii) Spectral or Harmonic analysis and cycle detection and (iii) Parametric analysis through modelling. We will consider successively these techniques and mention some recent developments concerning non linear model which might be useful for the study of rhythms.

§2. - Elementary analysis.

The first step in the analysis of a time series is usually to plot the series and look for features such as a long term trend or a cyclicial pattern. In biological series, one is mostly concerned with cyclicial variations (rythms). However, a long term trend, if exists, distort the estimation of cyclicial component and have to be removed. Also a long term trend might be just a long cycle and has its own interest. Usually trend and cyclicial components are extracted through filtering or through regression, which we shall discuss below.

2.1. Smoothing, trend and cyclicial component estimation.

A time series with trend and cyclicial variation can be modelled by

$$X(t) = T(t) + C(t) + \epsilon(t)$$

where $X(t)$, $t = 0, 1, \ldots, n-1$ is the observed series, $T(t)$ is a slowly varying function called trend, C(t) is a periodic function with a known period p called cyclicial component and $\epsilon(t)$ is a sequence of zero mean random variables called noise. We will assume $C(1) + \ldots + C(p) = 0$, since we can absorb any constant into T(t) .

In the absence of cyclicial variation the trend of time t can be estimated by a simple moving average around t :

$$\{ X(t-m) + \ldots + X(0) + \ldots + X(t+m) \} / (2m+1) .$$

More generally, one can use a weighted average $W(-m) X(t-m) + \ldots + W(m) X(t+m)$, with the weighs W(j) choosen be some method (Kendall, 1971, p.47, Anderson 1971, p.48).

In case of constant trend, the cyclicial variation can be easily extract through a Buy-Ballot scheme as follows (see for ex. Anderson 1971, p.112). Assume there are exactly $mp = n$ observations. We can arrange them is a rectangular array of m rows and p columns. Then the C(j) are estimated by the deviation of the mean of the j-th column and the overall mean.

The above methods are not applicable when trend and cyclicial variation are simultanously present. In this case, one can proceed as follows. One first removes the cyclicial component by a moving average with weighs : $W(j) = 1/p$, $|j| < p/2$ if p is odd, $W(j) = 1/p$, $|j| < p/2$, $W(-p/2) = W(p/2) = 1/2p$ if p is even. Hopefully, the trend is not much distorted. It is then extracted through a second appropriate moving average. The initial series is then detrended by substracting from it the above estimated trend. The Buy-Ballot scheme is then used to estimate the cyclicial variation.

The above operations are linear time invariant on the original time series. They are call filtering. Specifically, a filter transforms a series into another series with the propreties that if $X_1(t)$, $X_2(t)$ are transformed into $Y_1(t)$, $Y_2(t)$ then $a_1 X_1(t) + a_2 X_2(t)$ is transformed into $a_1 Y_1(t) + a_2 Y_2(t)$ and $X_1(t+1)$ is transformed into $Y_1(t+1)$. The action of such filter can be described by considering a complexe sinusoidal $\exp\{i(\lambda t + \varphi)\}$ which is transformed into $|g(\lambda)| \exp\{i(\lambda t + \varphi + \theta)\}$. The function $g(\lambda) = |g(\lambda)| \exp(i\theta)$ is called the response function of the filter. For a low pass filter, $g(\lambda)$ is small for large $|\lambda|$ and close to one for small $|\lambda|$, so that the sinusoidals of high frequency will be eliminated but those of low frequency will be untouched. Since a trend, when decomposed into Fourrier series contains mostly of low frequency components, it is little affected by a low pass filter whereas the noise is greatly reduced. The Buy-Ballot filter, on the otherhand has a response function equal to one at periods k p and small outside these periods, which explains why it is useful for extracting cyclicial variation. For more details on filtering see Brillinger (1975).

2.2. - Regression methods.

The regression method can be used for various purposes, including the estimation of trend and cyclicial variation. One exemple of regression in biological series can be found in Solberger and Davis (1972). The advantage of regression is that it provides good estimate of parameter. The drawback is that it requires the assumption of a specific model. Typically, the regression model is written as

$$(2.1) \qquad X(t) = \theta_1 \, g_1(t) + \ldots + \theta_k \, g_k(t) + \epsilon(t)$$

where $g_1(t), \ldots, g_k(t)$ are known functions, $\epsilon(t)$ are independent identically distributed random variables (white noise) and $\theta_1, \ldots, \theta_k$ are unknown parameters. For exemple, to model a cyclicial phenomenon, one might try the simple model :

$$(2.2) \qquad X(t) = A \cos(\lambda t + \varphi) + B + \epsilon(t)$$

$$= A \cos \varphi \, \cos \lambda t - A \sin \varphi \, \sin \lambda t + B + \epsilon(t)$$

which is of the form (2.1) with $g_1(t) = \cos \lambda t$, $g_2(t) = -\sin \lambda t$, $g_3(t) = 1$. Note that λ is assumed known. In general, several sines or cosines, in particular the harmonics of the cycle period, can be used, and a polynomial term can be added to account for a possible trend.

The parameter θ_j of (2.1) can be estimated by least squares method, which consists of minimising the sum of squares of the residuals $\Sigma \, [X(t) - \theta_1 \, g_1(t) - \ldots - \theta_k \, g_k(t)]^2$. Confidence interval for θ_j , or confidence region for $(\theta_{j_1}, \ldots, \theta_{j_r})$ can be constructed, under Gaussian assumption. For exemple, in the model (2.2), one can construct a confidence region for $\theta_1 = A \cos \varphi$, $\theta_2 = A \sin \varphi$ which is an ellipse and by passing to polar coordinates, one obtains confidence region for (A, φ) , jointly or seperately. Note that in time series situations, the noise $\epsilon(t)$ may be correlated but it has been shown that, at least in case of polynomial and trigonometric regression, the least squares method is still valid.

§3. - <u>The spectral approach</u>.

This approach can be viewed as a combination of Fourier analysis and statistical techniques. It is a powerful tool for the detection and the study of periodicities in time series. We will consider principal relevant techniques : estimation of power spectra, periodogram analysis, complex demodulation and per-gressive Fourier analysis.

3.1. - <u>Estimation of power spectra</u>.

The spectrum of a time series is a characteristic of the series related to its decomposition into various cyclicial components of different frequencies. It can be used to discriminate series of different behaviours as well as to detect cyclical variation within a series. Spectral analysis have been widely used in the study of the EEG (Walter and Brazier, 1968, Dumernuth and Flühler, 1967,...) and of the ECG (Frome and Frederickson, 1974,...). Exemples of applications of spectral analysis in the study of biorhythms include Campbell and Shipp (1974), Reynold, London and York (1978), Kruzberg, Richter Martin and Betz (1977)... This list is by no mean restrictive.

One can view a time series as a realisation of some stochastic process $X(t)$. In many situations, it is reasonable to assume that this process is statio-nary, that is, its character is unaffected by a time shift. Specifically, the mean $E\,X(t)$ and the autocovariance $\text{cov}\,\{X(t), X(t+k)\}$ do not depend on t , they will be denoted by m and γ_k . The γ_k is of particular interest since it mea-sures the degree of dependence of values of the process $|k|$ time units apart. Now, a way to look for periodicities in $X(t)$ is to consider the sequence γ_k since the former is random whereas the latter is not. Note that the theoretical autocovariance γ_k should not be confounded with its sample counterpart c_k , which is the average mean corrected lagged product of the $X(t)$. Thus one con-siders the Fourrier transform of the sequence γ_k

$$(3.1) \qquad f(\lambda) = \frac{1}{2\pi} \sum_{k=-\infty}^{\infty} \gamma_k \, e^{-i\lambda k}$$

which admits the inverse transform

$$(3.2) \qquad \gamma_k = \int_{-\pi}^{\pi} e^{i\lambda k} f(\lambda) \, d\lambda$$

provided $\gamma_k \to 0$ fast enough as $|k| \to \infty$. The function f is called the (power) spectral density of the process. To interprete f , consider the extreme case when f is very large in the neighborhood of $\pm \lambda_1, \ldots, \pm \lambda_m$, say, and is very small outside. Then γ_k is approximately $a_1 \cos(\lambda_1 k) + \ldots + a_m \cos(\lambda_m k)$ with a_j being proportional to $f(\lambda_j) = f(-\lambda_j)$. Thus a sharp peak of f at λ indicates the presence of a periodicity of period $2\pi/\lambda$ in the sequence γ_k . Another interpretation of f is provided by the spectral representation of the series $X(t)$ itself (Cramer Theorem). Roughly speaking, let the angular frequency range $[-\pi, \pi]$ be partitioned into narow bands $\Delta_1, \ldots, \Delta_m$ with mid points $\lambda_1, \ldots, \lambda_m$ then, $X(t)$ can be approximately expressed as $Z_1 \exp(i\lambda_1 t) + \ldots + Z_m \exp(i\lambda_m t)$ where the Z_j are uncorrelated complex random variables with square modulus having expectation approximately equal $f(\lambda_j) \Delta_j$.

A natural estimate of $f(\lambda)$ is obtained by replacing the γ_k in (3.1) by their sample counterpart c_k . But the resulting estimate has large statistical variability due to the presence of a large number of estimated value c_k of γ_k . To reduce the statistical fluctuation, one uses fewer lag than the maximum possible, M-1 instead of n-1 , by introducing a lag window W :

$$\hat{f}(\lambda) = \frac{1}{2\pi} \sum_{k=-M+1}^{M-1} W(\frac{k}{M}) e^{-ik\lambda} c_k$$

Commonly used lag windows are : (i) Tukey-Hanning window : $W(x) = (1+\cos \pi x)/2$, (ii) Bartlett window : $W(x) = 1-|x|$ and Parzen window : $W(x) = 1-6x^2 + 6|x|^3$ if $|x| < 1/2$, $= 2(1-|x|)^3$ if $1/2 \le x \le 1$.

An alternative approach is to start from the discrete Fourier transform of the series $X(1), \ldots, X(n)$ itself :

$$d(\lambda) = \sum_{t=1}^{n} e^{i\lambda t} X(t) .$$

Usually $d(\lambda)$ is computed at angular frequency $2\pi k/n$, using a fast Fourier

transform algorithm (Bingham, Godfrey and Tukey, 1967). The Fourier transform
of a time series can be expected to provide an estimate of its periodic components. In particular, one might try to estimate the spectral density by
$I(\lambda) = |d(\lambda)|^2 / (2\pi n)$. Note that, the above quantity which we call periodogram
is the same as the natural estimate of $f(\lambda)$ obtained from (3.1) when γ_k are
replaced by c_k . As has been said earlier, $I(\lambda)$ has large statistical fluctuation.
However, the $d(\lambda_k)$ and hence the $I(\lambda_k)$, $\lambda_k = 2\pi k/n$ are known to be approximately independent, so a mean of reducing the variability of $I(\lambda)$ is to average
it over neighboring frequency. Thus we estimate $f(\lambda)$ by the smoothed periodogram:

$$\frac{1}{m} \{ I(\lambda_1) + \ldots + I(\lambda_m) \}$$

where $\lambda_1, \ldots, \lambda_m$ are distinct angular frequencies of the form $2\pi k/n$, nearest
to λ .

The above spectral estimates, strictly speaking, are not estimates of
the spectral density at a particular angular frequency λ , but rather an estimate
of the average density of a frequency band centered at λ . The bandwidth is
proportional to $1/M$ for the windowed estimate and to m for the smoothed periodogram estimate. Thus, it is unnecessary to compute the spectral estimate at
all points, a frequency spacing of $1/2M$ or $n/2$ could be enough. The choice
of M or n depend on the desired frequency resolution, but one should bear
in mind that a high frequency resolution leads to a high statistical variability
and vice versa, so a compromise between them is needed.

The spectral density estimate can be improved by data tapering and
by prewhitening. For more details on spectral analysis, see Anderson (1971),
Brillinger (1975), Granger and Hanataka (1964), Hannan (1960), Jenkins and Watts
(1968), Kendall (1971), Koopman (1974), Parzen (1970),..., among others.

3.2. - Periodogram analysis and cycle detection.

The spectral density estimate could give range of frequencies which
may correspond to oscillations in the observed series. But because of limited
frequency resolution, it does not alow a precise estimate of the period of the
probable oscillation and could confound close but distinct frequencies. The perio-

dogram, having a maximum frequency resolution, is more suitable for periodicities detection ; hence its name. Exemple of periodogram analysis for biological series can be found in Kreuzberg, Richter, Martin and Betz (1977) Vaganucci, Wong and Liw (1973),...

A test for periodicities based on the periodogram, due to Fisher, is the following. Assume that the periodicities are divisors of the sample length, one is led to the model

$$X(t) = A_o + \sum_k [\alpha(k) \cos (\frac{2\pi kt}{n}) + \beta(k) \sin (\frac{2\pi kt}{n})] + \epsilon(t)$$

where $\epsilon(t)$ is a white noise. We assume that q periodicities, corresponding to $k = k_1,\ldots,k_q$ are in doubt, $r-q$ others corresponding to $k = k_{q+1},\ldots,k_r$ are certainly absent, and the remaining are certainly present. Let $A(k)$ be the amplitude of the periodicity n/k , that is $A(k)^2 = \alpha(k)^2 + \beta(k)^2$, $1 \leq k < n/2$ and for even n , $A(n/2) = \alpha(n/2)$. Then, the hypotheses of interest are

$$H_o : A(k_1) = \ldots = A(k_q) = 0$$

$$H_i : A(k_i) > 0 , A(k_j) = 0 , j \neq i , j = 1,\ldots,q$$

$$H_{ij} : A(k_i) > 0 , A(k_j) > 0 , A(k_\ell) = 0 , \ell = i \neq j , \ell = 1,\ldots,q$$

... Now, the least squares estimate of $\alpha(k)$ and $\beta(k)$ can be seen to be the real and imaginary parts of $(2/n) d(2\pi k/n)$. Thus, a high value of $I(2\pi k_i/n)$ favors the hypothesis H_i . Therefore one introduce the statistic

$$x_i = I(2\pi k_i/n) / \sum_{j=1}^{r} I(2\pi k_j/n)$$

Suppose we have to decide between $H_o, H_1,\ldots,H_q$. The decision procedure is to choose H_o if $x_j < g_1$ for $j = 1,\ldots,q$, otherwise choose H_i , i being such that x_i is the greatest among $x_1,\ldots,x_q$. The cut off value g_1 is computed such that the probability of rejecting H_o when it is true, equals α , the significant level.

Likewise, the decision procedure between H_o, H_{ij} , $i=1,\ldots,q$, $j=1,\ldots,q$

is to choose H_o unless two of the $x_i \geq g_2$, $i = 1,...,q$, in this case choose H_{ij} , i,j being such that x_i , x_j are the greatest among $x_1,...,x_q$. As above g_2 is computed such that the significant level is α . One proceeds similarly in case of many periodicities. For more details see Anderson (1971, p.126), Van Cauter and Huyberech (1972). The g_p are given by :

$$q \begin{pmatrix} q-1 \\ p-1 \end{pmatrix} \sum_{j=p}^{m} (-1)^{j-p} \begin{pmatrix} q-p \\ q-j \end{pmatrix} \frac{1}{j} (1+jg_p)^{r-1} = \alpha$$

where m is the largest integer not greater than q and $1/g_p$.

If the periodicities $n/k_{q+1} > ... > n/k_r \geq 2$ are known to be absent, then the variance of $\epsilon(t)$ can be estimated by

$$s^2 = \frac{1}{mn} [\sum_{j=q+1}^{r-1} 2|d(2\pi k_j/n|^2 + \delta|d(2\pi k_r/n)|^2]$$

where $\delta = 1$ or 2 according to $k_r = n/2$ or not and $m = 2(r-q-1) + \delta$. Let $\hat{\alpha}(k)$, $\hat{\beta}(k)$ be the real and imaginary part of $(2/n) d(2\pi k/n)$, the confidence region for $\alpha(k)$, $\beta(k)$ is then a circle center at $\hat{\alpha}(k)$, $\hat{\beta}(k)$ and having radius $2(s/\sqrt{n}) \sqrt{F_{2,m}(\alpha)}$, $F_{2,m}(\alpha)$ being the $1-\alpha$ percentile point of the F distribution of $2,m$ degrees of freedom.

The above procedure does not provide a precise estimate of cycle length since we have restricted ourselves to periods of the form n , $n/2$, $n/3,...$. Walker (1971) has proposed to estimate the angular frequency when one periodicity is present by maximising $I(\lambda)$, $0 < \lambda < \pi$. In case q periodicity are present, one would consider q largest local maxima of $I(\lambda)$. The main difficulty is the numerical computation of these maxima. Once the cycle length is obtained, the amplitude and phased can be easily estimated by the usual regression.

3.3. - Other cycle detection methods.

A procedure widely used by biologists for cycle detection and evaluation of its amplitude and phase is the cosinor method introduced by Halberg, Tong and Johnson (1965). However as has been pointed out by Van Cauter and Huyberech (1972), this procedure has to be used cautiously, since several implicit assumptions have been made which may not alway be satisfied. Specifically, one consider a tranverse sample of m series $X_i(t_1),\ldots,X_i(t_n)$, $i = 1,\ldots,m$, obeying the model :

$$(3.2) \quad X_i(t_j) = C_i + C \cos(\omega t_j + \varphi) + \epsilon_i(t_j)$$

the $\epsilon_i(t_j)$ being independent zero mean normal variates with variance σ^2 . The important assumption is that only one periodicity could be present and it is the same in each series and are synchronised (C, ω and φ do not depend on i) . The synchronization condition is rather difficult to meet. Also when only a large sample is available, one usually cut it into shorter one, but the latter would not be synchronized and even be independent.

Assume the model (3.2), then $C \cos \varphi$, $C \sin \varphi$ can be estimated by least squares method as in §2.2, yielding the estimates x_i , y_i based on the i-th series. The (x_i, y_i) can be viewed as a sample from a bivariate normal population of mean $(C \cos \varphi, C \sin \varphi)$. From the theory of Hotelling test, one can obtain a confidence ellipse for this mean. If this ellipse does not contain the origin, one concludes that there is a cycle of period $2\pi/\omega$, and one can obtain confidence intervals for C and φ by passing to polar coordinates. By trying several angular frequencies ω , one can detect a periodicity in the series. How- ever,the repetition of trial period would increase the chance of a wrong detection of cycle. This chance could be much greater than α although the cosinor test, for each given ω is set at level α . By constrast, for the periodogram test, the probability of a wrong detection cannot exceed α . Simulation study (Van Cauter, 1974) also favoured the periodogram analysis over the cosinor method.

Another cycle detection technique is the Pergressive Fourier Analysis of Blume (1977, 1978). The method is closely related to the complex demodulation which is more general. The aim of complex demodulation is to produce images of more or less gross frequency components of a time series. This is achieved by shifting the frequency band of interest to zero and running the result through a low pass filter. Let $X(t)$ be the original series, its complex demodulated at λ is the series Z_λ obtained by low pass filtering the shifted series $X(t) \exp(-i\lambda t)$.

To understand the working of the complex demodulation, consider the extreme case of a sinusoidal series $C \cos(\omega t + \varphi) = C e^{-i\varphi} e^{-i\omega t}/2 + C e^{i\varphi} e^{i\omega t}/2$. The shifted series is then

$$(C e^{i\varphi}/2) e^{i(\omega-\lambda)t} + (C e^{-i\varphi}/2) e^{-i(\omega+\lambda)t}.$$

Assume $\lambda > 0$, $\omega > 0$ and ω not too close to zero, then the second term will be almost eliminated by the low pass filter, giving

$$Z_\lambda(t) \simeq g(\omega-\lambda)(C e^{i\varphi}/2) e^{i(\omega-\lambda)t}$$

where g is the response function of the filter. Thus, the amplitude of $Z_\lambda(t)$, that is $|Z_\lambda(t)|$, decays to zero as λ receeds from ω. Therefore if we compute the complex demodulated at various frequencies $\lambda_1, \ldots, \lambda_r$, then those corresponding to the λ_j near ω would have much higher amplitude than the other, indicating the presence of a periodicity. Moreover the phase (argument) of the former is approximately $(\omega-\lambda_j)t + \varphi$, which is a linear function of t with slope $\omega-\lambda_j$, so that the examination of these phase functions permits a determination of ω. For more details on complex demodulation, see Bingham, Godfrey and Tukey (1967), Granger and Hanataka (1964), ...

Blume's Pergressive Fourier Analysis correspond to the case where $\lambda_j = 2\pi j/p$ and the low pass filter is a simple moving average over p terms. Specifically, an analysing interval of length p is choosen and is moved stepwise along the time axis. At each step, a Fourier analysis is done with initial phase zero for each harmonics, that is, one computes $Z_j(t) = \Sigma_0^{p-1} X(t-k) \exp(-i 2\pi jk/p)$. If p is odd, $p = 2m+1$, one can show that, up to a factor $\exp\{-i2\pi j(t+m)\}$ the $Z_j(t)$ are the complex demodulated of $X(t)$ at $2\pi j/p$ using a simple moving average filter over p terms. If p is even, the same is still true, but the filter is "disymetric". Thus by plotting the amplitude and phase of the $Z_j(t)$, one can detect periodicities and estimate its frequency.

Finally we mention the method of Discrete Fourier Analysis (De Prins and Cornelissen, 1971, Cornelissen and De Prins, 1973) and the Numerical Signal Averaging (De Prins and Cornelissen, 1975). Martin and Brinkman (1976, 1977) have compared the last methods with the Pergressive Fourier Analysis and have found that no method seems to be superior than the other. They favored the Numerical Signal Averaging method on computational ground. However, this method requires a first guess of the period and hence a preliminary analysis is needed. Also, the computation in the Pergressive Fourier Analysis could be reduced (Bingham, Godfrey and Tukey, 1967).

§4. - Parametric Approach.

Time series analysis through parametric model has recently attracted attention. It consists of fitting an appropriate model which can then be used for various purposes : prediction, simulation, control, spectral estimation... One advantage of the parametric approach is that it performs reasonably well for short samples and is therefore more suitable to biological series. Of course, there is alway the risk of using an unappropriate model.

In the following, we will discuss the simplest and widely used model in time series, namely the autoregressive model. We only briefly consider the more general autoregressive moving average model and some recent non linear models which could be used as possible model for cyclicial phenomenon.

4.1. - Autoregressive modelling.

The appeal of autoregressive model lies in its ease of analysis and interpretation. It is particularly suitable for prediction purpose and furthermore the fitted model can be used to obtain spectral density estimate and to detect rhythms. Exemple of autoregressive modelling for biological series can be found in Benchetrit and Pham (1974), Kwok (1979), Matis, Kleerekkoper and Gensler (1973). Recently, Linkens in a series of papers (1979, a,b,c) has used the autoregressive model for the detection and estimation of rhythms (see also Linkens and Datadina, 1978). Autoregressive has also been used in the EEG analysis as a technique spectral estimation and a mean of feature detection (Gersh, 1970, Zetterberg, 1969,...).

The autoregressive model of order q , denoted by $AR(q)$, assumes that the current observation $X(t)$, up to an additive white noise $\varepsilon(t)$, can be expressed as a linear combination of q most recent observations :

$$X(t) = a_1 X(t-1) + \ldots + a_q X(t-q) + \varepsilon(t) .$$

The roots of the polynomial $1-\Sigma_1^q a_j z^j$ are supposed to have modulus strictly greater than one to ensure the existence of a stationary process satisfying the model, since otherwise, $X(t)$ would tend to explode.

Let σ^2 denote the variance of $\varepsilon(t)$. The spectral density of an $AR(q)$ process is given by

$$(4.1) \qquad f(\lambda) = \frac{\sigma^2}{2\pi} \frac{1}{|1-a_1 \exp(i\lambda) - \ldots - a_q \exp(iq\lambda)|^2}$$

and the autocovariance function γ_k is related to the coefficients a_j through the Yule-Walker equations

$$\gamma_o = a_1 \gamma_1 + \ldots + a_q \gamma_q + \sigma^2$$

$$\gamma_k = a_1 \gamma_{k-1} + \ldots + a_q \gamma_{k-q} , \quad k \geq 1 .$$

The last equation is a difference equation which admits the general solution

$$\gamma_k = A_1 \rho_1^{-k} + \ldots + A_q \rho_q^{-k}$$

where $\rho_1, \ldots, \rho_q$ are the roots, supposed to be distinct, of the autoregressive polynomial $1-\Sigma_1^q a_j z^j$. Now, suppose that there are two complex conjugate roots $\rho_1 = \rho e^{i\omega}$, $\rho_2 = \rho e^{-i\omega}$ say, then the sum $A_1 \rho_1^{-k} + A_2 \rho_2^{-k}$ can be rearranged into the form $C \rho^{-k} \cos(\omega k)$, indicating a cyclicial pattern of period $\omega/2\pi$ in the autocovariance sequence, provided that ρ is close to one. Also, the spectral density can be seen to contain a factor $1/|1-2\rho \cos(\lambda-\omega)+\rho^2|^2$, which in this case has a sharp peak at $\lambda = \omega$. Thus the presence of a pair of complex conjugate roots with modulus close to one suggests the existence of a cycle.

The parameters of an autoregressive model can be estimated by the maximum likelihood method. For large sample, this is equivalent to solving the first $q+1$ Yule Walker equations with the theoretical autocovariance γ_k replaced by their sample counterparts. The resulting estimate is called the Yule Walker estimates.

An important aspect of autoregressive modelling is the choice of model order. A criterion of choice should take into account not only the goodness of fit of the proposed model but also the number of involved parameters. It is clear that a model of higher order would have a better fit than a lower order model, but the former would have more parameters. A model with a large number of parameters is undesirable because of the difficulty of interpretation and moreover because the parameters are less accurately estimate and hence the fitted model is less reliable. A criterion which balances the need of a good fit and of a small number of parameters is the Akaike Information Criterion (Akaike, 1973), in abbreviation AIC. Let $\hat{\sigma}^2(q)$ denotes the estimate of the variance of $\epsilon(t)$, that is the mean squares of the residuals, based on the fitted AR(q) model, the AIC is :

$$n \ \log \ \hat{\sigma}^2(q) + 2(q+1)$$

n being the sample length. This quantity is to be minimised to select the order q of the model. An alternative criterion is the final prediction error criterion which turns out to be equivalent to the bove for large sample.

The application of the AIC requires the fitting of autoregressive model of successive orders. Fortunately, there exists an algorithm, due to Levinson and Durbin which greatly reduces the computation (see for ex. Box and Jenkins, p.82).

The fitted autoregressive model can be used to provide an estimate of the spectral density (Akaike, 1969). The advantage is that we need not to choose a bandwidth. This notion is replaced by the model order. Indeed, the higher order corresponds to more frequency resolution and statistical variability and vice versa. However, for autoregressive spectral estimate, the model order can be choosen objectively by the AIC.

Linkens (1979 a) has applied the autoregressive spectral estimation method to short biological series. The also computed the roots of the autoregressive polynomial of the fitted model to get a pricise estimate of cycle period. For short series, the Yule Walker estimates of model parameters may not be adequate,

Linkens (1979 b,c) considered Burg's maximum entropy (ME) method and the "covariance error filter" (CPEF) method to fit autoregressive model. He has compared by simulation autoregressive methods and periodogram analysis and his finding favoured the former for short series, when the ME and CPEF techniques are used.

4.2. - Autoregressive moving average modelling.

In the autoregressive moving average (ARMA) model the current observation $X(t)$ is expressed as a linear combination of past observation and a error term which is a moving average of a white noise $\epsilon(t)$:

$$X(t) = \sum_{j=1}^{q} a_j X(t-j) + \epsilon(t) + \sum_{j=1}^{p} b_j \epsilon(t-j) .$$

Here p,q are the orders of the model. The advantage of the ARMA model is that it could provide a better fit than the AR model without requiring a larger number of parameters. However, because of the complexity of the analysis, the ARMA model has not been used for biological series as widely as the AR model. An exemple of application is the study of the EEG (Wenneberg and Zetterberg, 1971, Gersh and Yonemoto, 1970,...).

Parameter estimation for ARMA model can be achieved by maximum likelihood method. For large sample, there exists approximate procedures (par ex. Box and Jenkins, 1976) which require much less computation. The choice of model order can be made through the AIC criterion. The last is formally defined as

2 log (max likelihood) + 2(number of parameters)

which are to be minimised among various fitted model. The computation task is however heavy since no algorithm of the Levinson-Durbin type is available.

An equivalent form of the ARMA model is the Markovian model, which is most suitable for Kalmal filtering. The last technique can be used to analyse changing system (Bohlin, 1976, Gustafon, Willsky, Wang, Lancaster and Triebwasser, 1978).

4.3. - Non linear model.

The linear models are not quite adequate to describe cyclicial behaviour, because the oscillations in the model decay naturally and are sustained only by noises, acting as a driving force. The amplitude of oscillations is thus directly link to the noise level. Non linear model, in constrast, could have sustain oscillations by itself. This is well known for non linear differential system and one hopes that the same is still true for appropriate discrete non linear stochastic system. For this kind of model, the noises act only as perturbations masking the cyclicial character of the underlying process. Such behaviour have been usually modelled by a periodic function corrupted with noise. The non linear stochastic model is more satifactory since it provides more insight on the underlying mechanism generating the rhythm.

As exemples of non linear models, we mention the amplitude dependent exponential autoregressive (ADEAR) model introduced by Haggan and Ozaki (1980) and the threshold autoregressive (TAR) model introduced by Tong and Lim (1980, and this issue). Essentially, they are autoregressive models with autoregressive coefficients depending on past values of the observed process. A general formulation for these models is

$$X(t) = \sum_{j=1}^{q} a_j (X(t-d)) \, X(t-j) + \epsilon(t)$$

with $d \le q$ and the $a_1, \ldots, a_q$ being real functions of a real variable. Assume that the instantanous autoregressive polynomial $1 - \Sigma_1^q \, a_j(x) \, z^q$ has pair of conjugated roots which are inside the unit circle for small x and outside it for large x . Then if the past values of the process are small, it future values tend to explode. On the otherhand, if these past values are large, the future values tend to decay. This suggests that the process would settle into sustained oscillation for which $X(t)$ is neither too small nor too large. The above argument is only a henristic one, however, the oscillatory behaviour have been actually observed in both ADEAR and TAR models. For more details about these models see the above authors.

BIBLIOGRAPHY

AKAIKE, H. (1969) Power spectrum estimation through autoregressive model fitting. Ann. Inst. Statist. Math. 21:407-419

AKAIKE, H. (1973) Information theory and an extension of the maximum likelihood method. In 2nd International Symposium on Information Theory, 267-281. Pretrov and Csaki eds. Budapest : Akademiai Kiaido

ANDERSON, T.W. (1971) The statistical analysis of time series. New-York : Wiley

BENCHETRIT, G. PHAM, D.T. (1974) Un essai d'analyse statistique des séries de données respiratoires. Revue de Statistique Appliquée, 22 :51-68

BOHLIN, T. (1976) Four cases of identification of changing system. In System identification, advances and case studies, 422-518. Mehra and Lainiotis eds. New-York : Academic Press

BINGHAM, C., GODFREY, M.D., TUKEY, J.W. (1967) Modern techniques of power spectrum estimation. IEEE Trans. Audio Electroacoustic AU-15 : 56-66

BLUME, J. (1977) Pergressive analysis of plants, animals and man. J. Interdiscipl. Cycle Res. 8,3-4 : 403-408

BLUME, J. (1978) Theory and practice of pergressive Fourier analysis. J. Interdiscipl. Cycle Res. 9,1 : 3-28

BOX, G.E.P., JENKINS, G.M. (1976) Time series analysis, forecasting and control. San-Francisco : Holden-Day

BRILLINGER, D.R. (1975) Time series, data analysis and theory. New-York : Rinehart and Winston

CAMPBELL, D.J., SHIPP, E. (1974) Spectral analysis of cyclic behaviour with examples from the field cricket : TELEOGRYLLUS COMMODUS (walk). Anim. behav. 22 : 862-875

CORNELISSEN, G., DE PRINS, J. (1973) Cycle detection. J. Interdiscipl. Cycle Res. 6,1 : 159-177

DE PRINS, J.,CORNELISSEN, G. (1971) Analyse spectrale discrète. Bull. de la classe Sci. Acad. Roy. Belgique, 57,11 : 1243-1266

DE PRINS, J.,CORNELISSEN, G. (1975) Numerical signal averaging for cycle detection. J. Interdiscipl. Cycle Res. 6,1 : 59-102

DUMERMUTH, G., FLUHLER, H. (1967) Some modern aspects in numerical spectrum analysis of multichanel electroencephalographic data. Med. Biol. Eng. 5 : 329-331

FROME, E.L., FREDERIKSON, E.L. (1974) Digital analysis of the first and second heart sounds. Computer and Biomed. Res. 7 : 421-431

GERSH, W. (1970) Spectral analysis of EEG's by autoregressive decomposition of time series. Math. Biosci. 7 : 205-222

GERSH, W., YONEMOTO, J. (1977) Parametric time series models for multivariate EEG analysis. Computer and Biol. Res. 10 : 113-125

GRANGER, C.W.J., HANATAKA, M. (1964) Spectral analysis of economic time series. New Jersey : Princeton University press

GUSTAFSON, D., WILLSKY, A.S., WANG, J.Y., LANCASTER, M.C., TRIEBWASSER, J.H. (1978) ECG/VEG rhythm diagnosis using statistical signal analysis, I, II. IEEE Trans. Biomed. eng. BME-25,4 : 344-361

HAGGAN, V. (1977) The detection of circardian cycle in physiological data with missing observation points. J. Interdiscipl. Cycle Res. 8,3 : 161-174

HAGGAN, V., OZAKI, T. (1980) Amplitude dependent exponential AR model fitting for nonlinear random vibrations. In Time series, 57-71. Anderson ed., Amsterdam : North-Holland

HAON, C. (1980) Les méthodes du cosinor et de Tong. In Biométrie et temps, 128-147. Jolivet, Legay and Tomasone eds. Paris : Société Française de Biométrie

HALBERT, E., TONG, Y.L., JOHNSON, E.A. (1965) Circardian system phase, an aspect of temporal morphology : procedures and illustrative examples. In the cellular aspect of biorhythms. Von Meyerbash ed., Berlin : Springer

HANNAN, E.J. (1960) Time series analysis. London : Methuen

HUET, S. (1980) Etude du périodogramme. In Biométrie et temps, 148-170. Jolivet, Legay and Tomassone eds. Paris : Société Française de Biométrie

JACOB.,C. (1980) Aperçu sur les séries chronologiques périodiques. In Biométrie et temps, 88-127. Jolivet, Legay and Tomassone eds. Paris : Société Française de Biométrie

JENKINS, G.M., WATTS, D.G. (1968) Spectral analysis and its applications. San-Francisco : Holden-Day

JONES, R.H. (1971) Spectrum estimation with missing observations. Ann. Inst. Statist. Math. 23,3 : 387-398

KOOPMANN, L.H. (1974) The spectral analysis of time series. New-York : Academic Press

KENDALL, M.G. (1971) Time series. London : Charles Griffin

KREUZBERG, K.H., RICHTER, O., MARTIN, W., BETZ, A. (1977) Statistical analysis of NADH oscillations in the yeast saccharomyces carlbergensis fermenting on different sugars. J. Interdiscipl. Cycle Res. 8,2 : 135-146

KWOK, H.H.L. (1979) Autoregressive analysis applied to surface and serosal measurements of the human stomach. IEEE Trans. Biomed. Eng. BME-26,7 : 405-409

LINKENS, D.A. (1979 a) Estimation of circardian rhythms component using auto-regressive modelling methods. J. Interdiscipl. Cycle. Res. 10,1 : 1-40

LINKENS, D.A. (1979 b) Maximum entropy analysis of short time series. Biomedical rhythms. J. Interdiscipl. Cycle Res. 10,2 : 142-162

LINKENS, D.A. (1979 c) Covariance prediction error filter (CPEF) tracking of time varying biomedical rhythms. J. Interdiscipl. Cycle Res. 10,4 : 273-295

LINKENS, D.A., DATADINA, S.P. (1978) Estimation of gastrointestinal electrical rhythms using autoregressive modelling. Med. and Biol. Eng. and Comput. 16 : 262-268

MATIS, J., KLEEREKOPER, H., GENSLER, P. (1976) A time series analysis of some aspects of locomotor behaviour of godfish, CARASSIUS AURATUS L. J. Inter-discipl. Cycle Res. 4,2 : 145-158

MARTIN, W., BRINKMANN, K.(1976) Detection and measurement of periodicities in time series. Int. J. Chronobiology 4 : 185-195

MARTIN, W., BRINKMANN, K. (1977) A comparison of Numerical Signal Averaging of De Prins and Cornelissen and Blume's Pergressive Fourrier Analysis

PARZEN, E. (1970) Empirical multiple time series analysis. Fifth Berkeley Sympo-sium on Mathematical Statistics and Probability I, 305-340. Berkeley : Berkeley Univ. Press

REYNOLDS, T.D., LONDON, W.P., YORKE, J.A. (1978) Behavioural rhythms in shizophrenia. J. Nervous Ment. dis. 166, 7 : 489-499

SOLBERGER, A. (1970) Problems in the statistical analysis of short periodic time series. J. Interdiscipl. Cycle Res. 1,1 : 49-88

SOLBERGER, A. (1973) Statistical aspect of autorhythmometry. J. Interdiscipl. Cycle. Res. 3,3 : 313-325

SOLBERGER, A., DAVIS, M. (1972) Diurnal rhythm of the startle response : a statistical analysis. J. Interdiscipl. Cycle Res. 3,3-4 : 313-325

TONG, H., LIM, K.S. (1980) Threshold autoregression, limit cycles and cyclial data. J. Roy. Statist. Soc. B 42,3 : 245-292

VAGANUCCI, A.H., WONG, A.K.C., LIU,T.S. (1974) Time series analysis of hormonal patterns in human plasma. Computer and Biomed. Res. 7,5 : 513-532

VAN CAUTER, E. (1974) Method for the analysis of multifrequential biological time series. J. Interdiscipl. Cycle Res. 5,2 : 131-148

VAN CAUTER, E., HUYBERECH, S. (1972) Problem in the statistical analysis of biological series : the cosinor test and the periodogram. J. Interdiscipl. Cycle Res. 3,4 : 41-57

WALKER, A.M. (1971) On the estimation of a harmonic component of a time series
with stationary independent residuals. Biometrika 58,1 : 21-36

WALTER, D.O., BRAZIER, A.B. (1968) The method of complex demodulation. In
Advances in EEG analysis. Electroencephalogr. Clin. Neurophysiol., suppl.
27 : 53-57

WENNBERG, A., ZETTERBERG, L.H. (1971) Application of a computer based model
for EEG analysis. Electroencephalogr. Clin. Neurophysiol. 31 : 457-468

ZETTRBERG, L.H. (1969) Estimation of parameters for a linear difference equation
with application to EEG analysis. Math. Biosci. 5 : 227-275

LARGE DEVIATIONS AND MORE OR LESS RARE EVENTS IN POPULATION DYNAMICS

Gabriel RUGET.

*ils détiennent le secret des attitudes les
plus significatives que j'aurai à prendre
en présence de tels rares évênements qui
m'auront poursuivi de leur marque ...*

André BRETON.

1. SUMMARY.

We look at spatial branching processes, with the same accuracy which,
in the case of an ordinary branching process, would bring the idea of
Malthus parameter : let $N_t(\omega)$ be the (random) size of a population at
time t ; we get $N_t(\omega) \underset{\sim}{p.s.} e^{\mu t}$, or even better stated, $\frac{d}{dt} \log N_t \underset{\sim}{} \mu$.
Our way of extending the class of processes in consideration is the
following :

1) spatiality : instead of giving the probability law of the number of
children of an individual, we start with a probability lax $P(d\emptyset)$ on
the set $\mathcal{M}$ of integer atomic measures on some space $(X \ni x)$ (discrete
time case) or space x time (continuous time case) ; we will proceed
to some renormalisation operations, which suppose on X a vectorial
structure.

2) inhomogeneity : P is allowed to depend explicitely on time t
and locus x where father has appeared, but in such a way that P
changes smoothly frome one birth to the following ones : ϵ (intended
to be small) given, we contract time and space by the same factor ϵ ;
then, "$1/\epsilon$" generations are needed to observe a significative change in
$P_{x,t}(d\emptyset)$.

3) non linearity : if the process is a supercritical one
$(\mu = \int \mu(dx) = \iint \emptyset(dx) \ P(d\emptyset) > 1)$, population blows up exponentially.
Regularisation with a Cst.ε wide kernel allows to define population
density, whose logarithm we denote $\frac{1}{\varepsilon} \alpha(x,t,\omega)$. We introduce some non
linearity (saturation affect) in the process by assuming that P de-
pends explicitly on α :

$$P = P_{x,t,\alpha(x,t,\omega)}$$

4) for completeness, we can kill people after a random time whose law,
if it is reasonable, doesn't effect the results.

We will prove that $\alpha(x,t)$ has a deterministic way of life ; similar to $\log N_t$ for a branching process, α obeys a first order partial
differential equation. One can gets information about the propagation
speed of the process, and, in the case where subcritical P tend to
stop, for some values of x, the spread of the population, the same
formalism will give some indications about the probability of occurrence of individuals in a region which is, with probability almost one,
forbidden.

In the last section, in accordance with the title of the conference,
we will indicate how the multitype case, though our asymptotic reduces
it to a scalar first order equation, can induce (hysteretical) oscillations.

This whole lecture will be in a heuristic manner ; precise hypotheses and proofs are to be found in several papers by Alain Rouault and
Catherine Laredo.

2. PRELIMINARIES (discrete time only).

Let μ be a probability measure on X, to be interpreted first as
a probability measure P on $\mathcal{M}$, for which Dirac masses only are loa-
ded : the process is simply a random walk. Let's denote ξ the generic point of the space Ξ dual to X, and $L(\xi)$ the logarithm of the
Laplace transform of μ . We will call the probability measure
$d\mu^\xi(x) = \exp(\xi x - L(\xi)) \ d\mu(x)$ an exponential modification of μ ; its
expectation is $L'(\xi)$, and $\xi \to L'(\xi)$ maps bijectively the domain of
L into the inside of the convex hull of μ's support. Cramer's theorem [4] says that if X_i are i.i.d. random variables, with law μ,
$\varepsilon \log P(\varepsilon(X_1 + \ldots + X_{t/\varepsilon}) \sim x)$ tends, as ε goes to 0, to $-th(x/t)$,
where

$$h(v) = \sup_{\xi}(\xi v - L(\xi))$$

We notice that one gets the supremum for $\xi=0$ such that $L'(\theta)=v$. Indeed, any good proof of Cramer's theorem gives more : conditionnally to the fact that $\epsilon(X_1+...+X_{t/\epsilon}) \sim x$, the X_i resemble i.i.d.r.v. with law μ^θ, $L'(\theta) = x/t$.

Suppose now μ to be a positive measure of mass less than one ; one can naturally see μ as a P on $\mathcal{M}$ giving mass $1-|\mu|$ to zero, and, aside from that, loading only Dirac masses;the process associated to such a P is a random walk with extinction. Previous definitions and results remain of interest (note that μ^θ is a probability) : $\exp(-\frac{t}{\epsilon}h(x/t))$ approximates the probability of finding the process alive at time t, near x .

Let's look again at a spatial branching process, with law P, of intensity μ ; we suppose that the process is a supercritical one, i.e. $|\mu| > 1$. Biggins proved (see [2] for needed hypotheses) that, if $h(x/t) > 0$, at time t and near x , one can find, with a probability close to 1 when ϵ is small, a number of individuals whose order of magnitude is $\exp(-\frac{t}{\epsilon}h(x/t))$; the precise statement gives an equivalent for $\epsilon \log$ (number of individuals), which, obviously, is almost insensitive to the size of the neighbourhood of x we look at. Rouault [10] gives a description of the genealogy of a guy one supposes to be near X at time $t(t/\epsilon = n)$: let $x_1,...,x_n$ the displacements of the successive ancesters of this fellow $(\epsilon(x_1+...+x_n) = x)$, and let $\varphi_1,...,\varphi_n$ the sets from which the x_i are extracted (displacements of the brothers of the successive ancesters). There are two descriptions available for the law of the (x_i, φ_i) :

1) φ_i are independently drawn according to P^θ

$$P^\theta(d\phi) = [\int \exp(\theta x - L(\theta)) \phi(dx)] P(d\phi) ,$$

and then, x_i is chosen according to φ_i^θ .

2) x_i are independently drawn according to μ^θ, and then φ_i following Palm's measure associated to P, i.e. under P knowing that $x_i \in \text{supp } \varphi_i$.

These descriptions remain true when $h(x/t) \geq 0$, for instance for a subcritical process. Moreover, in the description of a genealogical tree such that there is a child at (t,x), one can say that, with a probability close to one, broods which do not lead to the given child behaves as predicted by P. One can deduce from this remark that, when one finds a guy near (t,x), if $h(x/t) > 0$, may be, there are a few other guys near (t,x), but their number cannot be exponentially big ($\epsilon \log (\text{number}) \xrightarrow[\epsilon \to 0]{} 0$), so that, if $h(x/t) > 0$, not only $-th(x/t)$ approximates

$$\epsilon \log E \text{ (number of individuals near } (t,x))$$

but also

$$\epsilon \log P \text{ (there is an individual near } (t,x))$$

3. SOME GENERAL RESULTS.

Consider now continuous time case : P is a probability measure on the set $\mathcal{M}$ of atomic measures on $X \times \mathbb{R}^+$; we denote μ for the intensity of P, and we suppose it has a Laplace transform whose logarithm we call $L(t,\xi)$; $h(t,x)$ will be the Legendre's transform of L.

Let's look at the displacements (t_i,x_i) of the successive ancesters of some people sitting near (t,x) : one can proove [9] that (for $\epsilon \to 0$), (t_i,x_i) are empirically independent, with some law which is an exponential modification of μ, the one whose expectation $(\underline{t},\underline{x})$ is homothetic to (t,x) and which minimizes $\frac{t}{t} h(\underline{t},\underline{x})$; see at fig.1.

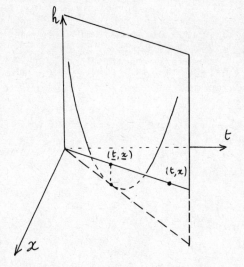

Fig. 1

The number of generations leading to people near (t,x) is close to $\frac{1}{\epsilon} \frac{t}{t}$, and the number of individuals near (t,x) , with a probability close to one, of the order of magnitude of

$$\exp - \frac{1}{\epsilon} \frac{t}{t} h(\underline{t},\underline{x})$$

The "ϵ-log-density" of individuals

$$\alpha(x,t) = - \frac{t}{t} h(\underline{t},\underline{x})$$

verifies the equation

$$L(- \frac{\partial \alpha}{\partial t} , - \frac{\partial \alpha}{\partial x}) = 0 \quad .$$

Taking now into account possible inhomogeneities, P depends on t and x, so that $L = L(t,x ; \tau, \xi)$. It seems reasonable to guess that the process, for ϵ small, has a deterministic ϵ-log-density verifying equation

$$L\left(t,\dot{x} \; ; \; -\frac{\partial\alpha}{\partial t} \; , \; -\frac{\partial\alpha}{\partial x}\right) = 0$$

which here can always be written into the form

$$\frac{\partial\alpha}{\partial t} = F\left(t,x \; ; \; \frac{\partial\alpha}{\partial x}\right).$$

This is not quite true : besides, this equation, with initial conditions, does not determines a unique α . To get a precise result, we have to guess at the most probable way the ancesters of a guy at (t,x) followed : a bit of knowledge of large deviation theory ([13], [1], [12]) makes plausible the fact that, if the population starts concentrated at $(0,0)$, the most prolific generations ending at (t,x) follow the path

$$\varphi_i[0,T] \rightarrow \mathbb{R}^{+} \times X \;\; (\text{free } T)$$

such that $\varphi(T) = (t,x)$ and which minimizes

$$I_T(\varphi) = \int_0^T h(\varphi(u);\dot{\varphi}(u))\,du$$

Looking back to the homogeneous case, we see that the optimal way is given by $T = t/\underline{t}$, $\varphi(u) = (u\underline{t}, u\underline{x})$.

The "action integral" $I_s(\varphi)$ gives the size ($\sim \exp\frac{1}{\varepsilon}I_s(\varepsilon)$) of the population which, standing in locus $\varphi_2(s)$ at time $\varphi_1(s)$, will contribute almost alone to people to be found at (t,x) ; this is true at least when $I_s(\varphi) < 0$, in which case, thanks to Biggins'result, everything looks deterministic. But, were $I_s(\varphi) > 0$, it would only be related to the (tiny) probability to see someone at $\varphi(s)$, so that, with probability "1" , branches of the genealogical tree near φ died before time $\varphi_1(s)$, and $I_T(\varphi)$, even if negative, could only give the expectation of the size of the population at (t,x). We conclude that we must carefully distinguish between

$$\beta(t,x) = \varepsilon \log E \,(\text{number of individuals at } (t,x))$$

and

$$\alpha(t,x) = \varepsilon \log \,(\text{number of individuals at } (t,x) \text{ for a set of}$$
$$\text{genealogies of probability "1").}$$

It's true that

$$\beta(t,x) = - \inf_{\varphi} I_T(\varphi) \; ,$$

and that β is one of the solutions of $L(t,x \; ; \; -\frac{\partial\beta}{\partial t}, \; -\frac{\partial\beta}{\partial x}) = 0$, the one satisfying the entropy condition [7], which indicates what numerical scheme is to be used [5]. As to α, its value is

$$\alpha(t,x) = - \inf (I_T(\varphi),\varphi|\forall s \in [0,T], I_s(\varphi) \le 0) .$$

Notice that β may be negative, whereas α, if strictly negative, can only be $-\infty$. We give finally, as an exercise for the reader, the formula for

$$\gamma(t,x) = \epsilon \log P \text{ (someone is present at } t,x)$$

$$\gamma(t,x) = - \inf_{\varphi} \sup_{s} I_s(\varphi), \quad \varphi(T)=(t,x), \quad 0 \le s \le t$$

This gives the probability of getting through something like an "immunological barrier" (a region where the process is an subcritical one).

The case when P depends on α (it would have no sense to make it depend on β!), seems hardly more complicated, though we haven't written it down, the population behaves deterministically, with an ϵ-log density α which must verify

$$\alpha(t,x) = - \inf_{\varphi/\ldots} I_T (\varphi,\alpha)$$

But one can see that, at least for small values of T, the mapping $\alpha \mapsto - \inf_{\varphi/\ldots} I_T(\varphi,\alpha)$ is a contraction of $L^\infty ([0,T]xX)$, so that the preceding equation determines a unique α.

4. SPEEDS OF PROPAGATION.

The homogeneous case, with no saturation, is clear : population occupies the cone in the space x time domain generated by the convex region where h is negative, which can be translated in terms of propagation speeds in the different spacial directions. Consider now a homogeneous process, but whith saturation : I think that the multidimensional (space) case will only be clear when we will be able to say what partial differential inequation $\alpha(t,x)$ is a solution f, so that we will here look only at the one-dimensional case ; on the other hand, we will be more precise, putting a little more distance from the case $\epsilon=0$.

To show simply what happens, let's suppose that the population 's density affect the reproduction process's intensity only by a multiplicative factor, so that β's equation is

$$\frac{\partial \beta}{\partial t} = S(\beta) + L(-\frac{\partial \beta}{\partial x}) \qquad L(0) = 0.$$

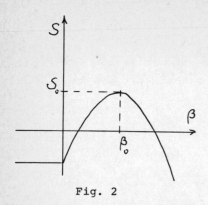

Fig. 2

As shown in fig. 2, the process is supposed to be supercrital when the (ϵ-log) density of population belongs to some intervall around β_o , where rate of reproduction is the highest.

If we look formally at a wave ($\beta = \beta (x-ct)$) solution of the evolution equation, denoting $\frac{\partial \beta}{\partial x} = u$, and searching β via a differential equation $\beta = f(u)$, one see that, necessarily

$$\frac{\partial u}{\partial t} = \frac{\partial u}{\partial x} \frac{\partial}{\partial u} [S (f(u)) + L(-u)] \quad ,$$

whence we deduce easily, because of a priori constraints about the shape of the wave, that we must have

$$S(f(u)) + L(-u) = -c_o u \quad ,$$

whith c_o given by $h(c_o) = S_o$. This result has a clear interpretation in terms of optimal ways of growth : the part of the wave of ϵ-log density β_o is, so to speak, self sufficient to propagate at speed c_o, that speed being, thanks to Biggins'theorem, the highest obtainable here. The same argument leads to the slope of the wave at level β_o , which could equally have been given by calculus : it is $-h'(c_o)$.

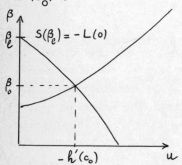

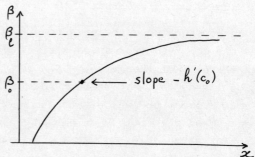

Fig. 3 : graph of $S(\beta)+L(-u) = -c_o u$ and graph of the wave (from both solutions of $h(c_o)=S_o$, we selected the smallest, so that we look at the left side of the contamined domain.

Simulations of the process, with moderate sizes of population (discrete space, a few dozen people at a locus, and propagation speed of

the order of 1), show that the preceding formula systematically over-
estimates the speed , which has an obvious reason, giving a methode
for calculating a corrective term : people at ϵ-log-density β_o, who
push the wave, have a fluctuating position with respect to the theoretical wave, so that, really, they never are immerged inside an op-
timally sized population (for small ϵ, this phenomenon is far more
important than the fluctuations of the shape of the wave).

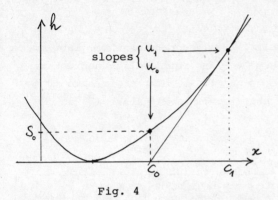

Fig. 4

To determine the true speed
v, let us write that an individual who maintains itself near
the level β_o of the wave during
a unit of time (which event,
were S=0, would have a probabi-
lity $\sim \exp -\frac{1}{\epsilon} h(v)$) comes back
after that time with multipli-
city 1 :

$$0 = -\frac{1}{\epsilon} h(v) + \log E \exp \int_0^1 [S_o + \frac{1}{2} S''(\beta_o) u_o^2 y^2(t,\omega)] \frac{dt}{\epsilon} ,$$

where $y(t,\omega)$ denotes the discrepancy between the trajectory ω and
the wave propagating with speed v, this discrepancy evaluated conditionnally to the fact that the individual survives near the front.
Since $\frac{1}{\epsilon} \int_0^1 y^2 dt$ is small with ϵ, this equation can be replaced by
the simpler one

$$0 = S_o - h(v) + \frac{1}{2} S''(\beta_o) u_o^2 E \int_0^1 y^2 dt$$

Conditioning does not affect individuals before the front of propagation, who move then according to a random walk with increments of
law μ . People behind the front, given that they come back to the
front, move according to a random walk with increments of law μ^{u_1}
and mean speed $c_1 > c_o$ (see Fig. 4, and [3]). We would now like to
apply an ergodic theorem, and to replace $E \int_0^1 y^2 dt$ by $\int_{-\infty}^{\infty} y^2 d\nu(y)$,
where ν denotes the invariant measure of the conditioned walk ; gene-
rally speaking, there are not simple formulas for this measure (except
from the case of -1,0 + 1 valued increments [6]) ; but, we can at least
get the right order of magnitude by accepting near 0 the exponentially
decreasing behavior predicted by large deviation theory (or Wald identity) for away from 0 : that is, here, ν happens to be symmetrical,

homothetic with $\exp - \frac{u_1}{\epsilon} |y|$. Whence this final (approximated) equation determining v

$$h(v) = S_o + \epsilon^2 S'' (\beta_o) (\frac{u_o}{u_1})^2$$

Besides a precise determination of v, a pertinent way of getting a better result is to replace this equation by an implicit one, making every expansion around v, no more c_o, so that, for instance, u_o and u_1 depend on v.

Let's give a few numerical results [8] : here, everything happens on $\mathbb{Z} \subset \mathbb{R}$, μ is $pS_o + (1-p) S_1$, and e^S is a parabolic function of the size of the population at a locus (it is in fact preferable to take a mean on a neighbourhood) ; e^S gets its maximum value e^{S_o} at $e^{\beta_o} = N_o$, and reach value 0 at N_1

	Process			Speeds			
p	e^{S_o}	$N_o = e^{\beta_o}$	N_1	reaction diffusion approximation	large deviations approximation	large deviation with rough corrective term	observed
0,4	1,5	30	60	1,04	0,98	0,95	0,93
0,5	1,5	100	200	0,95	0,92	0,77	0,86
0,5	1,2	50	170	0,80	0,79	0,75	0,76
0,35	1,05	50	280	0,80	0,79	0,76	0,78
0,4	1,5	30	80	1,04	0,98	0,97	0,97
0,65	1,2	100	350	0,64	0,65	0,58	0,60

First a few words about a saturation of a more general form : suppose that $L(\beta, -u)$, which is convex with respect to u, is concave with respect to β (for $\beta > 0$), but not necessarily of the form $S(\beta) + L(-u)$. The same formal manipulation of the propagation equation shows that the slopes of the two planes containing axis $O\beta$ and tangent to the graph of L give the speeds of propagation ; the differential equation determining the wave for large times remains

$$L(\beta, - \frac{d\beta}{dx}) = -c \frac{d\beta}{dx}$$

the coordinates of the contact point give the level of population responsible for the propagation, and the slope of the wave near that level.

5. THE MULTITYPE CASE.

Once again, time will be discrete, and space monodimensional ; there are several types of individuals , indexed by $i=1,...,R$; the process is an homogeneous one, without saturation ; it is defined by a collection of point processes of intensities μ_{ij} ($\mu_{ij}(u)$ is the expectation of the number of children of type j, lying in u , of an individual of type i sitting at 0). Let

$$\hat{\mu}_{ij} (\xi) = e^{\xi x} \mu_{ij}(dx) ,$$

and let $p(\xi)$ be the biggest eigenvalue of $M(\xi) = (\hat{\mu}_{ij} (\xi))$, the right and left eigenvectors associated with $\rho(\xi)$ being $u(\xi)$ and $v(\xi)$ respectively ; $L(\xi) = \text{Log } \rho(\xi)$ is a convex function, whose Legendre's dual we denote $h(x)$.

Let $z_i^j (t,U)$ the (random) number of children of type j, lying in U at time t, issued from a i-guy at $(0,0)$. If $L'(\theta) = c/t$ and γ are small, it is proven in [11] that

$$E \, z_i^j (t; [c, c+\gamma]) = \gamma \, u_i(\theta) \, v_j(\theta) \sqrt{\frac{t}{2\pi \, L''(\theta)\epsilon}} \, e^{- \frac{t}{\epsilon} h(\frac{c}{t})} (1+o(1))$$

We proven that this result in the mean gives also the time size of $z_i^j (t; I)$ with probability "1". So that, independently from the initial repartition of the types, the proportion of types observed in the part of the genealogical tree corresponding to a propagation speed v converges to $v_j(\theta)$ for $L'(\theta) = v$; this remark in mind, one can say that the population, all types together, developpes as it was a unitype process whose intensity would have $\rho(\xi)$ as its Laplace transform. We can so come back to the results of § 3 (inhomogeneity, and saturation depending only of the size of the population as a whole) : knowing at each time the mean speed of people sitting at (t,x) (it is $\dot{\varphi}(t)$, for the optimizing φ), we can say which are the types present in the population, but we essentially have a scalar first order evolution equation, whence no oscillation phenomenon.

Such oscillations can only appear if the law of the process does depend on types proportions, but we aren't interested in small oscillations of the relaxation type (with wave length of magnitude $\sqrt{\epsilon}$) which could appear and be studied by a reaction-diffusion asymptotic, whereas large diffusion theory is a bad tool for that. Sufficiently strong mixing hypotheses do imply that the dynamic of the process can be described with two time scales :

1) Locally, one gets an equilibrium point for the repartition of types: this seems to be true, for instance, for a two-types population (with some spread condition about the support of μ) ; let's denote $\pi = (\pi_j)$, $\sum\limits_{j=1}^{R} \pi_j = 1$, the vector of types proportions, and α the global ε-log-density ; now, we suppose $L = L(\alpha,\pi;\xi)$ and $h = h(\alpha,\pi;x)$. For a given global level α of the population, and a mean speed c, one must have

$$\begin{cases} \pi_j = v_j \ (\alpha,\pi;\xi) \\ \\ L' \ (\alpha,\pi; \ \xi) = c \end{cases}$$

This gives at least one and perhaps several possibilities for π , to each corresponds a different $h(\alpha,\pi;c)$, whence a different rate of growth. Our program of work is to show (perhaps beginning with the non spatial continuous time case) that the process behaves deterministically in accordance with a solution of π-equation (in the non spatial continuous time case, this equation would be $\pi_j = v_j \ (\alpha,\pi;\tau)$, $L \ (\alpha,\pi;\tau) = 0$) .

2) Slow dynamic : when α changes, some bifurcations may appear on the set of π-solutions. We proceed now to construct a rather natural example where such bifurcations induce hysteretical oscillations of α (fig. 5)

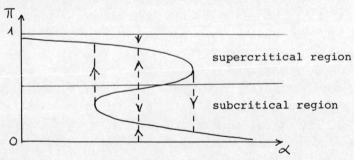

Fig. 5 : Quick dynamic is shown by interrupted vertical lines.

[1]   Azencott-Ruget : Mélanges d'équations différentielles et grands
       écarts à la loi des grands nombres. Zeit. für War. vol. 38,
       (1977), p. 1.

[2]   Biggins : Chernoff's theorem in the branching random walk.
       Jour. of Appl. Prob. 14 (1977), p. 630

[3]   Cottrell-Fort-Malgouyres : Large deviations and rare events in
       the study of stochastic algorithms. To appear in IEEE A.C.
       (1982).

[4]   Cramer : Sur un nouveau théorème limite de la théorie des pro-
       babilités. Colloquium on the theory of Probability. Paris :
       Hermann, 1937.

[5]   Harten-Hyman-Lax : On finite-difference approximations and
       entropy conditions for shocks. Comm. on pure and appl. Math.
       Vol. 29 (1976), p. 297.

[6]   Kennedy : Some martingales related to cumulative-sum tests and
       single-server queues. Stoch. proc. and their appl. Vol. 4
       (1976), p. 261

[7]   Keyfitz : Solutions with shocks an example of an L'-contrac-
       tive semigroup. Comm. on pure and appl. math. Vol. 24 (1971),
       p. 125.

[8]   Laredo : thèse de 3ème cycle, Orsay 1981.

[9]   Laredo-Rouault : Une généralisation du paramètre de Malthus
       pour les processus de Crump-Mode-Jagers spatiaux. Note aux
       C.R.A.S. du 26 Octobre 1981.

[10]   Rouault : Lois empiriques dans les processus de branchement
       spatiaux homogènes supercritiques. Note aux C.R.A.S. du 1er
       juin 1981 (t. 292).

[11]   Rouault : Etude asymptotique des processus de branchement
       spatiaux homogènes supercritiques à temps discret. Prépubli-
       cation mathématiques d'Orsay, 1982.

[12]   Ventsel : Rough limit theorems on large deviations for Markov
         stochastic processes. Th. Prob. and Appl. vol. 21 (1976),
         p. 227 et p. 499.

[13]   Ventsel-Freidlin : On small random perturbations of dynamical
         systems. Russian Math. Survey, t. 25 (1970), p. 1.

Bio-mathematics

Managing Editor: S. A. Levin

Volume 8
A. T. Winfree

The Geometry of Biological Time

1979. 290 figures. XIV, 530 pages
ISBN 3-540-09373-7

The widespread appearance of periodic patterns in nature reveals that many living organisms are communities of biological clocks. This landmark text investigates, and explains in mathematical terms, periodic processes in living systems and in their non-living analogues. Its lively presentation (including many drawings), timely perspective and unique bibliography will make it rewarding reading for students and researchers in many disciplines.

Volume 9
W. J. Ewens

Mathematical Population Genetics

1979. 4 figures, 17 tables. XII, 325 pages
ISBN 3-540-09577-2

This graduate level monograph considers the mathematical theory of population genetics, emphasizing aspects relevant to evolutionary studies. It contains a definitive and comprehensive discussion of relevant areas with references to the essential literature. The sound presentation and excellent exposition make this book a standard for population geneticists interested in the mathematical foundations of their subject as well as for mathematicians involved with genetic evolutionary processes.

Volume 10
A. Okubo

Diffusion and Ecological Problems: Mathematical Models

1980. 114 figures, 6 tables. XIII, 254 pages
ISBN 3-540-09620-5

This is the first comprehensive book on mathematical models of diffusion in an ecological context. Directed towards applied mathematicians, physicists and biologists, it gives a sound, biologically oriented treatment of the mathematics and physics of diffusion.

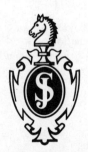

Springer-Verlag
Berlin
Heidelberg
New York

Journal of Mathematical Biology

ISSN 0303-6812

Title No. 285

Editorial Board:
H.T.Banks, Providence, RI; **H.J.Bremermann,** Berkeley,
CA; **J.D.Cowan,** Chicago, IL; **J.Gani,** Lexington, KY; ·
K.P.Hadeler (Managing Editor), Tübingen;
F.C.Hoppensteadt, Salt Lake City, UT; **S.A.Levin**
(Managing Editor), Ithaca, NY; **D.Ludwig,** Vancouver; .
L.A.Segel, Rehovot; **D.Varjú,** Tübingen in cooperation
with a distinguished advisory board.

The **Journal of Mathematical Biology** publishes papers in
which mathematics leads to a better understanding of biological phenomena, mathematical papers inspired by biological research and papers which yield new experimental data
bearing on mathematical models. The scope is broad, both
mathematically and biologically and extends to relevant
interfaces with medicine, chemistry, physics, and sociology.
The editors aim to reach an audience of both mathematicians
and biologists.

Contents:

Subscription information and sample copy upon request

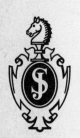

Springer-Verlag
Berlin
Heidelberg
New York

Lecture Notes in Biomathematics

This series reports new developments in biomathematics research and teaching – quickly, informally and at a high level. The type of material considered for publication includes:

1. Preliminary drafts of original papers and monographs

2. Lectures on a new field or presentations of new angles in a classical field

3. Seminar work-outs

4. Reports of meetings, provided they are

   a) of exceptional interest and

   b) devoted to a single topic.

Texts which are out of print but still in demand may also be considered if they fall within these categories.

The timeliness of a manuscript is more important than its form, which may be unfinished or tentative. Thus, in some instances, proofs may be merely outlined and results presented which have been or will later be published elsewhere. If possible, a subject index should be included. Publication of Lecture Notes is intended as a service to the international scientific community, in that a commercial publisher, Springer-Verlag, can offer a wide distribution of documents which would otherwise have a restricted readership. Once published and copyrighted, they can be documented in the scientific literature.

Manuscripts

Manuscripts should be no less than 100 and preferably no more than 500 pages in length.
They are reproduced by a photographic process and therefore must be typed with extreme care. Symbols not on the typewriter should be inserted by hand in indelible black ink. Corrections to the typescript should be made by pasting in the new text or painting out errors with white correction fluid. Authors receive 75 free copies and are free to use the material in other publications. The typescript is reduced slightly in size during reproduction; best results will not be obtained unless the text on any one page is kept within the overall limit of 18 x 26.5 cm (7 x 10½ inches). On request, the publisher will supply special paper with the typing area outlined.

Manuscripts in English, German or French should be sent to Prof. Simon Levin, Ecology and Systematics, Corson Building, Cornell University, Ithaca, NY 14853-0239, USA

Springer-Verlag, Heidelberger Platz 3, D-1000 Berlin 33
Springer-Verlag, Tiergartenstraße 17, D-6900 Heidelberg 1
Springer-Verlag, 175 Fifth Avenue, New York, NY 10010/USA

ISBN 3-540-12302-4
ISBN 0-387-12302-4